Clinical Management of Salivary Gland Disorders

Louis Mandel, DDS
Oral and Maxillofacial Surgery
Columbia University /New York
Presbyterian Hospital
New York, NY, USA

Clinical Management of Salivary Gland Disorders

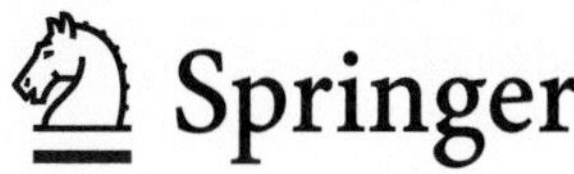 Springer

Louis Mandel, DDS
Oral and Maxillofacial Surgery
Columbia University /New York Presbyterian Hospital
New York, NY, USA

ISBN 978-3-031-50014-5   ISBN 978-3-031-50012-1   (eBook)
https://doi.org/10.1007/978-3-031-50012-1

This Springer imprint is published by the registered company Springer Nature Switzerland AG
The registered company address is: Gewerbestrasse 11, 6330 Cham, Switzerland

Paper in this product is recyclable.

Dedication

The seeds for this book have been germinating within my mental field for many years. Its materialization was made possible only through the genes that I inherited from my Hungarian immigrant parents. Their nurturing, direction, work ethic, and sacrifices paved the way for me to achieve a professional education. Simultaneously, it facilitated my recognition of these indispensable qualities in the woman I courted and married, Mary Damiani. In turn, Mary and I endeavored to implant these values into our two children, Susan and Richard. The results have not been disappointing. They both have meaningful lives and successful careers. I have taken pride in their principles and accomplishments, and it is to Susan and Richard that I dedicate this book. It is one avenue made available to me, albeit insufficient, to express my love for them, something that I may not have always adequately demonstrated.

Although in truth the family always comes first, there are individuals whose interactions with me served as a continued inspiration and incentive for my writing, teaching and study, my students. Their thirst to learn galvanized my patient investigations. Standouts include, but are not limited to, Drs. David Alfi, Ashley Houle, Daria Vasilyeva, and Vicky Yau. In addition, I will be forever grateful for the opportunities afforded to me by my superior, Dr. Sidney Eisig, and for my friendships with Murray Slochover, Carl Nelson, Ian Hu, and George Minervini. They all contributed to making my life complete.

Preface

My interest in salivary gland disorders originated when I was a graduate student many years ago. Consequently, I have had ample opportunity to evaluate patients victimized by a wide variety of salivary gland diseases. Inevitably, I developed "smarts" or what is referred to as clinical expertise. In addition to my examinations of the more familiar salivary gland afflictions, my experiences have allowed me to become familiar with a group of salivary gland conditions that nowadays are seen infrequently. Surgical (acute) parotitis and HIV lymphoepithelial cysts represent examples of this cohort of salivary gland problems. Furthermore, the passage of time has allowed me to accumulate and evaluate a collection of false/positive patients. I have attempted to incorporate into this text the knowledge that I have acquired from my exposure to the full gamut of salivary gland disorders and to those entities (the false/positives) that mimic salivary gland pathology.

A huge step forward in my ability to evaluate salivary gland disorders occurred in 1988 with the establishment of the Columbia University Salivary Gland Center. The impetus for its establishment came from Dr. Irwin Mandel (no relation of mine, just a coincidence in names) who had a background in biochemistry and was interested in the biochemistry of saliva. I am a clinician and he thought that we would make a perfect team, we did. As you peruse this book, you will note that some chapters allude to salivary chemistry, a reflection of Dr. Irwin Mandel's influence upon me.

In addition, the continued value of sialography in the diagnosis of salivary gland disease has been recognized. Examples of its place in diagnosis have been sprinkled throughout the chapters. Sialography is a venerable diagnostic technique whose scope has gradually been impinged upon by other imaging (CT scan, MRI, etc.) approaches. Nevertheless, it has a significant place in the salivary gland diagnostic armamentarium. It is unrivaled in its ability to image normal/abnormal ductal patterns as they relate to glandular disorders. Mastering the technique will reward the clinician.

The reader should look upon this book's compendium of salivary gland disorders as only opening the door to the subject. The text should serve as a guide in attaining a diagnosis and in mastering pathophysiology. Digestion of this information should be followed by a pivot to current scientific journals for recent updates. The derived information should then be filed away in the reader's intellectual memory bank. Clinical expertise will now develop and can be added to the investigator's diagnostic abilities.

New York, NY, USA   Louis Mandel, DDS

Contents

Editor and Contributor

Editor

Louis Mandel, DDS Oral and Maxillofacial Surgery, Columbia University/New York Presbyterian Hospital, New York, NY, USA

Contributors

Kevin C. Lee, DDS, MD Department of Head, Neck/Plastic and Reconstructive Surgery, Roswell Park Comprehensive Cancer Center, Buffalo, NY, USA

Letty Moss-Salentijn, DDS, PhD Vice Dean for Curriculum Innovation and IPE, Columbia University, College of Dental Medicine, New York, USA

Chapter 1
Anatomical Considerations

Letty Moss-Salentijn

Abstract The general anatomy and histology of human major and minor salivary glands are described. The sublingual glands and all minor glands develop in the submucosa close to the sites of the oral mucosa where the openings of their excretory ducts are located. Particular attention is paid to the development of the submandibular and parotid glands. The final anatomical location and morphology of these glands, as well as the lengths of their excretory ducts, are influenced by the rapid facial growth and development, and the spatial restrictions imposed by the developing muscles, nerves, and organs that are present in this shared connective tissue space.

Introduction

Saliva is the product of a collection of major and minor salivary glands, which by their secretory activity contribute to the maintenance of a healthy oral environment.

Saliva plays a key role in maintaining oral health under normal conditions. If conditions change, for example, in sedated patients in intensive care, a rapid shift in oral flora may occur to Gram-negative species. This may subsequently spread into the respiratory tract, causing pulmonary afflictions.

While a detailed description of the composition and role of the salivary constituents is beyond the scope of this chapter, we note here the principal functions of these constituents (Fig. 1.1):

- Affecting the processing of food prior to swallowing.
- Protecting mineralized tissues against demineralization and stimulating remineralization.
- Providing innate and acquired immune protection against micro-organisms.

L. Mandel, *Clinical Management of Salivary Gland Disorders*,
https://doi.org/10.1007/978-3-031-50012-1_1

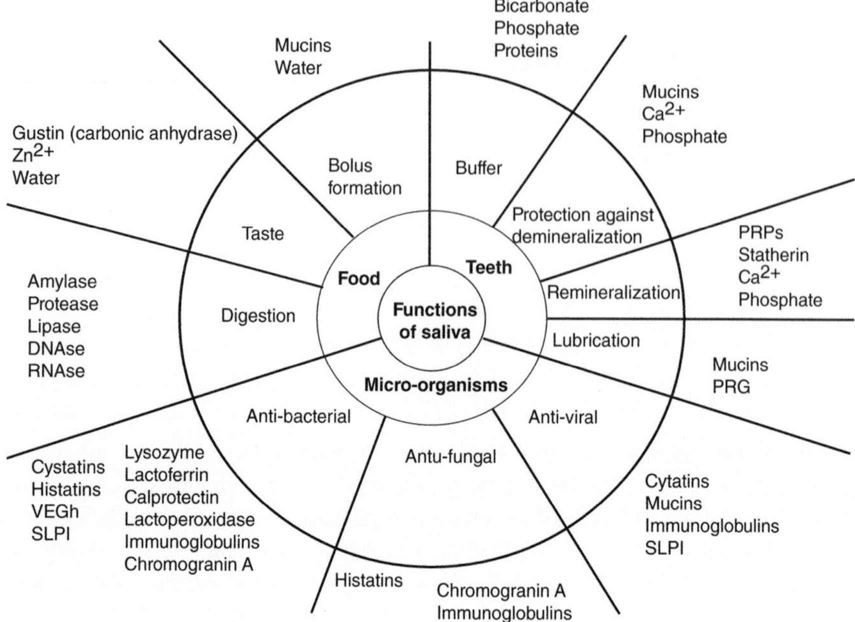

Fig. 1.1 Functions of saliva [1]

Traditionally, a distinction has been made between three pairs of *major* glands, the parotid, submandibular, and sublingual glands, and numerous *minor* salivary glands.

While these glands all have in common that they release their product into the oral cavity, the parotid and submandibular glands are not located directly below the oral mucosa, but at some distance, which necessitates the transport of saliva via lengthy excretory ducts: of the parotid (Stensen) with an opening on a papilla of the buccal mucosa near the second maxillary molar and of the submandibular gland (Wharton) which opens on the surface of the sublingual papilla. The smallest of the major salivary glands, the sublingual glands, are well developed in only about 65% of cases where a distinct anterior "major sublingual gland" is present [2]. The anterior major sublingual gland and a collection of minor sublingual glands that are located immediately below the sublingual oral mucosa have separate excretory ducts that open along the top of the sublingual fold (Rivinus). If an excretory duct of the major sublingual gland is well developed (Bartholin), it may join the submandibular duct (Wharton) and open on the sublingual papilla [3, 4].

Numerous minor salivary glands are found immediately below the oral mucosa in almost every location of the oral cavity. These glands are named according to their respective locations: **sublingual**: 8–20 in the floor of the mouth, **lingual**: directly below the ventral lining mucosa of the tongue and the dorsal specialized mucosa—particularly numerous near the lingual tonsil, **labial**: in the submucosa below the lining mucosa of the lips, **buccal**: directly below the lining mucosa of the cheeks, **palatine**: directly below the masticatory mucosa of the hard palate and the lining mucosa of soft palate, and **glossopalatine**: particularly rich near the tonsil. Finally, a rare developing gingival gland has been described [5].

In many of these locations, no submucosa is present. If a submucosa is present, the minor salivary glands are located in that layer.

General Structure

Salivary glands are organs that consist of epithelial and connective tissue components. The epithelial components are responsible for the production, modification, and transport of saliva, while the connective tissue components provide physical support and carry the neurovascular supply needed for the function of the glands.

Epithelial Component

The *epithelial component* resembles a tree in which the major branches and the "trunk" are the largest (excretory) ducts. The principal excretory duct opens into the oral cavity, while the "leaves" are the acini where the production of saliva begins. The intervening "branches" and "twigs" are part of the ductal system, through which the secretory product is moved and modified until it reaches the oral cavity as saliva [6] (Fig. 1.2). This epithelial structure is most visible during the fetal period when the salivary glands are still developing. When cytodifferentiation of the epithelial cells of the acini and the ductal system is completed, the epithelial components seem to dominate the histology of the lobules.

A well-known diagram that was published in 1924 by Braus [7] (Fig. 1.3) illustrates the principal cellular details of the epithelial components of a salivary gland (mixed seromucous):

- Acini—these may be serous or seromucous in nature.
- Intercalated ducts—long in serous glands and short or non-existent in seromucous glands.
- Striated ducts—longer in serous glands.
- Excretory ducts.

In the major salivary glands, the acini, intercalated ducts, and most of the striated ducts constitute the *parenchyma* of the lobules of the salivary gland and are therefore described as intralobular.

The remaining lengths of the striated ducts and the excretory duct system run in the connective tissue between the lobules and are therefore described as interlobular.

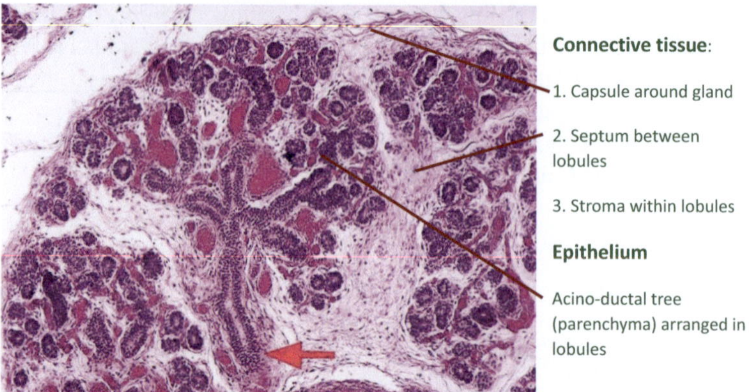

Fig. 1.2 Developing major salivary gland in a human fetus showing the distal epithelial components forming an acino-ductal tree intralobularly and one of the excretory ducts (red arrow) interlobular in a connective tissue septum. Original magnification 32 × [6]

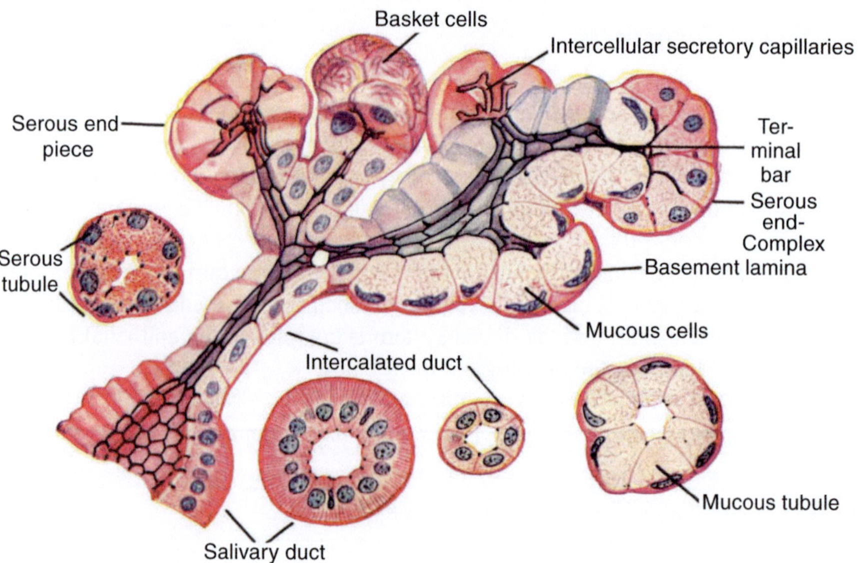

Fig. 1.3 Diagram. After a reconstruction by Vierling: Braus H (1924). Anatomie des Menschen. Berlin, Springer Verlag. Adjusted nomenclature: basket cells: myoepithelial cells: Mucous tubule: seromucous acinus (sectioned). Salivary duct: striated duct. Serous tubule: serous acinus (sectioned). Serous end piece: serous acinus (in 3D)

Connective Tissue Component

The *connective tissue component* forms a connective tissue *capsule* around the entire glandular mass. From this capsule, several *connective tissue septa* extend into the mass of the gland, between the lobules. These septa contain the interlobular ducts and the major neurovascular supply of the glands. A fine *connective tissue stroma* is present within the lobules and surrounds all the intralobular epithelial components. The stroma carries an abundant capillary supply and the afferent and autonomic nerves that supply the glandular tissue.

The epithelial components of the minor salivary glands generally are limited to seromucous acini and excretory ducts. A few cells resembling striated duct cells may be present in the excretory ducts. As will be discussed below, most minor salivary glands have seromucous acini, except for the purely serous von Ebner glands that are associated with the circumvallate and foliate papillae of the tongue.

The minor glands do not have distinct connective tissue capsules. In most cases, the connective tissue of these glands is limited to connective tissue stroma that surrounds the epithelial parenchyma and carries the vascular and neural elements needed for the epithelial functions.

Salivary Gland Development

The major glands start to develop during the embryonic period: the parotid glands (4–6 weeks) are first, and the sublingual glands are the last (8 weeks). The minor salivary glands begin their development slightly later, during the third prenatal month.

The salivary glands develop as the result of a series of epithelio-mesenchymal interactions that lead to an initial ingrowth of *solid epithelial strands* into the underlying mesenchyme, at the future site of the opening of the excretory duct into the oral cavity. The ductal system continues to expand by forming a series of successively smaller branches that will become striated ducts, intercalated ducts, and finally the terminal buds: the future acini. Thus, the pattern of development runs in a direction that is opposite to the production, flow, and secretion of saliva.

The pattern of development is characterized by several stages:

1. **Morphodifferentiation stages:** pre-bud, bud, and pseudoglandular: epithelial cord growth and successive rounds of branching of the solid cord [8–10].
2. **Canalicular stage**: During this stage, a hollowing or cavitation of the solid cord [11] leads to the formation of lumina in the developing glandular ducts.
3. **Terminal stage**: cytodifferentiation [12].

Eventually, *bulbous terminals (acini) are formed* at the ends of the strands during the third prenatal month. These terminals are the future acini.

The complexity of the growth and differentiation of the components of salivary glands has been studied by many investigators during recent decades. The selected references will provide some insight into the current literature on this topic. However, a full picture of the signaling cascades that are required in salivary gland development is still incomplete [13].

Finally, stabilizing effects of elements of the extracellular matrix: fibroblasts and collagen, and the basal lamina components: laminin and nidogen, are needed to support branching morphogenesis [13]. While the stages of morphogenesis have been well-studied, little is known about the factors that control cell differentiation in the terminal stage. Those factors differ from the ones that control the morphogenesis stages.

Salivary Gland Anatomical Relationships

Developmentally, a salivary gland starts proliferating from the future site of the oral opening of its excretory duct to become the tree-like structure that was described above. This process of growth and development occurs during the same period during which the surrounding tissues are proliferating and establishing their respective territories. So, the final "space" in which a fully developed gland is located is a compromise between the domains that are needed by the gland and its neighboring structures, tissues, and organs. Notably, it is subject to individual variation. The differences in thickness of the connective tissue fasciae which serve as packing structures between the salivary glands and the surrounding tissues and organs reflect these compromises in the establishment of such domains.

The patterns of vasculature and innervation of the salivary glands similarly need to be considered within the frame of the glandular development. Thus, while the function of the salivary glands usually is described from the distal-most acini to the oral openings of the excretory ducts, the arterial supply and venous drainage of the glands follow the pattern of the duct system in reverse, with the blood vessels entering the mass of the gland near the excretory ducts in a way that is somewhat like a hilum [4].

As noted before, there is no consensual agreement in the literature concerning some gross structural details that are potentially important in surgical procedures [3]. The descriptions that follow are general. Detailed studies based on extensive dissections may be found in [14, 15] and to a lesser extent in [2].

Parotid Gland

The parotid gland is the largest of the three major salivary glands. The shape of this gland is variable, and more than those of the other major glands, it is determined by the neighboring structures that define the space into which the gland has grown. The gland occupies the space between the posterior surface of the mandibular ramus and the sternocleidomastoid muscle. It extends vertically from a level below the external auditory meatus to a level below the angle of the mandible and extends anteriorly, covering the posterior part of the masseter muscle, where it is wedged between the skin and the muscle. The excretory duct (Stensen) of the gland runs in an anterior direction across the external surface to the anterior border of the masseter muscle, where it curves medially and crosses the buccinator muscle before opening near the second maxillary molar on the buccal mucosa (Fig. 1.4).

The fetal development of the acinotubular structure of the parotid gland occurs during intensive growth of the facial region in the late embryonic and fetal stages, in a limited anatomical space, simultaneously with the development of the future facial muscles. The muscles are formed by myoblasts that have migrated from the second pharyngeal arch to their locations in the developing face along with related branches of the facial nerve which undergo variable branching as needed by the developing muscles. This fetal jigsaw puzzle results in a gland that has a more complicated gross anatomical organization than that of other salivary glands and with less fascial definition.

The peripheral connective tissue capsule around the parotid, if present, is of minimal thickness. The skin and the other surrounding structures, that form the walls of this tight parotid space, supply the deep cervical fascia which provides connective tissue packing material for biomechanical protection and support.

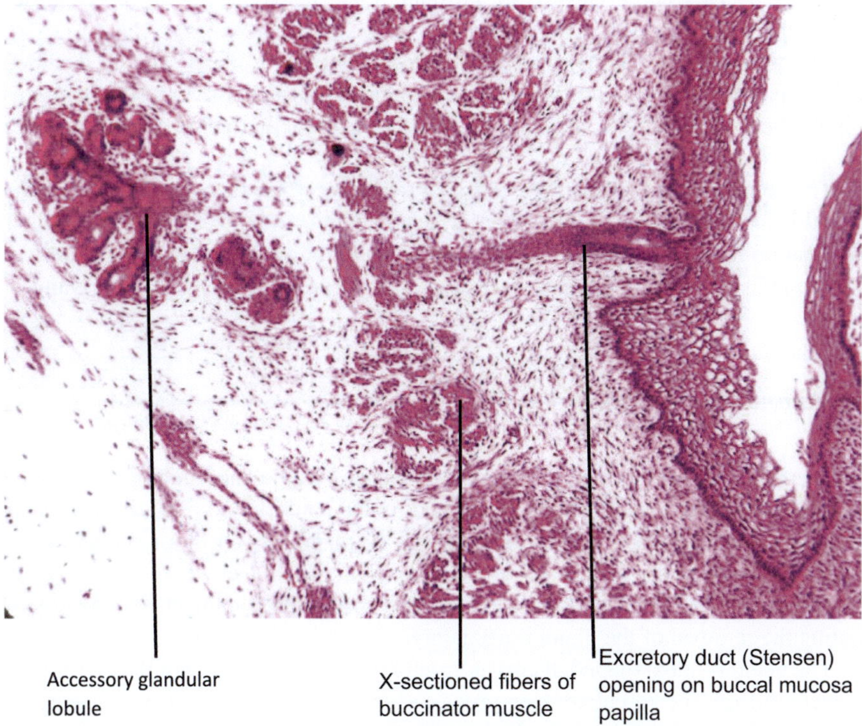

Fig. 1.4 Parotid excretory duct (Stensen) in human fetus (5 months). Coronal section. The duct crosses the buccinator muscle, the fibers of which are seen in this view in cross section. Original magnification 25 × [6]. A small accessory glandular lobule may be associated with the excretory duct

In addition to the poorly defined connective tissue capsule of the parotid, a well-recognized complicating factor in the surgery of the parotid gland is the presence of the five principal branches of the facial nerve (N VII) that run through the parotid space and supply the muscles of facial expression. The variability of the branching pattern and the relationships between the branches [16] may lead to facial nerve palsy during facial surgery.

Vascular and Nerve Supply

The parotid gland lies superficial to the external carotid artery and the external jugular vein and some of their branches. While the facial artery, which branches off the external carotid artery, and the retromandibular vein, which drains into the external jugular vein, are considered the principal vessels that provide the arterial supply and the venous drainage of the gland, these functions may also be carried out opportunistically by other branches of these principal vessels.

The parotid gland receives its afferent nerve supply from the auriculotemporal nerve (V3). This nerve carries the postganglionic parasympathetic (cholinergic) nerve fibers.

The preganglionic parasympathetic (cholinergic) nerve fibers that are destined for the parotid gland accompany the glossopharyngeal nerve (IX) to the otic ganglion where they synapse and travel from there with the auriculotemporal nerve to the parotid.

The preganglionic sympathetic (adrenergic) nerve fibers that are destined for the parotid gland synapse in the superior cervical ganglion and travel from there to their destination in the gland along the vascular coats of the arteries that travel there.

See [17, 18] for detailed studies on anatomical variations of the parotid gland.

Submandibular Gland

The larger and well-defined part of this gland lies in the superficial (close to the skin) submandibular triangle that is formed by the anterior and posterior bellies of the digastric muscle and the inferior border of the mandible. The floor of the triangle is the mylohyoid muscle. The submandibular gland has a distinct connective tissue capsule, which is relatively non-adherent to the surrounding connective tissue, facilitating the removal of the gland if necessary.

The gland is hook-shaped. It curves around the posterior border of the mylohyoid muscle to form the so-called deep process (Figs. 1.5 and 1.6). This is the smaller, more variable part of the gland which lies on the oral side of the mylohyoid muscle. This part of the gland was the earliest to develop. Space restrictions imposed by the surrounding tissues forced the further development of the gland into the

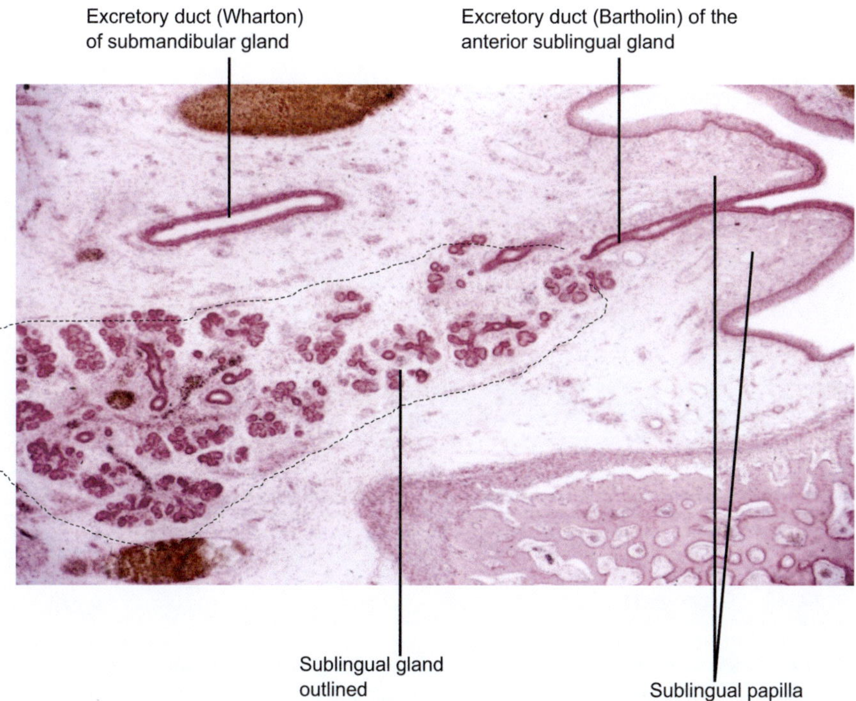

Fig. 1.5 Developing sublingual gland in human fetus (5 months). Sagittal section of the sublingual region. The lingual surface of the developing mandible is shown in the lower right-hand corner. Original magnification 6 ×. Author's slide collection

submandibular triangle. The excretory duct (Wharton) runs anteriorly from the deep process to open on the summit of the sublingual papilla. Along its path, the duct crosses the lingual nerve that runs in a medial direction to innervate the tongue.

Sublingual Gland

The sublingual gland is the smallest of the major salivary glands. It is located on the oral side of the mylohyoid muscle, in the sublingual fossa of the mandible, and immediately below the sublingual mucosa which forms a sublingual fold. As noted before, a distinct anterior major sublingual gland with a well-developed excretory duct (Bartholin) may be present in 65% of the cases. A group of minor sublingual glands is located along the sublingual fold with a variable number [1, 9–20] of small excretory ducts (Rivinus). While they are separate, they are considered part of the total mass of the sublingual gland.

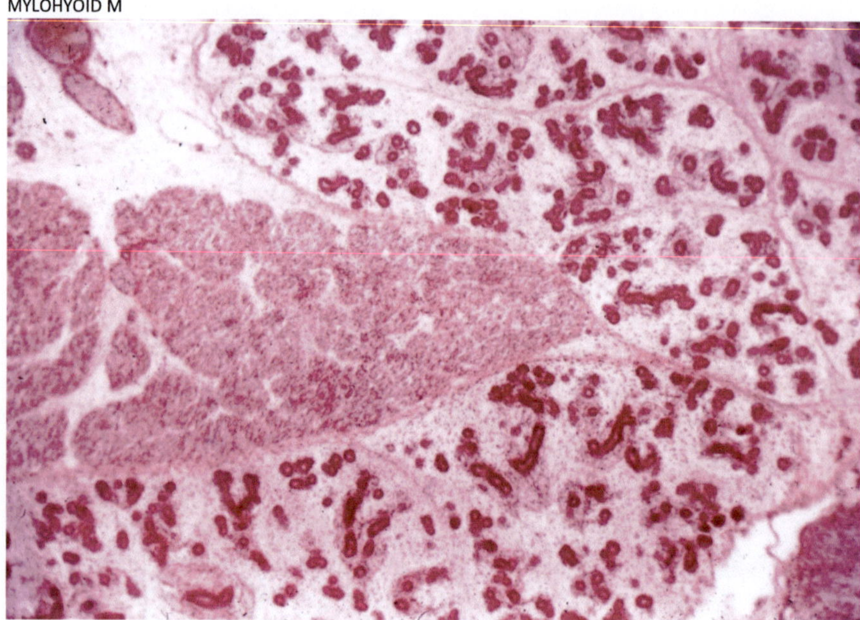

Fig. 1.6 Developing submandibular gland in human fetus (5 months). Sagittal section. Original magnification 6 ×. Author's slide collection. The larger and well-defined part of this gland lies in the superficial submandibular triangle (bottom of this image). The gland is hook-shaped. It curves around the posterior border of the mylohyoid muscle the fibers of which are cross-sectioned in this image

On occasion, portions of the developing sublingual gland may slip between two developmentally distinct parts of the mylohyoid muscle. Both parts initially attach to Meckel's cartilage. During the early fetal period, the anterior part of the attachment is transferred to the developing mandible at the superficial side (skin side) of Meckel's cartilage, while the attachment of the posterior part moves to the mandible at the deep side (oral side) of Meckel's cartilage. The resulting slit-like space between the anterior and posterior muscle components allows the developing sublingual gland to grow from the deep to the superficial side [19, 20] (Fig. 1.7).

Vascular and Nerve Supply

The submandibular and sublingual glands receive their vascular supplies from branches of the facial and lingual arteries.

Their afferent nerve supply is from the lingual nerve (V3). The preganglionic parasympathetic (cholinergic) nerve fibers that are destined for the submandibular and sublingual glands accompany the facial nerve until they are carried by the chorda tympani to the lingual nerve. They synapse in the submandibular ganglion. The postganglionic fibers rejoin the lingual nerve to supply the glands.

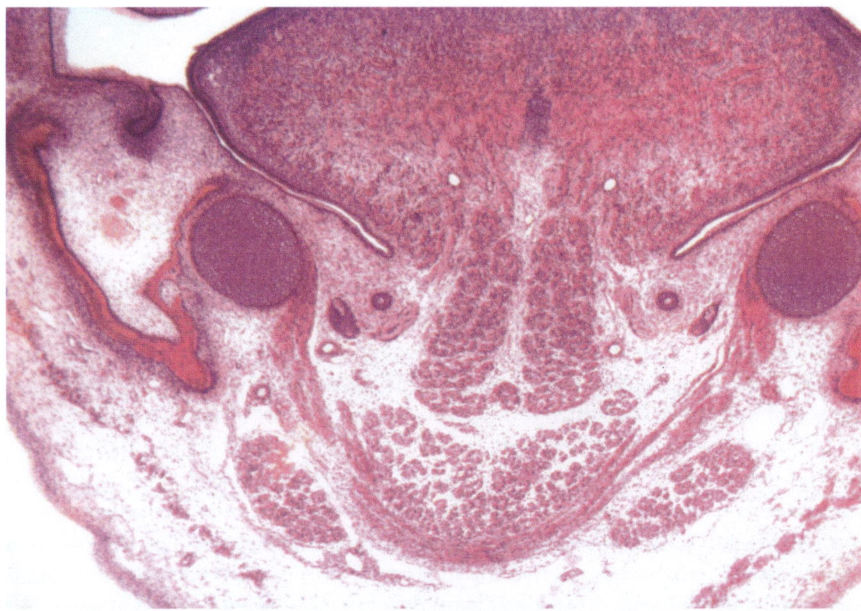

Fig. 1.7 Initial attachment of the mylohyoid muscle to Meckel's cartilage. Human fetus 8 weeks, original magnification 6 ×. Author's slide collection. The attachment of the anterior portion of the muscle will subsequently migrate to the mandible on the superficial (skin) side of the lower jaw, while the attachment of the posterior portion of the muscle will migrate to the mandible on the deep (oral) side of the lower jaw. Developing sublingual glands occasionally slip between the anterior and posterior portions of the mylohyoid muscle from the deep side to the superficial side of the mylohyoid muscle, as described in [19]

The postganglionic sympathetic (adrenergic) nerve fibers reach the glands with the branches of the facial and lingual arteries.

Morphology and Function of the Acino-Ductal Tree of Major Salivary Glands

Saliva is a product that is secreted and modified throughout the length of the acino-ductal system. Saliva is a product that is secreted and modified throughout the length of the acino-ductal system.

With the exception of the excretory ducts, the other ducts and the acini are characterized by simple epithelia. Their epithelial cells are supported by a basal lamina at the interface with the connective tissue stroma; their apical ends face the central lumina of the acini and ducts. All cells are attached apically by tight junctional complexes (terminal bar system), which prevent the salivary product from moving into the intercellular spaces and start digesting the gland itself.

Acini

Acini may be spherical (serous) or sausage-shaped (seromucous). Even in purely seromucous glands, a seromucous acinus frequently has a cap of serous cells *(serous crescent: Gianuzzi; serous demilune: Heidenhain)* that occupies the terminal face of the acinus. The acinar cells form a *simple cuboidal-pyramidal epithelium* that surrounds a narrow lumen. Their apical cytoplasm is filled with secretory granules, whose contents may be discharged into the lumen upon stimulation.

In serous cells, these granules contain *zymogen,* the precursor of a watery enzyme product, composed of α-amylase: an enzyme for digesting starches, histatins, positively charged glycoproteins, proline-rich proteins, and secretory protein. The contents of the zymogen granules are visible in the light microscope. Prior to discharge, the acinar cells look well-filled.

In mucous cells and serous acinar cells of (sero)mucous glands, the granules contain *mucin (MUC5B and MUC7),* the precursors of a heavy, viscous product, composed of negatively charged, high-molecular-weight sialomucins, which tend to form aggregates and a mucous coat on the oral mucosal surfaces. The mucous coat may serve not only as a protective shield but may also provide key immunoregulatory signals that educate dendritic cells to develop tolerance toward food and commensal antigens, like the function of MUC2 that is found in the GI tract [21].

In addition to the zymogen/mucigen product, salivary glands are the most important source for secretory IgA antibodies in the upper respiratory and digestive tracts.

Secretory IgA coats oral epithelium and limits colonization of micro-organisms, thereby reducing an influx of soluble antigens. It also mediates immune responses such as phagocytosis and antibody-dependent, cell-mediated cytotoxicity through a specific IgA receptor that is expressed by monocytes, eosinophils, neutrophils, and macrophages [22]. Importantly, IgA permits a response to harmless commensal bacteria in the oral cavity by limiting inflammation, thus preventing damage to the epithelial barrier.

The serous acinar cells of all major salivary glands and the von Ebner glands secrete **histatins** in the saliva. Histatins are low-molecular-weight histidine-rich proteins that are bactericidal and fungicidal. They are a major component of the innate host non-immune defense system [23].

Also added to the saliva are several growth factors [24, 25].

Intercalated Ducts

Intercalated ducts are the narrowest of the salivary ducts. They are lined by a single layer of *low cuboidal cells,* whose cytoplasm stains relatively neutral and whose volume is occupied mostly by a nucleus. Like the acinar cells, intercalated duct cells are also involved in the *production of secretory IgA,* which is added to the salivary product. The cells are *mitotically active* and may serve as a source of renewal for adjacent acini (although this point has been contested [26]) and striated ducts. Small groups of stem cells have been identified in murine intercalated ducts [27]. Certain salivary gland tumors first develop in these ducts.

Myoepithelial cells surround all intercalated ducts, as well as the acini and parts of the striated ducts (in humans only). Myoepithelial cells are dendritic. They have a cell body in which the nucleus is located and several dendritic cell extensions that surround the acino-ductal components. For this reason, they are sometimes called *basket cells*.

The cell extensions contain *myofibrils* and are contractile. Myoepithelial cells have an epithelial origin and are located on the epithelial side of the basal lamina. Myoepithelial cells have dual sympathetic and parasympathetic innervation. Upon stimulation by either, they contract and assist in the discharge and movement of the salivary product. Myoepithelial cells communicate through gap junctions whose gap junctional protein, connexin 43, is different from the proteins, connexin 32/26, which are found in gap junctions between alveolar cells and are more characteristic for secretory and resorptive epithelia, among others. This suggests separate communication compartments: myoepithelial cells communicate with each other and are related to contraction, and the alveolar cells are related to secretion [28, 29].

Striated Ducts

Striated ducts are lined by a simple, (tall) columnar, epithelium. The epithelial cells are *eosinophilic and highly refractile. In their basal cytoplasm, rows of mitochondria are aligned parallel to the long axis of the cell, between deep infoldings of the basal cell membrane.* This arrangement gives the impression of a striated basal cytoplasm, which gives this duct its name. The histology of striated ducts resembles that of the distal convoluted tubules of the kidney—for a similar functional reason: the *salivary product is altered by a modification of the electrolytes*: the removal from the saliva of NaCl (essentially without water, thereby making the final saliva hypotonic) and secondarily addition of K-ions and HCO_3 ions.

Salivary fluid secretion in the alveolar cells is driven by an electrolyte co-transport system, which results in a net increase of Cl^- ions as well as water in the initial saliva product. Ion transport is necessary to restore the electrolyte balance. Carbonic anhydrase, an enzyme associated with Cl^- ion transport, is prominently present in striated and excretory ducts. Striated duct cells are also implicated in the transport of secretory IgA and release of growth factors into the saliva [30].

Excretory Ducts

Excretory ducts are lined near the lobules by simple, tall columnar epithelium. The epithelium gradually changes to the pseudostratified epithelium. Near the oral cavity, the lining changes to stratified squamous epithelium [31]. These ducts are by no means passive conduits. They *further modify the salivary product by the following:*

Apocrine secretion from the principal epithelial cells (product unknown).

Secretion products of associated sebaceous glands.

Secretion product (mucins) of goblet cells, which are present in the epithelium [21].

Absorption of Cl^- ions.

Release of secretory IgA into the lumen [32].

Once the salivary product is discharged into the oral cavity, it is *further modified* by growth factors, as well as IgG, all of which are added through the gingival crevice.

Morphology and Function of Minor Salivary Glands

All minor salivary glands are mixed, predominantly seromucous in nature, except for *the purely serous von Ebner* glands, which are associated with the vallate and foliate papillae of the tongue. Minor salivary glands have the following:

- *Mucous acini with serous or seromucous demilunes.*
- *Short, intercalated ducts (frequently only some isolated cells).*
- *Intralobular ducts without striations (frequently only some isolated cells).*
- *Short excretory ducts.*

In contrast to the major glands, which must be stimulated to secrete, the minor glands produce a continuous flow of saliva at a rate of about 0.1 μL/minute/gland. Their product is rich in highly glycosylated mucins (MUC5B and MUC7) for tissue lubrication and bacterial aggregation. Minor salivary glands play a critical role in maintaining oral health by secretion of secretory IgA as well as the production by ductal cells of human β defensins. A few additional proteins have been identified in the proteomes of human minor salivary gland secretions that are not present in the secretions of the major salivary glands. This finding suggests that the minor salivary gland may have specific functions in the oral cavity.

The purely serous Von Ebner glands that are associated with circumvallate and foliate papillae have recently been shown to produce a significant amount of histatins, which may suggest that they have an important role in preventing microbial assaults on the tissues of the posterior region of the tongue [23].

References

1. van Amerongen A, Veerman ECI. Saliva—the defender of the oral cavity. Oral Dis. 2008;8(1):12–22. https://doi.org/10.1034/j.1601-0825.2002.1o816.x.
2. Castelli WA, Huelke DF, Celis A. Some basic anatomic features in paralingual space surgery. Oral Surg. 1969;27:613–21.
3. Moss-Salentijn L, Moss ML. Chapter 2: Developmental and functional anatomy. In: Rankow RM, Polayes IM, editors. Diseases of the salivary glands. Philadelphia: W.B. Saunders; 1976.

4. Young JA, van Lennep EW. The morphology of salivary glands. In: 2. Gross anatomy. London: Academic Press; 1978. p. 8–21.
5. Moss-Salentijn L, Applebaum E. A minor salivary gland in human gingiva. Arch Oral Biol. 1972;17:1373–4.
6. Moss-Salentijn L, Applebaum E, Lammé A. Orofacial histology and embryology. A visual integration. Philadelphia: F.A. Davis; 1972.
7. Braus H. Anatomie des Menschen. Berlin: Springer; 1924.
8. Koyama N, Hayashi T, Ohno K, Siu L, Gresik EW, Kashimata M. Signaling pathways activated by epidermal growth factor receptor or fibroblast growth factor receptor differentially regulate branching morphogenesis in fetal mouse submandibular glands development. Growth Differ. 2008;50(7):565–76. https://doi.org/10.1111/j.1440-169x.2008.01053.x.
9. Kashimata M, Hayashi T. Regulatory mechanisms of branching morphogenesis in mouse submandibular gland rudiments. Jpn Dent Sci Rev. 2018;54(1):2–7. https://doi.org/10.1016/j.jdsr.2017.06.002.
10. Musselmann K, Green JA, Sone K, Hsu JC, Bothwell IR, Johnson SA, Harunaga JS, Wei Z, Yamada KM. Salivary gland gene expression atlas identifies a new regulator of branching morphogenesis. J Dent Res. 2011;90(9):1078–84. https://doi.org/10.1177/0022034511413131.
11. Martín-Belmonte F, Yu W, Rodríguez-Fraticelli AE, Ewald AJ, Werb Z, Alonso MA, Mostov K. Cell-polarity dynamics controls the mechanism of lumen formation in epithelial morphogenesis. Curr Biol. 2008;18(7):507–13.
12. Mellas RE, Kim H, Osinski J, Sadibasic S, Gronostajski RM, Cho M, Baker OJ. NFIB regulates embryonic development of submandibular glands. J Dent Res. 2015;94(2):312–9. https://doi.org/10.1177/0022034514559129.
13. Miyazaki Y, Nakanishi Y, Hieda Y. Tissue interaction mediated by neuregulin-1 and ErbB receptors regulates epithelial morphogenesis of mouse embryonic submandibular gland. Dev Dyn. 2004;230(4):591–6. https://doi.org/10.1002/dvdy.20078.
14. Grodinsky M, Holyoke EA. The fascia and fascial spaces of the head, neck and adjacent regions. Am J Anat. 1938;63:367–408.
15. Som PM, Brandwein-Gensler MS. Anatomy and pathology of the salivary glands. In: Som PM, Curtin HD, editors. Head and neck imaging E-Book. ProQuest Ebook Central; 2011. http://ebookcentral.proquest.com.
16. De Bonnecaze G, et al. Variability in facial-muscle innervation: a comparative study based on electrostimulation and anatomical dissection. Clin Anat. 2019;32:169–75.
17. Davis RA, Anson BJ, Budinger JM, Kurth LE. Surgical anatomy of the facial nerve and parotid gland based upon a study of 350 cervicofacial halves. Surg Gynecol Obstet. 1956;102:385–412.
18. Gaughran GRL. The parotid compartment. Ann Otol. 1961;70:31–52.
19. Moss-Salentijn L. Reattachment of the mammalian mylohyoid muscle during late embryonic development. Craniofacial growth series, vol. 10. Ann Arbor: University of Michigan; 1981. p. 145–64.
20. Moss-Salentijn L, Hendricks-Klyvert M. A bilateral superficial location of human sublingual glands. A case report. J Oral Maxillofac Surg. 1987;45:983–6. https://doi.org/10.1016/0278-2391(87)90456-3.
21. Shan M, Gentile M, Yeiser JR, Walland AC, Bornstein VU, Chen K, He B, Cassis L, Bigas A, Cols M, Comerma L, Huang B, Blander JM, Xiong H, Mayer L, Berin C, Augenlicht LH, Velcich A, Cerutti A. Mucus enhances gut homeostasis and oral tolerance by delivering immunoregulatory signals. Science. 2013;342(6157):447–53. https://doi.org/10.1126/science.1237910.
22. Herr AB, Ballister ER, Bjorkman PJ. Insights into IgA-mediated immune responses from the crystal structures of human FcαRI and its complex with IgA1-Fc. Nature. 2003;423:614–20.
23. Piludu M, Serenella Lantini M, Cossu M, Piras M, Oppenheim FG, Helmerhorst EJ, Siqueira W, Hand AR. Salivary histatins in human deep posterior lingual glands (of von Ebner). Arch Oral Biol. 2006;51(11):967–73. https://doi.org/10.1016/j.archoralbio.2006.05.011.

24. Bläuer M, Wichmann L, Punnonen R, Tuohimaa P. Measurement of activin B in human saliva and localization of activin subunits in rat salivary glands. Biochem Biophys Res Commun. 1996;222(2):230–5. https://doi.org/10.1006/bbrc.1996.0727.
25. Cossu M, Perra MT, Piludu M, Lantini MS. Subcellular localization of epidermal growth factor in human submandibular gland. Histochem J. 2000;32(5):291–4. https://doi.org/10.1023/a:1004036929006.
26. Taga R, Sesso A. Cell population growth in the rat parotid gland during postnatal development. Arch Oral Biol. 2001;46(10):909–18. https://doi.org/10.1016/s0003-9969(01)00056-5.
27. Kwak M, Alston N, Ghazizadeh S. Identification of stem cells in the secretory complex of salivary glands. J Dent Res. 2016;95:776–83.
28. Shimono M, Young Lee C, Matsuzaki H, Ishikawa H, Inoue T, Hashimoto S, Muramatsu T. Connexins in salivary glands. Eur J Morphol. 2000;38(4):257–61. https://doi.org/10.1076/0924-3860(200010)38:4;1-o;ft257.
29. Chitturi RT, Veeravarmal V, Nirmal RM, Ramana Reddy BV. Myoepithelial cells (MEC) of the salivary glands in health and tumours. Clin Diagn Res. 2015;9(3):ZE14–8.
30. Tandler B, Gresik EW, Nagato T, Phillips CJ. Secretion by striated ducts of mammalian major salivary glands: review from an ultrastructural, functional, and evolutionary perspective. Anat Rec. 2001;264(2):121–45. https://doi.org/10.1002/ar.1108.
31. Tandler B, Pinkstaff CA, Phillips CJ. Interlobular excretory ducts of mammalian salivary glands: structural and histochemical review. Anat Rec A Discov Mol Cell Evol Biol. 2006;288(5):498–526. https://doi.org/10.1002/ar.a.20319.
32. Perra MT, Puxeddu R, Maxia C, Sirigu P. Immunohistochemical localization of secretory immunoglobulins in the main excretory duct of the human submandibular gland. Arch Histol Cytol. 1998;61(5):427–32. https://doi.org/10.1679/aohc.61.427.

Chapter 2
Saliva

Louis Mandel

Abstract Salivary volume measurements are an integral part of any investigation of a salivary gland (SG) disorder. Abnormal SG conditions brought about by intrinsic and extrinsic factors usually impact upon salivary production. Mechanisms for the assessment of changes in salivary volume, a key element in diagnosing a SG problem, are available. However, the evaluation must be objectively based. Subjective complaints of decreased saliva (xerostomia) or increased saliva (sialorrhea) are unreliable and prove to be anecdotal in nature. Objective techniques for salivary volume collection and study have been established while standardized values have been accepted for the presence of hyposalivation or hypersalivation. The aim of this chapter is to review those conditions that impinge upon SG volume production. Medications, organophosphates and some medical conditions can lead to hypersalivation, while neurodegenerative diseases cause drooling, often misinterpreted as hypersalivation. Hyposalivation is the more common salivary entity that is encountered. Systemic diseases, many medications and radiation are causes of hyposalivation.

Normal

The overall responsibilities of saliva are to aid in the digestive process by breaking down starch, maintain a stable ecologic environment in the mouth and throat, promote oral health, participate in taste sensation, and moisturize the oral mucosa [1]. Because of these very important functions, saliva plays an intimate role in maintaining patient well-being. Consequently, an increased interest by a variety of investigators has focused on all aspects of normal qualitative and quantitative saliva. Additionally, it has become apparent to them that some systemic abnormalities can directly affect saliva and the salivary gland structure. The information that has been obtained has been applied to the study of saliva and salivary gland disease (SGD) with no systemic manifestations, those associated with systemic disease, and as a

© The Author(s), under exclusive license to Springer Nature Switzerland AG 2024

L. Mandel, *Clinical Management of Salivary Gland Disorders*,
https://doi.org/10.1007/978-3-031-50012-1_2

tool in some conditions to monitor patient progress. Diagnosis of a salivary problem and SGD requires a multifaceted approach. Determining a patient's salivary flow rate is usually a key factor in diagnosis, but the result must be integrated into the information gained from the patient's medical history, physical and clinical examinations, imaging, serology, and, if necessary, a surgical biopsy. Only when the collection of these data is completed can a confident firm diagnosis be reached.

Normally 500–1500 mL of saliva, whose pH varies from 6.0 to 7.5, is produced in a 24-h period [1, 2]. This volume includes the combined unstimulated and stimulated whole saliva flow rates. Unstimulated (resting) saliva is that portion of saliva produced while there is nothing in the mouth acting as a stimulant. Stimulated saliva is that fraction of saliva produced when an oral stimulant (food, gum, etc.) is present. At rest, the submandibular salivary glands produce approximately 65% of the whole unstimulated saliva, while the parotid glands (PG) secrete 20% of the total volume, and the sublingual salivary glands function to produce 5–7% with the minor salivary glands serving to contribute about 10% to the unstimulated salivary flow [3]. However, with salivary gland stimulation, the PG secretory share increases to approximately 50% of the total secretory volume [4]. Although some modest divergences exist in the acknowledged measurements of whole salivary flow and its effect on oral dryness, it is generally accepted that approximately 0.3–0.5 mL/min represents a normal flow rate for unstimulated whole saliva. Hyposalivation becomes a problem when unstimulated whole saliva of <0.1 or <0.5 mL/min of stimulated whole saliva (normal 1.0–2.0 mL/min) is produced [4–9]. Saliva has a circadian rhythm such that during sleep the salivary flow rate decreases to 0.1 mL/min. This fact combined with some patients' tendency to mouth breathe (snoring) probably explains the frequent complaint of oral dryness upon awakening.

Saliva is 99% water. It also contains electrolytes such as sodium, potassium, calcium, bicarbonate, chloride, iodine, and phosphate. The salivary enzymes such as lipase and amylase serve to begin fat and starch digestion. Antimicrobial substances (lysozyme, IgA, lactoferrin) and mucus (glycoprotein) are also present in saliva.

Clear definitions of terminology are essential elements in understanding the results of the numerous studies that center around normal and abnormal salivary flow rates. Standardized language is an absolute requirement for communication between professionals. Hypersalivation is the accepted term now used to describe an objectively measured increase in salivary flow, while hyposalivation refers to an objective decrease in measured flow rate. Xerostomia is not to be used to describe an objective decrease in salivary volume. It is a term best used to describe the patient's subjective sensation of oral dryness. Drooling represents a failure in the management of what is usually a normal salivary volume. It is mainly caused by a defect in the neuromuscular swallowing mechanism. Swallowing is activated when the oral salivary volume reaches a level of 1.1 mL [10]. An inability to create a competent lip seal contributes to the drooling problem. Confusion arises because sialorrhea is a word often used to describe extraoral salivary drooling or increased salivation. To avoid confusion, "sialorrhea" should probably be scrapped and replaced by hypersalivation or drooling as indicated.

Hypersalivation

Overview

Hypersalivation is defined as an increase in salivary production. The term "sialorrhea" is frequently used in the literature, and although used as a synonym for hypersalivation, its use should be avoided. Typically, salivary volume in a 24-h period totals between 500 and 1500 mL. Normal unstimulated whole salivary volume is in the range of 0.3–0.5 mL/min, while stimulated whole salivary volume in the range of 1.0–2.0 mL/min is considered normal [4–9]. A circadian rhythm is also present with salivary production during sleep dropping sharply. Often if there is an increase in salivary production, or if saliva becomes unmanageable because of neurodegenerative or neuromuscular problems, drooling will develop. Drooling is the involuntary extraoral spilling out of saliva caused by the failure of its oral clearance.

Known causes of hypersalivation include medications (cholinergics and anticholinesterases), heavy metal poisoning, rabies, some forms of seizure disorders, and oral irritating factors such as teething or dentures. Additionally, the subjective complaint of excessive salivation often is perceptual (somatoform) in origin with these patients representing a high percentage of those seeking care in the Columbia University Salivary Gland Center (SGC).

Hyposalivation

Medications

With an expanding and aging population and the constant arrival of new effective therapeutic pharmaceuticals, the use of prescription medications has grown considerably. Remarkably, there were 5.8 billion prescriptions dispensed in the United States in 2018 [11] with adverse drug reactions increasing in direct proportion to the number of drugs that the patient uses. Medication dosage and duration of use also play roles in the onset of drug complications. A review of the 200 most frequently prescribed drugs in the USA revealed dry mouth to be the most common oral adverse reaction (Fig. 2.6) [12]. There are hundreds or even thousands of drugs that can be xerogenic [13]. Age, accompanied by multiple medication use, can also play a role in the development of objective hyposalivation, while female gender and psychologic factors are other key elements in complaints of subjective dryness [14].

The elderly have a reported prevalence of subjective dry mouth that ranges up to 72% [15]. At this point, it again should be re-stated that hyposalivation is an objective decrease in salivary volume that creates a sense of oral dryness, while xerostomia represents the subjective sense of oral dryness. Normal unstimulated whole resting flow rate measures 0.3–0.5 mL/min with values <0.1 mL/min considered abnormal and indicative of hyposalivation. Stimulated whole saliva normally measures in the range of 1–2 mL/min with values <0.5 mL/min requiring prompt attention regarding a true dryness [12, 14].

A patient's complaint of oral dryness is not to be regarded as a trivial issue. Difficulties that can develop include dental caries, halitosis, candidiasis, dysgeusia, periodontal disease, oral burning, tongue fissuring, eating, and speaking. All may result from the simultaneous use of multiple xerogenic drugs. Pharmaceuticals such as antidepressants, antipsychotics, antihistamines, antihypertensives, bronchodilators, diuretics, appetite suppressants, skeletal muscle relaxants, drugs of abuse, and drugs to treat reflux disease or an overactive bladder have been implicated as causes of hyposalivation and xerostomia. Reference guides regarding the multitude of drugs involved in hyposalivation, as well as hypersalivation, have been published and are available for the practitioner's perusal [14, 16].

Once more, it should be stated that it is the experience of the Columbia University Salivary Gland Center that the use of one anticholinergic medication is not sufficient to cause subjective symptomatology. The modest salivary decrease that occurs with one medication is difficult for the patient to subjectively recognize and is readily compensated when eating stimulates the salivary glands to increase their output. It is the use of multiple xerogenic drugs that cause a subjective and objective oral dryness.

Hypersalivation

Myasthenia Gravis Treatment

Myasthenia gravis (MG) is an autoimmune disorder of the neuromuscular junction, mainly characterized by fatigue, respiratory difficulties, and weakness of a wide range of skeletal muscles, particularly the ocular muscles. MG can develop at any age, but it is most commonly seen in women under 40 years of age and in men over 60 years old [17, 18]. It has an estimated annual incidence of 0.25–2.0 per 100,000 people [19].

The MG problem develops from a disruption in neuromuscular transmission that results when circulating autoantibodies bind to proteins involved in the signaling mechanism at the neuromuscular junction [17]. A thymoma or thymus hyperplasia is present in a high percentage of MG patients. Therefore, the thymus is suspected as the source of these autoantibodies. Because these antibodies interfere with the activity of the acetylcholine (ACH) receptors, they discourage the release of ACH. A failure to adequately stimulate muscarinic and nicotinic receptors occurs. The muscarinic receptors have secretory stimulation, salivary and lacrimal, as one of their major responsibilities [20]. When the nicotinic receptors are involved, nerve impulses are prevented from triggering muscle contractions. Consequently, patients develop muscular defects that include muscle weakness, muscle fasciculations, respiratory difficulties, dysphagia, and limb weakness [21].

Because the pathophysiology of untreated MG involves interference with ACH activity, hyposalivation should be anticipated as one of its clinical features. However, a literature review failed to uncover any data relative to measurements of salivary flow rates in untreated MG patients. Of interest is the fact that even in the presence of an assumed decrease in salivation, drooling may still occur. The drooling results from the weak oro-facial musculature, associated with MG, failing to provide an adequate sealing of the lips. Alternatively, increases in salivary flow can be expected with the therapeutic introduction of cholinergic medications, particularly pyridostigmine, for the treatment of MG. The therapeutic regimen for MG is varied, and it also includes immunosuppressives, plasmapheresis, immunoglobulins, thymectomy when indicated, and rituximab [22]. Nevertheless, pyridostigmine is utilized as MG's therapeutic pillar. Acetylcholinesterase (ACHE) is the enzyme responsible for the degradation of ACH. The therapeutic agent pyridostigmine functions as an inhibitor of ACHE. This inhibitor derives its potent cholinergic effect from its ability to prevent the breakdown of any released ACH by the enzyme ACHE. Therefore, the clinician should be aware that hypersalivation, from overstimulation of the muscarinic receptors during inappropriate therapy, may become collateral damage.

Prescribed dosages for MG of the ACHE inhibitors must be carefully monitored. Overdosage is not unusual and will result in a cholinergic crisis [20]. The crisis develops from the medication's overstimulation of the muscarinic and nicotinic receptors. A significant elevation in the salivary flow rate is one of the consequences of the increased stimulation of muscarinic receptors. Miosis, urinary frequency, diaphoresis, bradycardia, emesis, and lacrimation are some of the other clinical findings related to excessive stimulation of the muscarinic receptors during a cholinergic crisis.

Atropine has proven to be an effective agent to combat overstimulation by the muscarinic effects of ACH. It binds to the muscarinic receptor and thereby prevents further action of ACH [20]. It has become the drug of choice for the treatment of a medication-induced cholinergic crisis.

Hypersalivation

Organophosphates

Organophosphates (OP) are a group of chemicals used in the manufacture of insecticides and herbicides. However, their use comes with some caveats. The OP have a deleterious effect in humans derived from their ability to inhibit the enzyme acetylcholinesterase (ACHE), which is the key agent involved in the breakdown of the neurotransmitter acetylcholine (ACH). Exposure to the OP may result from inhalation, ingestion, or dermal contact. Factories involved in the production of OP continually monitor their employees for any adverse event that may result from exposure to these inhibitors of ACHE. In addition to the factory employees, agricultural workers and gardeners using OP in their work represent other individuals who may be exposed to the effects of OP.

The failure of ACH breakdown by ACHE causes an overabundance of ACH. Excessive stimulation of the muscarinic receptors present in the sympathetic and parasympathetic nervous systems is the end result. Hypersalivation represents one of the symptoms associated with the resulting increased cholinergic activity. The hypersalivation can be sufficient to initiate the patient's concern and request for medical attention. Over the years, two such patients (a factory-employed chemical engineer and a gardener) have been seen in the Salivary Gland Center. Their hypersalivation was readily confirmed when measurements of their whole unstimulated and whole stimulated salivary flows were obtained. The exposure to OP may be life-threatening, with increased salivation representing one of the harbingers of OP toxicity.

Atropine inhibits acetylcholine activity at the muscarinic receptor site. Therefore, it has been successfully prescribed for OP toxicity as a counter to the increased salivation and for the systemic effects of the OP.

Hypersalivation

Gastroesophageal Reflux Disease (GERD)

The esophagus contains afferent nerve fibers that travel with the vagus and spinal splanchnic nerves on their way to the salivary nuclei located in the pons. These nerves function as the basis of the esophageal salivary reflex (ESR). The afferent receptors within the esophageal wall are either chemoreceptors or mechanoreceptors. Activation by gastric chemical irritation of a chemoreceptor will stimulate salivary flow [1]. The mechanoreceptors are stimulated to increase salivation when there is esophageal distention caused by the physical presence of a foreign body or neoplasm. These irritations that develop within the esophageal lumen, be they chemical or physical, can initiate an increased salivary flow via the ESR. The increased slightly alkaline saliva finds its way to the esophagus where it dilutes/neutralizes the chemical irritant or attempts to flush away any mechanical obstruction [1].

Gastroesophageal reflux disease (GERD) represents a common cause of hypersalivation that is episodic in nature. GERD is the end result of the backward flow of gastric contents (acid, pepsin, bile) into the esophagus [23, 24]. The acidic gastric regurgitation irritates the mucosal wall of the esophagus and causes GERD and the symptoms of heartburn [25, 26]. Hiatus hernia (HH) and pregnancy serve as major causes of GERD [27]. The reflux is made possible either because of a mechanical problem, as is thought to occur in relation to an HH, or associated with a defective sphincter tone that may develop during pregnancy.

Obesity and aging are considered general risk factors for HH, while increased abdominal pressure from violent coughing, emesis, or straining during defecation acts as immediate precipitants. HH occurs because of loss of diaphragmatic muscle tone or increased intra-abdominal pressure that allows a pouch of the stomach to herniate through the diaphragm's normal anatomic esophageal hiatus [28]. The herniated stomach segment comes to rest in the thorax. It is this herniated segment that then acts to mechanically compromise the gastroesophageal sphincter. The impaired malfunctioning sphincter allows acidic stomach contents in the herniated segment to flow backward into the esophagus and cause significant esophageal irritation that often manifests itself with heartburn symptomatology [29]. It is the anatomic changes caused by the HH that physically affect the mechanics involved in sphincter function [30]. Sphincter incompetency with more severe GERD usually occurs in HH patients when the size of the herniated segment measures 2 cm or more [31].

In addition, GERD has been recognized as a common occurrence (30–80%) in pregnant women [32, 33]. Probably, the increase in circulating estrogen and progesterone hormones lessens the contractility of the gastroesophageal sphincter. The sphincter consisting of smooth muscle, guarding against retrograde movement of gastric contents, can lose its tautness and become somewhat flaccid, thus facilitating the reflux of gastric contents into the esophagus [34, 35]. Serious esophageal problems do not have time to develop because, after fetus delivery, sphincter tone returns and regurgitation ceases.

GERD is estimated to occur in 20–50% of the general population and there seems to be an increasing incidence [36–38]. Reflux of gastric contents can occur as much as 20 or more times each day with each episode lasting 2–3 min [39], and in these circumstances will cause episodic heartburn and GERD. Heartburn is recognized as a midline retrosternal burning sensation that may extend from the throat to the xiphoid process. It becomes most pronounced after meals, especially if spicy or citric foods, caffeine, or fatty foods have been ingested. Gravity, as in assuming a prone position during sleep or when bending, is also a facilitator of reflux and the onset of GERD. Oral regurgitation may develop and result in a bitter taste, while the acidic reflux chronicity can lead to hoarseness, constant coughing, and dental corrosion. A loss of dental enamel represents the end product of persistent orally regurgitated gastric acid and is compounded by the gastric acid contents present in any associated emetic episodes.

Repeated and frequent incursions of reflux containing acid, pepsin, and bile can result in inflammatory injury to the esophageal mucosa. Gastric acid, essentially hydrochloric acid, has an extremely low pH of 1.5–2.0. Regurgitated pepsin is a proteolytic enzyme that also has a deleterious effect on the esophageal mucosa. Esophageal erosions and ulcerations can develop, with inflammation and strictures that make swallowing painful. Acid-mediated injury may cause dysplastic changes in the lower esophagus such that the squamous epithelial lining becomes columnar (Barrett's esophagitis). This process makes the patient more susceptible to the onset of an adenocarcinoma [38, 40, 41]. Consequently, in order to avoid this tendency toward esophageal damage, it has become imperative to clear the lower esophagus from invasion by gastric contents.

Normally, esophageal clearance is accomplished by one or two peristaltic waves that serve to eliminate the bulk of the reflux. Primary peristalsis is initiated by a swallow and triggered at pH 4.0, while secondary peristalsis results from local esophageal stimulation [42]. However, peristalsis alone is not sufficient to clear residual gastric contents clinging to the mucosal wall of the esophagus. Even a small amount of residual gastric material is sufficient to damage tissue. Therefore, the need for further esophageal acid clearance is obvious.

Final and effective clearance and mucosal wall protection results from a combination of factors. As stated, the ESR is mediated through vagus and splanchnic nerves that have receptors in the esophageal wall. Although the neurophysiologic basis of esophageal sensation is not well understood, it is accepted that stimulation of the ESR by GERD causes a hypersalivation known as water brash. With the inevitable swallow following the water brash episode, saliva with its contained bicarbonate acts to neutralize any residual gastric acid present in the esophagus [42]. Simultaneously, the increased salivary volume serves to prevent esophageal wall damage through its diluting and lavaging actions. Further protection of the esophageal mucosa is expedited by the epidermal growth factor contained within the saliva. Mucus within the saliva and the increased mucus secreted by inflamed esophageal mucous glands represent additional means to inhibit esophageal wall damage.

Medications represent the mainstay of GERD treatment. Antacids, histamine-2 receptor antagonists, and proton pump inhibitors have all been prescribed [43]. They serve to neutralize and reduce the refluxed gastric volume and its acid content that incites GERD and its consequences. Avoiding large meals and the consumption of alcohol and spices have proven to be helpful. Elevating the head during sleep discourages nocturnal reflux. Oral drooling from water brash during sleep may cause a wet pillow and serve as a clue regarding the presence of GERD. Skin excoriations at the angle area of the mouth develop from chronic drooling on the side to which the head is constantly tilted while sleeping (Figs. 2.1 and 2.2).

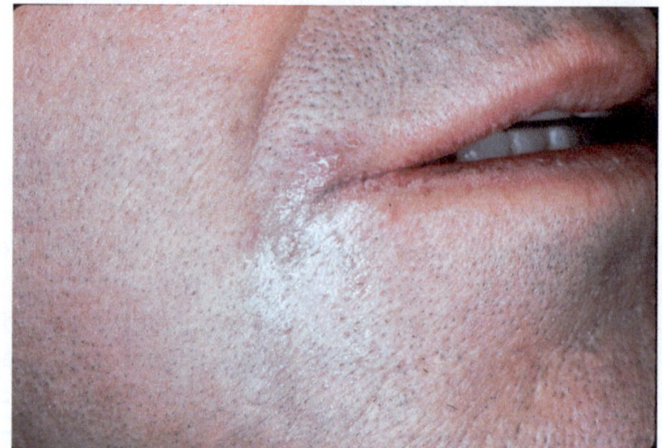

Fig. 2.1 Hypersalivation. GERD with chronic nocturnal drooling causing a commissural cheilitis. Patient had a hiatal hernia. (Mandel L, JADA 1995; 126:1537)

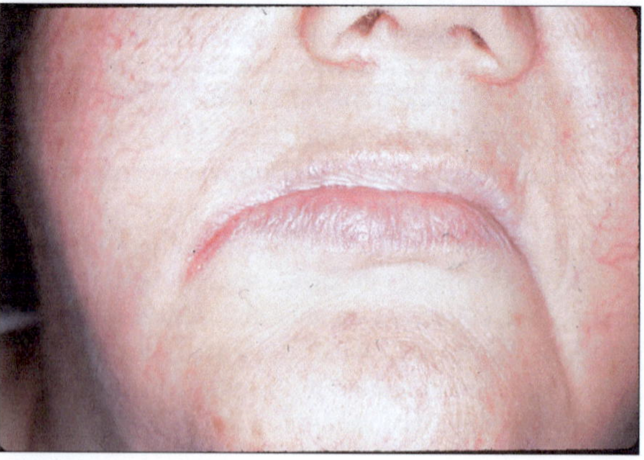

Fig. 2.2 Hypersalivation with chronic nocturnal drooling from an unknown cause. Commissural cheilitis is present (right side)

Hypersalivation

Self-Limited Epilepsy with Centrotemporal Spikes

Self-limited epilepsy with centrotemporal spikes (SLECTS), formerly called benign epilepsy with centrotemporal spikes, is an idiopathic benign epileptic syndrome that affects children but remits spontaneously by the age of 18 years [44]. Patients develop focal seizures, accompanied by periods of excessive salivation, that usually occur during sleep. In some unusual cases, seizures and hypersalivation occur during awake periods [45].

SLECTS is a rare cause of episodic hypersalivation. The Columbia University Salivary Gland Center has only seen one such patient since the Center's establishment in 1987. Because SLECTS involves children, a more detailed review of the entity can be found in Chap. 12 ("Salivary Gland Disease in Children").

Drooling

Overview

Drooling results from an upset in the coordinated control mechanism of the orofacial and palatal–lingual musculatures. Because this musculature dysregulation impairs the swallowing mechanism, saliva accumulates in the mouth floor. Often, an accompanying inadequate lip seal allows the pooled saliva to unintentionally exit the mouth and cause visible drooling. Drooling is considered a normal manifestation in infants up to the age of 30 months, but, in older children and adolescents, drooling usually represents a secondary condition arising from a developmental neuromuscular defect. In the elderly, it usually is an issue associated with neurodegenerative disease. Sialorrhea is a term often used both as a synonym for drooling and for an increased salivary production. Nonetheless, the proper term for a raised salivary production is hypersalivation. Clarification and standardization require that sialorrhea be discarded as a diagnostic word and replaced by drooling or hypersalivation as indicated.

Drooling demands attention because it has a significant effect on the patient's quality of life in that it has physical, psychological, and social implications. The drooled saliva soils the clothing, requires excessive and constant caregiving, causes perioral skin macerations, affects speech and eating, can cause pulmonary complications, and can have serious psychologic consequences not only for the patient but also for the family.

Patients who drool are often misdiagnosed with hypersalivation (excessive production of saliva). Hypersalivation is the misdiagnosis often made for patients who are victims of a variety of neurodevelopmental or neurodegenerative diseases. Patients with Parkinson's disease (PD), Alzheimer's disease (AD), and all other forms of dementia, amyotrophic lateral sclerosis (ALS), and cerebral palsy (CP) often display drooling. The primary common denominator uniting these disparate neurologic disorders is a disturbance in the patient's neuromusculature with a consequent failure of normal swallowing activity, usually abetted by an open mouth. A normal swallowing process can be disrupted in two ways: from neurodevelopmental/neurodegenerative conditions or structurally from trauma and masses [46].

Definitive therapy for drooling should be directed at the cause. However, treatment of the underlying cause often is not possible. In such situations, palliative care is indicated. A variety of approaches for the control of drooling is available [47, 48]. Oral motor training to increase muscle tone and stabilize head position represents a conservative first option. It can be supplemented with behavioral therapy and biofeedback. A proactive approach involves reducing cholinergic activity with the administration of medications such as glycopyrrolate, atropine, or benztropine. Surgical duct ligation or surgical redirection of the submandibular duct has met with some success [49], but the surgeon should be aware that the postoperative development of a ranula is always a threat when performing submandibular duct surgery. Botulinum toxin injections are beneficial, but repeated injections after 4–6 months are required [50]. Sclerotherapy results in salivary gland ablation and its use has been suggested for refractory drooling [51]. Irradiation to the salivary glands can cause decreases in the salivary volume that accumulates in the anterior mouth floor. Unfortunately, the decrease in salivary return comes with a price. The emissions have the potential to incite pre-malignancies in irradiated tissues.

Drooling

Alzheimer's Disease

Alzheimer's disease (AD) is a progressive fatal neurodegenerative disorder characterized by a cognitive deterioration that manifests itself with a loss of intellectual function, memory, problem-solving ability, language skills, and abstract reasoning [52]. It was estimated in 2014 that five million Americans were affected by AD with an expectation of 13 million victims by the year 2050 [53].

Cholinergic neurons in the forebrain degenerate in the early stages of AD leading to a significant decrease in acetylcholine (ACH) levels [54]. Therefore, treatment is directed at increasing ACH levels. Cholinesterase (ChE) is the enzyme responsible for the hydrolytic breakdown of ACH. Acetylcholinesterase inhibitors (AChEI) increase ACH levels and temporarily slow the progression of AD. Their use has demonstrated moderate improvements in the cognitive function of AD patients [54, 55]. Currently, donepezil is widely used as the AChEI of choice because it has proven to be centrally effective with minimal peripheral side effects [56].

The synaptic dysfunction and death of cholinergic nerve cells in AD lead to decreased cholinergic stimulation of the salivary glands. However, only a modest

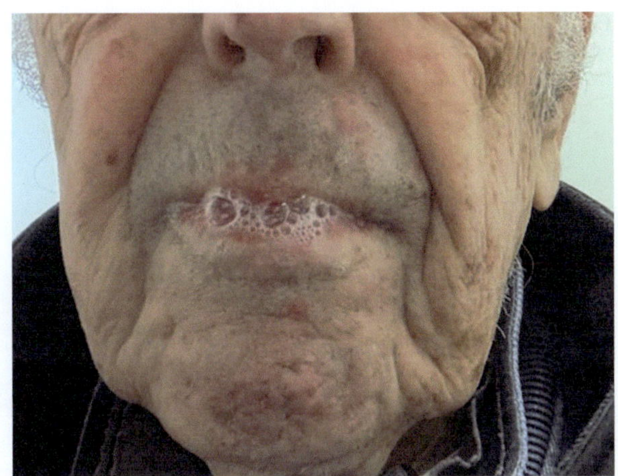

Fig. 2.3 Drooling. Patient with Alzheimer's disease

decrease in the submandibular gland flow rate and no changes in the parotid flow rate have been observed in untreated AD patients [53, 57]. Nevertheless, drooling develops despite the decreased submandibular flow (Fig. 2.3). The problem originates from the fact that even the decreased salivary volume cannot be adequately managed by AD patients. Defective swallowing from neurodegenerative disease, an issue in AD patients, is generally improved with an increase in the ACH concentration. With the administration of donepezil, the salivary secretory volume approaches normality. Furthermore, donepezil's ability to increase ACH concentration contributes to more effective swallowing because it also improves the activity of the swallowing musculatures [53]. Regardless, donepezil is not sufficient to negate the salivary pooling and drooling that occurs in AD.

Drooling

Parkinson's Disease

Parkinson's disease (PD) is an idiopathic slowly progressive neurodegenerative disease caused by neuron loss in the substantia nigra of the midbrain. The gradual destruction of dopaminergic nerve cells results in the development of symptoms of dopamine deficiency [58]. PD has a prevalence of 0.3% in the general population. It occurs in 1% of those over 60 years of age [58, 59] making it the second most common, after dementia, neurodegenerative disease. The diagnosis of PD is based on the presence of bradykinesia and one of the three following cardinal signs: rigidity, resting tremors, and loss of postural reflexes [60]. In addition to these motor disturbances, there is an autonomic nerve system dysfunction, particularly involving the digestive system with manifestations of dysphagia, gastrointestinal disorders, and constipation [60, 61].

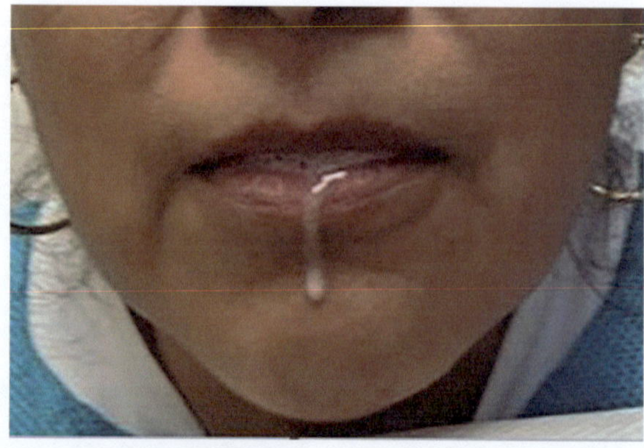

Fig. 2.4 Drooling. Patient with Parkinson's disease. Inadequate lip seal

Salivary flow rate during resting and stimulated secretory states is decreased in PD as a result of the autonomic dysfunction [58, 62–65]. Surprisingly, drooling is an issue despite the presence of this decreased salivation (Fig. 2.4). Hyposalivation with drooling occurs in 70–84% of a mostly male PD population [59, 62, 63] for a variety of reasons. Primarily, PD patients have difficulty with swallowing (dysphagia) because of their oropharyngeal bradykinesia [58, 59, 64]. In addition, the dysphagia is associated with a reduced frequency of swallows [63, 64]. Although swallowing difficulties are the main cause of drooling, other factors play important roles. Hypomimia, a manifestation of akinesia in PD patients, promotes the presence of an open mouth with an inadequate lip seal and a forward flexing of the head. These conditions encourage drooling [47, 59, 62, 63, 66].

Standard systemic treatment for PD involves the use of levodopa, a dopaminergic medication. A modest increase in salivary production occurs, but no beneficial effect regarding dysphagia has been observed with the medication's use [67]. A multi-pronged therapeutic regimen for drooling, as outlined under the previous section "Drooling-Overview," is also a treatment approach that has been utilized with some success.

Drooling

Amyotrophic Lateral Sclerosis

Amyotrophic lateral sclerosis (ALS) is a fatal progressive neurodegenerative disease affecting the motor neurons in the anterior horn of the spinal cord, the brainstem, and the motor cortex [68]. These neurons control voluntary muscle activity, and with their destruction, the abilities to eat, speak, and use the respiratory muscles to breathe are eventually lost. The mean age for patients with ALS has been reported to be 56 years. It has a prevalence of 4–6 people per 100,000 in the general population, with males mostly affected [69]. Most cases initially present with spinal disease that involves the limbs. The majority of ALS patients eventually develop bulbar symptomatology, characterized by a progression to generalized muscle weakness, muscle atrophy, and muscle spasticity [70]. Respiratory problems lead to death in 3–5 years [68].

Drooling is one of the significant disabling symptoms of ALS. It has a reported incidence in ALS that varies from 31 to 67% [68–71] and is a manifestation of the bulbar involvement that causes a swallowing defect from weaknesses in the oro-facial and palate/lingual musculatures [69, 70]. Therefore, drooling is caused by an impairment in the mechanics of swallowing with salivary flow rate being in the normal range rather than increased in volume [72, 73]. The constant drooling causes patient embarrassment, problems with speaking and eating, soiling of the clothing, increased caregiving, and perioral tissue maceration. Aspiration pneumonia becomes a serious complication because patients cannot swallow their secretions effectively. Patients also develop a cough defect due to progressive diaphragm and respiratory muscle weaknesses [68]. The end result is that the most frequent cause of death is respiratory failure, while the second is pneumonia [69].

Effective pharmacologic treatment for ALS is not available, but riluzole and eda-ravone have some limited therapeutic value [69]. Palliative care is all that can be offered for the vexing problem of drooling. Several therapeutic regimens have been advocated for the drooling. Initial treatment includes anticholinergics: atropine, benztropine, scopolamine, glycopyrrolate, and amitriptyline [68–70, 74]. If these agents prove to be ineffective or cause complications, botulinum toxin injections can be administered [74]. Duct or gland surgery should be avoided because ALS patients have a short life expectancy and an inability to tolerate surgery [69]. Low-dose radiotherapy (7–20 Gy) is advised when the anticholinergics and botulinum toxin injections have proven ineffective [74, 75]. The lifespan of the ALS patient is such that radiation's pre-malignant effect is not a concern.

Drooling

Cerebral Palsy

Cerebral palsy (CP) is the most common cause of motor disability in children. It affects 2–2.5 children per 1000 born in the United States [76]. CP results from a brain injury before the neurologic completion of cerebral development. Because brain development continues during the first 2 years of life, the injury may have occurred in the prenatal, perinatal, or postnatal periods [76]. The symptomatology of CP includes a group of movement and posture disorders caused by brain injury [77]. The clinical complications of CP feature the presence of muscle spasticity, dyskinesia, ataxia, feeding difficulties, and drooling, with spasticity being the most common problem [78].

The prevalence of drooling has been variously estimated to occur in 10–58% of CP patients [77, 79, 80]. As with other neurologic patients who drool, the problem is not hypersalivation. Rather, drooling represents a defective swallowing mechanism. Swallowing demands a series of sequential reflexes and coordinated movements of the muscles of the mandible, lips, tongue, palate, pharynx, larynx, and esophagus [81] and consists of two muscular stages. The oral stage requires coordination of the oro-facial musculature, while the palate/lingual/pharyngeal stage is concerned with the propulsion of food, saliva, and debris into the stomach [79]. Therefore, it should not be surprising that CP patients accumulate saliva in their mouth from defective swallowing originating from the inadequate function of the musculature. Furthermore, drooling is aided by a dependent head position and abetted by inefficient labial sealing that results in an open mouth.

Saliva pooling in the posterior oropharyngeal area can lead to aspiration with consequent respiratory infection. Respiratory illness is the primary cause of the morbidity and mortality observed in CP patients [82]. The intensity of dysphagia and drooling correlates directly with the severity of CP [83].

A primary aim of the medical team is to control drooling. Success eliminates poor hygiene and constant soiling of clothing, elevates patient esteem, and lessens the burden for caregivers. Treatment of the drooling problem in CP has followed many avenues. Conservative therapy involves training in speech therapy, sensory awareness, and oral motor skills. Anticholinergic medications can be used as adjuncts to the conservative regimen. Botox injections into both submandibular glands, the source of most resting salivary flow, are effective. Surgery in the form of submandibular gland excision, duct rerouting, or duct ligation has been advocated [82]. Sclerotherapy to ablate the salivary gland has also been entered into the recommended therapeutic regimen.

Drooling

Intellectual Disability

Intellectual disability (ID), previously referred to as mental retardation, is an entity that is usually included in the range of conditions associated with neurodegenerative disease [84]. ID is a relatively common problem that becomes manifest in individuals who are less than 18 years old and who exhibit subaverage intellectual functioning and impairment of adaptive skills [85]. Patients with ID are limited in their cognitive functions and skills. They develop and learn slowly when compared with the typically developing normal child.

Drooling of saliva is common in children with ID [86] because they have a poor neuromuscular control that is caused by a faulty oromotor function [87]. The effective function of the oral and facial muscles is dependent upon the coordination of the muscles of the jaw, tongue, lips, and soft palate [87]. Dysfunction of this muscle group from inefficient neuromuscular control results in an impaired swallow that leads to drooling.

A conservative regimen represents the choice of therapeutic approach. Behavioral modification, medications, and botulinum toxin injections have been utilized to control the drooling.

Drooling

Infant Drooling

Drooling in the newborn is a common condition because total oral motor control has not had the time to develop. Drooling is considered normal up to the age of 30 months (Fig. 2.5). At this age, the oro-motor muscles will have matured and drooling usually ceases [88, 89]. Drooling while awake beyond 48 months is considered pathologic [89] and demands investigation as to the possible presence of a co-existing systemic neurodevelopmental/neurodegenerative disease process.

Although the major etiologic cause of infant drooling is generally accepted to be directly related to the development of the oro-motor musculature, other factors may play auxiliary roles. Deciduous teething begins at 6 months and has been demonstrated to be associated with drooling [90]. Infants with malocclusions, such as an open bite, and problems with effective sealing of the lips are also candidates for persistent drooling [88].

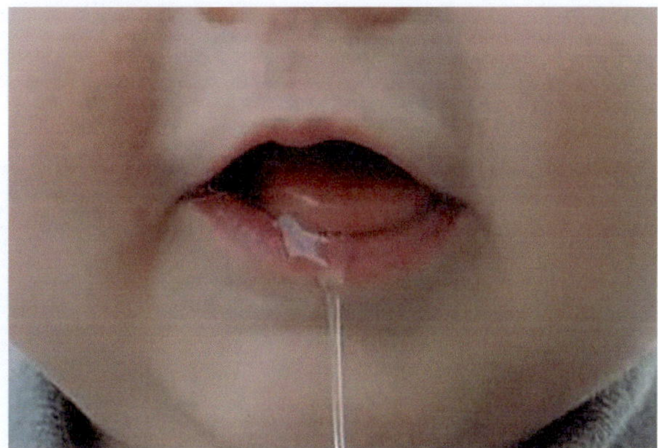

Fig. 2.5 Drooling. Infant 14 months old

Hyposalivation (Dry Mouth)

Overview

It must be emphasized again that xerostomia is a subjective feeling of a dry mouth, while hyposalivation is the objective presence of a decreased production of saliva. Normal whole stimulated salivary volume ranges from 1.0 to 2.0 mL/min, while whole unstimulated saliva has a normal range of 0.3–0.5 mL/min. Objectively, hyposalivation exists when whole stimulated saliva is <0.5 mL/min and unstimulated whole saliva is measured at <0.1 mL/min [91–93].

Dry mouth may develop from the hyposalivation caused by Sjögren syndrome, other autoimmune diseases, or irradiation to the salivary glands during treatment for head/neck cancer. However, these conditions are minor provocateurs in the overall incidence of a patient's subjective complaint of xerostomia. A frequent focus for the complaint is the prescribed medications that are being used by the patient. A large percentage of the more than 400 commonly prescribed medications (i.e., diuretics, anticholinergics, antihistamines, antidepressants, sedatives, antihypertensives, etc.) are known to cause decreased salivation [91, 93, 94]. The medications usually exert their ability to curb salivation by suppressing the release of acetylcholine or by occupying the muscarinic/adrenergic receptor sites [93]. The incidence of dry mouth increases in direct proportion to the number of prescribed medications [92, 95] (Fig. 2.6). Caution must be exerted in evaluating the role medications play in the patient's complaint of xerostomia. Although many medications reduce salivary flow, it is the experience of the Salivary Gland Center (SGC) that the use of one or two such agents is not sufficient to cause objective hyposalivation with subjective xerostomia. It is only when multiple prescribed xerogenic medications are used that hyposalivation with subjective xerostomia develops. The SGC believes that a systemic problem or a somatoform origin is more likely the root cause of a xerostomic complaint in those patients using only one or two xerogenic pharmaceuticals.

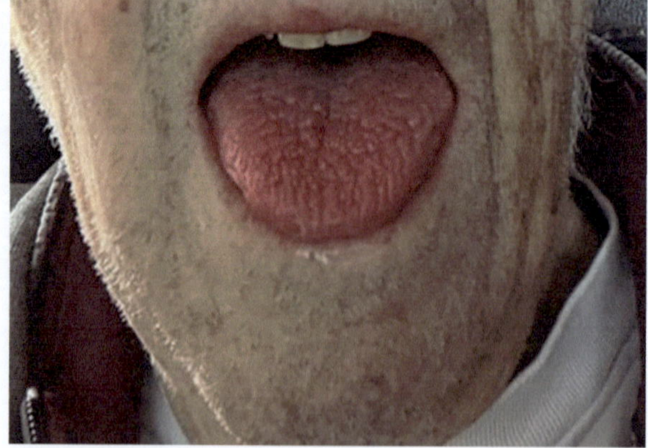

Fig. 2.6 Hyposalivation. Patient was using multiple systemic medications with xerogenic side effects (psychotherapeutics, cardiovascular agents, and antihistamine)

The prevalence of perceived and objective xerostomia as reported in previous studies varies between 5.5 and 46% in the general population [96]. Its incidence increases in older patients, probably because of their increased usage of multiple prescribed medications [91, 92, 97], which often are anticholinergic, and their acute awareness of the xerogenic effect of these prescribed medications. Furthermore, the prevalence of xerostomia is slightly skewed toward females [92, 98]. Regardless of the cause, dryness will lead to difficulties in swallowing, speaking, eating, and a decreased taste sensation. There will be an increased susceptibility to dental caries, periodontal disease, candidiasis, and halitosis. It is important to be aware that true oral dryness may also develop in the presence of normal salivary production. Examples include mouth breathing, smoking, and the use of alcohol, all of which contribute to rapid salivary evaporation [93] and the subjective xerostomia.

The clinical identification of actual oral dryness is facilitated by the presence of several helpful diagnostic signs proposed by Osailan [99]. These signs include adherence of an intraoral mirror to the buccal mucosa, fissured tongue, loss of papilla on the tongue dorsum, presence of debris adhering to the mucosa (Fig. 2.7), glassy appearance of the oral mucosa, and cervical dental caries. Nevertheless, objective salivary volume measurements are required to substantiate these clinical signs of oral dryness.

It has been reported and it has been the experience of the SGC that a significant number of patients with subjective xerostomia have psychologic issues (depression and anxiety) that may be related to their subjective complaint [92, 99]. They commonly have a classic symptomatology triad of oral burning, dysgeusia, and subjective, not objective, oral dryness. These patients do not demonstrate hyposalivation and are classified with somatoform disease. Somatoform disease is best defined as a physical complaint with no recognized organic basis that is initiated by the patient's abnormal mental state, often depression. They frequently have histories of psychiatric care and/or the use of a variety of psychotherapeutic medications. A review of somatoform disease will be found in Chap. 19.

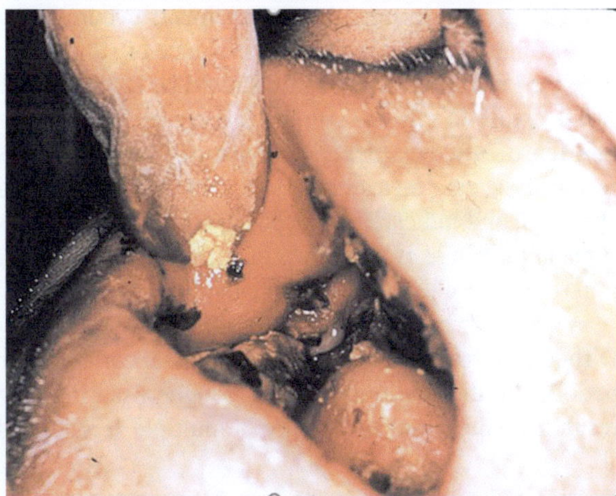

Fig. 2.7 Hyposalivation with debris adhering to the mucosa

Occasionally, it is difficult to evaluate the origin of a patient's xerostomic complaint. Is it objective from xerogenic medications or even somatoform in origin? The SGC approaches the problem by measuring whole unstimulated and whole stimulated saliva. When medications are the base cause of the xerostomic complaint, whole unstimulated salivary volume will be below the normal range of 0.3–0.5 mL/min. However, stimulation will overcome any existing anticholinergic effect of the drugs and normal volumes will be obtained when measured. If the somatoform disease is the cause of the trouble, collections of whole unstimulated and whole stimulated saliva will both be in a normal range. Therein lies a ready and significant means to differentially diagnose a medication-incited true hyposalivation from a subjective only xerostomia. Furthermore, patients with true systemic-related oral dryness will demonstrate decreased whole unstimulated and whole stimulated salivary returns when objectively measured.

Hyposalivation

Medications

With an expanding and aging population and the constant arrival of new effective therapeutic pharmaceuticals, the use of prescription medications has grown considerably. Remarkably, there were 5.8 billion prescriptions dispensed in the United States in 2018 [11] with adverse drug reactions increasing in direct proportion to the number of drugs that the patient uses. Medication dosage and duration of use also play roles in the onset of drug complications. A review of the 200 most frequently prescribed drugs in the USA revealed dry mouth to be the most common oral adverse reaction (Fig. 2.6) [12]. There are hundreds or even thousands of drugs that can be xerogenic [13]. Age, accompanied by multiple medication use, can also play a role in the development of objective hyposalivation, while female gender and psychologic factors are other key elements in complaints of subjective dryness [14].

The elderly have a reported prevalence of subjective dry mouth that ranges up to 72% [15]. At this point, it again should be re-stated that hyposalivation is an objective decrease in salivary volume that creates a sense of oral dryness, while xerostomia represents the subjective sense of oral dryness. Normal unstimulated whole resting flow rate measures 0.3–0.5 mL/min with values <0.1 mL/min considered abnormal and indicative of hyposalivation. Stimulated whole saliva normally measures in the range of 1–2 mL/min with values <0.5 mL/min requiring prompt attention regarding a true dryness [12, 14].

A patient's complaint of oral dryness is not to be regarded as a trivial issue. Difficulties that can develop include dental caries, halitosis, candidiasis, dysgeusia, periodontal disease, oral burning, tongue fissuring, eating, and speaking. All may result from the simultaneous use of multiple xerogenic drugs. Pharmaceuticals such as antidepressants, antipsychotics, antihistamines, antihypertensives, bronchodilators, diuretics, appetite suppressants, skeletal muscle relaxants, drugs of abuse, and drugs to treat reflux disease or an overactive bladder have been implicated as causes of hyposalivation and xerostomia. Reference guides regarding the multitude of drugs involved in hyposalivation, as well as hypersalivation, have been published and are available for the practitioner's perusal [14–16].

Once more, it should be stated that it is the experience of the Columbia University Salivary Gland Center that the use of one anticholinergic medication is not sufficient to cause subjective symptomatology. The modest salivary decrease that occurs with one medication is difficult for the patient to subjectively recognize and is readily compensated when eating stimulates the salivary glands to increase their output. It is the use of multiple xerogenic drugs that causes a subjective and objective oral dryness.

Hyposalivation

Psychologic Disorders and Medications

Depression

Depression is a complex disorder that causes feelings of sadness and loss of interest in everyday activity and relationships. It usually is a natural normal but temporary reaction to a life event such as the death of a loved one. It can also originate as a side effect of a drug or as a symptom of some physical illness. Major episodes of depression are more persistent and are characterized by at least 2 weeks of low mood, low self-esteem, and loss of pleasure from everyday normal enjoyable events. Depression usually appears in the late teens or early twenties with women being more vulnerable. It was estimated that, in the year 2020, psychiatric disturbances comprised 15% of the presenting global diseases with depression and anxiety representing the most common afflictions [100, 101].

Emotional alterations, particularly depression, can by themselves cause changes that lead to the subjective complaint of oral dryness (xerostomia) [102]. The prevalence of xerostomia in the general population is high: 5–26% for men and 20–46% for women [96]. A Japanese study [103] has substantiated the concept that a direct relationship exists between subjective oral dryness complaints (xerostomia) and objective findings (hyposalivation) seen in depressed patients. Conversely, other studies [104, 105] have contradicted this correlation. Although patients subjectively complained of oral dryness, these studies found no changes in the salivary flow rates of depressed patients. The apparent confusion probably originates from several factors. Different definitions (subjective or objective?) of oral dryness are used. Furthermore, investigative procedures vary. Salivary collection techniques differ, circadian rhythms are not considered, and studied patient groups (age, sex) have not been standardized. Definitive conclusions regarding the relationship between salivary volume and the mental state await further definitive studies.

The most effective therapy for depression is generally accepted to be a combination of psychotherapy and medication [106]. Medications such as selective serotonin reuptake inhibitors (SSRIs) block the reuptake of serotonin by neurons and make more serotonin available for message transmission. Tricyclic antidepressants (TCA) are also used therapeutically because they block the serotonin transporter and result in elevated serotonin synaptic concentrations with an enhancement of neurotransmission [107]. However, it is a noteworthy paradox that both the SSRI and TCA are anticholinergic agents that have the ability to block specific muscarinic receptors [108].

Hyposalivation

Psychologic Disorders and Medications

Bipolar Disease

Bipolar disease (BP), formerly known as manic-depressive disorder, is a psychiatric illness associated with recurrent cycles of mania and depression that are separated by remissions during which time the patient experiences periods of normal mood. The etiology of BP is thought to be derived from the interplay of several factors that include genetics, neurochemical influences, substance abuse, and stressful infant/childhood experiences [109]. BP is now considered the sixth leading cause of disability [109] among the general population.

The standard therapeutic pharmacologic agent used for BP treatment is lithium. Antipsychotics and antidepressants are often used as adjuncts with lithium. An early report indicated that salivary flow rates were normal in lithium-treated BP [110]. However, more recent studies have generally accepted the fact that lithium induces hyposalivation [109, 111, 112]. Decreased salivation has been observed in 71% of the BP patients receiving lithium [111]. Initially, it was believed that the hyposalivation resulted from lithium damage to the acini [111], but the hyposalivation may more likely be associated with a functional glandular change rather than a structural problem [112].

The associated prescribed BP medications (antidepressants, antipsychotics) also fractionally contribute to the decreased salivation observed in these patients. Furthermore, the depressed state may play a role in decreasing salivation [113–115]. Therefore, although lithium has been associated with dry mouth, the practitioner must be forewarned that the decreased salivation seen in BP may be related to the prescribed adjunctive medications or possibly even the depressed state of the patient.

Hyposalivation

Psychologic Disorders and Medications

Schizophrenia

Schizophrenia is a psychotic disorder characterized by hallucinations, delusions, and abnormal thinking and behavior. Problems with fetal brain development, imbalances in neurochemistry, and loss of connections between different brain areas are thought to be involved in the evolution of schizophrenia. Genetics, environmental factors, and substance abuse are considered risk factors for its onset. About 0.3–0.7% of the American population is diagnosed with schizophrenia during their lifetime [116]. Although there is no cure, schizophrenia can be effectively managed with medications and supportive therapy.

The mainstay of schizophrenia treatment is the first-generation antipsychotics (chlorpromazine, haloperidol, etc.). As with other psychotherapeutics, these antipsychotics initiate a decrease in unstimulated salivary flow. Unfortunately, a significant portion of schizophrenic patients do not respond mentally to these first-line antipsychotics. Clozapine has proven to be the drug of choice for patients with standard treatment-resistant schizophrenia. Although clozapine causes fewer extrapyramidal symptoms compared with other antipsychotics, it should be closely monitored regarding the possible onset of adverse complications such as myocardial problems, agranulocytosis, and alterations in salivary flow.

Reports regarding clozapine's effect on salivary flow have been contradictory. It has been generally accepted that hypersalivation develops and may serve as a possible drawback to clozapine's use. The hypersalivation is in contradistinction to Scully and Bagan's [117] premise that like most antipsychotics clozapine causes hyposalivation. There are also objective studies measuring whole unstimulated and whole stimulated salivary flow that have indicated clozapine users do not produce increased salivary volumes when compared to non-users [118–120]. Confusion arises from the fact that the study of Praharaj et al. [121] indicated an increase in salivary flow occurred only when the salivary glands were not being stimulated. Furthermore, Ekström et al. [122] reported that not all but about one-third of schizophrenics receiving treatment with clozapine complained of excessive salivation. Nocturnal salivation in clozapine users is an accepted fact [123] and is usually accompanied by drooling. Explanations as to the cause of hypersalivation and drooling, whether during the day or during sleep, have been attributed to agonistic action on muscarinic receptors [122, 124, 125]. The varied reports (is it hyposalivation, normal salivation, or hypersalivation?) have been brought together by the work of Ekström et al. [125]. They have indicated that clozapine has an affinity for several different receptor sites. Depending on which receptor site is affected, clozapine and/ or its metabolites may act to both stimulate and inhibit salivary secretions. Despite the controversy, the antipsychotic clozapine is generally considered a medication that causes hypersalivation. The mechanism of this action probably originates from the blockade of the alpha 2 adrenergic receptors, causing a reduced salivary gland sympathetic stimulation, combined with stimulation of the M3 muscarinic receptors that serve to induce increased parasympathetic stimulation of the salivary glands [126].

Hyposalivation

Psychologic Disorders and Medications

Panic Attacks/Seizures

Panic attacks are characterized by sudden periods of intense fear associated with palpitations, shortness of breath, sweating, numbness, confusion, and a feeling of impending doom [127]. Seizures can also develop and result from abnormal neuron brain activity that causes physical systemic symptoms that may last from a few seconds to several minutes. Confusion, vision changes, muscle spasms, loss of bladder and bowel control, and loss of consciousness are associated with the seizures. The difference between seizures and panic attacks rests in the fact that seizures are physiologic in nature, while panic attacks are considered to be psychologic in origin. Annually, about 11% of the USA population is affected by these panic attacks/seizures [128].

Clonazepam (a benzodiazepine) alone or combined with a selective serotonin reuptake inhibitor (SSRI) and/or behavioral therapy have been successfully prescribed for the treatment of panic attacks and seizures [129]. The SSRI makes more serotonin available for neuro-message transmission, while the benzodiazepines, central nervous system depressants, induce feelings of calm. Both the SSRI and benzodiazepines act to inhibit muscarinic receptors [130] and decrease salivary volume production.

Hyposalivation

Dry at Rest (Unstimulated Glands): Mouth Breathing

People normally breathe through their nose and/or mouth. In most cases, mouth breathing is a result of a reduction in the patency of the nasal airway [131]. Patients who mouth breathe are often seen with a subjective complaint of xerostomia. However, when the salivary flow rates of these patients are objectively measured, they will demonstrate normal salivary flows, both at rest and when the salivary glands are stimulated. No statistically significant differences have been found in the flow rates of mouth-breathing patients and controls [132].

The movement of air intraorally during mouth breathing causes oral dryness from the rapid evaporation of oral saliva, particularly during periods of salivary rest. Periods of unstimulated (resting) salivary flow occupy the major part of a 24-h day because increases in saliva production are essentially limited to stimulation during periods of eating. Decreased flow rates occur while sleeping because a normal physiologic drop in salivary production takes place [133–135] and accentuates the problem. The little saliva that is produced during sleep is subject to evaporation because of the constant air flow associated with mouth breathing. Not only is saliva lost by evaporation, but water absorption through the mucosa can occur. Saliva has one-sixth the osmotic pressure of extracellular fluid, thus creating a water gradient across the mucosa [7]. Oral dryness occurs, and mouth breathers become aware of their oral dryness upon awakening. Because snoring takes place only when the mouth is open, it can serve as a clue regarding a patient's tendency to mouth breathe during sleep.

References

1. Boyce HW, Bakheet MR. Sialorrhea: a review of a vexing, often unrecognized sign of oropharyngeal and esophageal disease. J Clin Gastroenterol. 2005;39(2):89–97.
2. Glickman S, Deaney CN. Treatment of relative sialorrhoea with botulinum toxin type a: description and rationale for an injection procedure with case report. Eur J Neurol. 2001;8(6):567–71. https://doi.org/10.1046/j.1468-1331.2001.00328.x.
3. de Almeida PDV, Grégio AM, Machado MA, de Lima AA, Azevedo LR. Saliva composition and functions: a comprehensive review. J Contemp Dent Pract. 2008;9(3):72–80.
4. Miranda-Rius J, Brunet-Llobet L, Lahor-Soler E, Farré M. Salivary secretory disorders, inducing drugs, and clinical management. Int J Med Sci. 2015;12(10):811–24. https://doi.org/10.7150/ijms.12912.
5. Saliva: its role in health and disease. Working Group 10 of the Commission on Oral Health, Research and Epidemiology (CORE) [published correction appears in Int Dent J 1992 Dec;42(6):410]. Int Dent J 1992;42(4 Suppl 2):287–304.
6. Sreebny LM, Zhu WX. The use of whole saliva in the differential diagnosis of Sjögren's syndrome. Adv Dent Res. 1996;10(1):17–24. https://doi.org/10.1177/08959374960100010201.
7. Dawes C. How much saliva is enough for avoidance of xerostomia? Caries Res. 2004;38(3):236–40. https://doi.org/10.1159/000077760.
8. Dawes C. Salivary flow patterns and the health of hard and soft oral tissues. J Am Dent Assoc. 2008;139(Suppl):18S–24S. https://doi.org/10.14219/jada.archive.2008.0351.
9. Dawes C. Rhythms in salivary flow rate and composition. Int J Chronobiol. 1974;2(3):253–79.
10. Iorgulescu G. Saliva between normal and pathological. Important factors in determining systemic and oral health. J Med Life. 2009;2(3):303–7.
11. IQVIA Institute for Human Data Science. Medicine use and spending in the U.S.—a review of 2018 and outlook to 2023. 2019.
12. Scully C. Drug effects on salivary glands: dry mouth. Oral Dis. 2003;9(4):165–76. https://doi.org/10.1034/j.1601-0825.2003.03967.x.
13. Sreebny LM, Schwartz SS. A reference guide to drugs and dry mouth—2nd edition. Gerodontology. 1997;14(1):33–47. https://doi.org/10.1111/j.1741-2358.1997.00033.x.
14. Bergdahl M, Bergdahl J. Low unstimulated salivary flow and subjective oral dryness: association with medication, anxiety, depression, and stress. J Dent Res. 2000;79(9):1652–8. https://doi.org/10.1177/00220345000790090301.

15. Villa A, Wolff A, Narayana N, et al. World workshop on oral medicine VI: a systematic review of medication-induced salivary gland dysfunction. Oral Dis. 2016;22(5):365–82. https://doi.org/10.1111/odi.12402.
16. Wolff A, Joshi RK, Ekström J, et al. A guide to medications inducing salivary gland dysfunction, xerostomia, and subjective sialorrhea: a systematic review sponsored by the world workshop on oral medicine VI. Drugs R D. 2017;17(1):1–28. https://doi.org/10.1007/s40268-016-0153-9.
17. Barber C. Diagnosis and management of myasthenia gravis. Nurs Stand. 2017;31(43):42–7. https://doi.org/10.7748/ns.2017.e10434.
18. Rabiou H, Haboubacar ID, Kaoutar EF, Musoni L, Ezzouine H, Charra B. Myasthenia gravis in an old woman discovered during sedation for diagnostic digestive fibroscopy: case report. Ann Med Surg (Lond). 2021;69:102809. https://doi.org/10.1016/j.amsu.2021.102809.
19. McIntyre K, McVaugh-Smock S, Mourad O. An adult patient with new-onset dysphagia. CMAJ. 2006;175(10):1203. https://doi.org/10.1503/cmaj.060488.
20. Adeyinka A, Kondamudi NP. Cholinergic crisis. In: StatPearls. Treasure Island (FL): StatPearls Publishing; 2022.
21. Binu A, Kumar SS, Padma UD, Madhu K. Pathophysiological basis in the management of myasthenia gravis: a mini review. Inflammopharmacology. 2022;30(1):61–71. https://doi.org/10.1007/s10787-021-00905-9.
22. Suresh AB, Asuncion RMD. Myasthenia gravis. In: StatPearls. Treasure Island (FL): StatPearls Publishing; 2022.
23. Ali MS, Parikh S, Chater P, Pearson JP. Bile acids in laryngopharyngeal refluxate: will they enhance or attenuate the action of pepsin? Laryngoscope. 2013;123(2):434–9. https://doi.org/10.1002/lary.23619.
24. Sharma P, Yadlapati R. Pathophysiology and treatment options for gastroesophageal reflux disease: looking beyond acid. Ann N Y Acad Sci. 2021;1486(1):3–14. https://doi.org/10.1111/nyas.14501.
25. Allison PR. Peptic ulcer of the oesophagus. Thorax. 1948;3(1):20–42. https://doi.org/10.1136/thx.3.1.20.
26. Korsten MA, Rosman AS, Fishbein S, Shlein RD, Goldberg HE, Biener A. Chronic xerostomia increases esophageal acid exposure and is associated with esophageal injury. Am J Med. 1991;90(6):701–6.
27. Azer SA, Reddivari AKR. Reflux esophagitis. In: StatPearls. Treasure Island (FL): StatPearls Publishing; 2022.
28. Smith RE, Shahjehan RD. Hiatal hernia. In: StatPearls. Treasure Island (FL): StatPearls Publishing; 2022.
29. Valdez IH, Fox PC. Interactions of the salivary and gastrointestinal systems. II. Effects of salivary gland dysfunction on the gastrointestinal tract. Dig Dis. 1991;9(4):210–8. https://doi.org/10.1159/000171305.
30. Holloway RH, Dent J. Pathophysiology of gastroesophageal reflux. Lower esophageal sphincter dysfunction in gastroesophageal reflux disease. Gastroenterol Clin N Am. 1990;19(3):517–35.
31. Shahsavari D, Smith MS, Malik Z, Parkman HP. Hiatal hernias associated with acid reflux: size larger than 2 cm matters. Dis Esophagus. 2022;35(8):doac001. https://doi.org/10.1093/dote/doac001.
32. Baron TH, Richter JE. Gastroesophageal reflux disease in pregnancy. Gastroenterol Clin N Am. 1992;21(4):777–91.
33. Olans LB, Wolf JL. Gastroesophageal reflux in pregnancy. Gastrointest Endosc Clin N Am. 1994;4(4):699–712.
34. Fisher RS, Roberts GS, Grabowski CJ, Cohen S. Altered lower esophageal sphincter function during early pregnancy. Gastroenterology. 1978;74(6):1233–7.

35. Van Thiel DH, Wald A. Evidence refuting a role for increased abdominal pressure in the pathogenesis of the heartburn associated with pregnancy. Am J Obstet Gynecol. 1981;140(4):420–2. https://doi.org/10.1016/0002-9378(81)90037-5.

36. Hershcovici T, Fass R. Pharmacological management of GERD: where does it stand now? Trends Pharmacol Sci. 2011;32(4):258–64. https://doi.org/10.1016/j.tips.2011.02.007.

37. Addo A, George P, Zahiri HR, Park A. Patients with ineffective esophageal motility benefit from laparoscopic antireflux surgery. Surg Endosc. 2021;35(8):4459–68. https://doi.org/10.1007/s00464-020-07951-4.

38. Schmidt M, Hackett RJ, Baker AM, McDonald SAC, Quante M, Graham TA. Evolutionary dynamics in Barrett oesophagus: implications for surveillance, risk stratification and therapy. Nat Rev Gastroenterol Hepatol. 2022;19(2):95–111. https://doi.org/10.1038/s41575-021-00531-4.

39. Gitnick G. Gastroenterology. New Hyde Park: Medical Examination Publishing Co.; 1985. p. 19–24.

40. Stein HJ, Siewert JR. Barrett's esophagus: pathogenesis, epidemiology, functional abnormalities, malignant degeneration, and surgical management. Dysphagia. 1993;8(3):276–88. https://doi.org/10.1007/BF01354551.

41. Lowe D, Kudaravalli P, Hsu R. Barrett metaplasia. In: StatPearls. Treasure Island (FL): StatPearls Publishing; 2022.

42. Frazzoni M, Frazzoni L, Ribolsi M, et al. Esophageal pH increments associated with post-reflux swallow-induced peristaltic waves show the occurrence and relevance of esophago-salivary reflex in clinical setting. Neurogastroenterol Motil. 2021;33(7):e14085. https://doi.org/10.1111/nmo.14085.

43. Dhar A, Maw F, Dallal HJ, Attwood S. Side effects of drug treatments for gastro-oesophageal reflux disease: current controversies. Frontline Gastroenterol. 2020;13(1):45–9. https://doi.org/10.1136/flgastro-2019-101386.

44. Han JY, Choi SA, Chung YG, et al. Change of centrotemporal spikes from onset to remission in self-limited epilepsy with centrotemporal spikes (SLECTS). Brain Dev. 2020;42(3):270–6. https://doi.org/10.1016/j.braindev.2019.11.005.

45. Galicchio S, Espeche A, Cersosimo R, et al. Self-limited epilepsy with centro-temporal spikes: a study of 46 patients with unusual clinical manifestations. Epilepsy Res. 2021;169:106507. https://doi.org/10.1016/j.eplepsyres.2020.106507.

46. Paine CC 2nd, Snider JW 3rd. When saliva becomes a problem: the challenges and palliative care for patients with sialorrhea. Ann Palliat Med. 2020;9(3):1333–9. https://doi.org/10.21037/apm.2020.02.34.

47. Scully C, Limeres J, Gleeson M, Tomás I, Diz P. Drooling. J Oral Pathol Med. 2009;38(4):321–7. https://doi.org/10.1111/j.1600-0714.2008.00727.x.

48. Varley LP, Gooney M, Denieffe S, Murphy A. Sialorrhoea management practices in residential older adults care settings: a qualitative study. J Nurs Manag. 2021;29(5):989–97. https://doi.org/10.1111/jonm.13236.

49. Bekkers S, de Bock S, van Hulst K, Kok SE, Scheffer ART, van den Hoogen FJA. The medium to long-term effects of two-duct ligation for excessive drooling in neurodisabilities, a cross-sectional study. Int J Pediatr Otorhinolaryngol. 2021;150:110894. https://doi.org/10.1016/j.ijporl.2021.110894.

50. Isaacson J, Patel S, Torres-Yaghi Y, Pagán F. Sialorrhea in Parkinson's disease. Toxins (Basel). 2020;12(11):691. https://doi.org/10.3390/toxins12110691.

51. Chow A, Peters K, Schrepfer T. A novel approach to treat pediatric sialorrhea using sialendoscopy for salivary gland directed sclerotherapy. Am J Otolaryngol. 2022;43(4):103489. https://doi.org/10.1016/j.amjoto.2022.103489.

52. Friedlander AH, Norman DC, Mahler ME, Norman KM, Yagiela JA. Alzheimer's disease: psychopathology, medical management and dental implications. J Am Dent Assoc. 2006;137(9):1240–51. https://doi.org/10.14219/jada.archive.2006.0381.

53. Nakamura K, Watanabe N, Ohkawa H, et al. Effects on caregiver burden of a donepezil hydrochloride dosage increase to 10 mg/day in patients with Alzheimer's disease. Patient Prefer Adherence. 2014;8:1223–8. https://doi.org/10.2147/PPA.S69750.

54. Sayer R, Law E, Connelly PJ, Breen KC. Association of a salivary acetylcholinesterase with Alzheimer's disease and response to cholinesterase inhibitors. Clin Biochem. 2004;37(2):98–104. https://doi.org/10.1016/j.clinbiochem.2003.10.007.

55. Jann MW. Rivastigmine, a new-generation cholinesterase inhibitor for the treatment of Alzheimer's disease. Pharmacotherapy. 2000;20(1):1–12. https://doi.org/10.1592/phco.20.1.1.34664.

56. Jackson S, Ham RJ, Wilkinson D. The safety and tolerability of donepezil in patients with Alzheimer's disease. Br J Clin Pharmacol. 2004;58(Suppl 1):1–8. https://doi.org/10.1111/j.1365-2125.2004.01848.x.

57. Ship JA, DeCarli C, Friedland RP, Baum BJ. Diminished submandibular salivary flow in dementia of the Alzheimer type. J Gerontol. 1990;45(2):M61–6. https://doi.org/10.1093/geronj/45.2.m61.

58. Baram S, Karlsborg M, Øzhayat EB, Bakke M. Effect of orofacial physiotherapeutic and hygiene interventions on oral health-related quality of life in patients with Parkinson's disease: a randomised controlled trial. J Oral Rehabil. 2021;48(9):1035–43. https://doi.org/10.1111/joor.13214.

59. Arboleda-Montealegre GY, Cano-de-la-Cuerda R, Fernández-de-Las-Peñas C, Sanchez-Camarero C, Ortega-Santiago R. Drooling, swallowing difficulties and health related quality of life in Parkinson's disease patients. Int J Environ Res Public Health. 2021;18(15):8138. https://doi.org/10.3390/ijerph18158138.

60. Nicaretta DH, Rosso AL, Mattos JP, Maliska C, Costa MM. Dysphagia and sialorrhea: the relationship to Parkinson's disease. Arq Gastroenterol. 2013;50(1):42–9. https://doi.org/10.1590/s0004-28032013000100009.

61. Cersósimo MG, Tumilasci OR, Raina GB, et al. Hyposialorrhea as an early manifestation of Parkinson disease. Auton Neurosci. 2009;150(1–2):150–1. https://doi.org/10.1016/j.autneu.2009.04.004.

62. Chou KL, Evatt M, Hinson V, Kompoliti K. Sialorrhea in Parkinson's disease: a review. Mov Disord. 2007;22(16):2306–13. https://doi.org/10.1002/mds.21646.

63. Kalf JG, Munneke M, van den Engel-Hoek L, et al. Pathophysiology of diurnal drooling in Parkinson's disease. Mov Disord. 2011;26(9):1670–6. https://doi.org/10.1002/mds.23720.

64. Karakoc M, Yon MI, Cakmakli GY, et al. Pathophysiology underlying drooling in Parkinson's disease: oropharyngeal bradykinesia. Neurol Sci. 2016;37(12):1987–91. https://doi.org/10.1007/s10072-016-2708-5.

65. Mito Y, Yabe I, Yaguchi H, et al. Relationships of drooling with motor symptoms and dopamine transporter imaging in drug-naïve Parkinson's disease. Clin Neurol Neurosurg. 2020;195:105951. https://doi.org/10.1016/j.clineuro.2020.105951.

66. Reynolds H, Miller N, Walker R. Drooling in Parkinson's disease: evidence of a role for divided attention. Dysphagia. 2018;33(6):809–17. https://doi.org/10.1007/s00455-018-9906-7.

67. Tumilasci OR, Cersósimo MG, Belforte JE, Micheli FE, Benarroch EE, Pazo JH. Quantitative study of salivary secretion in Parkinson's disease. Mov Disord. 2006;21(5):660–7. https://doi.org/10.1002/mds.20784.

68. Banfi P, Ticozzi N, Lax A, Guidugli GA, Nicolini A, Silani V. A review of options for treating sialorrhea in amyotrophic lateral sclerosis. Respir Care. 2015;60(3):446–54. https://doi.org/10.4187/respcare.02856.

69. Garuti G, Rao F, Ribuffo V, Sansone VA. Sialorrhea in patients with ALS: current treatment options. Degener Neurol Neuromuscul Dis. 2019;9:19–26. https://doi.org/10.2147/DNND.S168353.

70. Wang Y, Yang X, Han Q, Liu M, Zhou C. Prevalence of sialorrhea among amyotrophic lateral sclerosis patients: a systematic review and meta-analysis. J Pain Symptom Manag. 2022;63(4):e387–96. https://doi.org/10.1016/j.jpainsymman.2021.12.005.

71. Cooper-Knock J, Ahmedzai SH, Shaw P. The use of subcutaneous glycopyrrolate in the management of sialorrhoea and facilitating the use of non-invasive ventilation in amyotrophic lateral sclerosis. Amyotroph Lateral Scler. 2011;12(6):464–5. https://doi.org/10.3109/1748296 8.2011.584195.

72. Percival RS, Challacombe SJ, Marsh PD. Flow rates of resting whole and stimulated parotid saliva in relation to age and gender. J Dent Res. 1994;73(8):1416–20. https://doi.org/10.117 7/00220345940730080401.

73. Andersen PM, Grönberg H, Franzen L, Funegård U. External radiation of the parotid glands significantly reduces drooling in patients with motor neuron disease with bulbar paresis. J Neurol Sci. 2001;191(1–2):111–4. https://doi.org/10.1016/s0022-510x(01)00631-1.

74. Tysnes OB. Treatment of sialorrhea in amyotrophic lateral sclerosis. Acta Neurol Scand Suppl. 2008;188:77–81. https://doi.org/10.1111/j.1600-0404.2008.01037.x.

75. Slade A, Stanic S. Managing excessive saliva with salivary gland irradiation in patients with amyotrophic lateral sclerosis. J Neurol Sci. 2015;352(1–2):34–6. https://doi.org/10.1016/j.jns.2015.02.008.

76. Krigger KW. Cerebral palsy: an overview. Am Fam Physician. 2006;73(1):91–100.

77. Dias BL, Fernandes AR, Maia Filho HS. Sialorrhea in children with cerebral palsy. J Pediatr. 2016;92(6):549–58. https://doi.org/10.1016/j.jped.2016.03.006.

78. Vitrikas K, Dalton H, Breish D. Cerebral palsy: an overview. Am Fam Physician. 2020;101(4):213–20.

79. Tahmassebi JF, Curzon ME. The cause of drooling in children with cerebral palsy—hypersalivation or swallowing defect? Int J Paediatr Dent. 2003;13(2):106–11. https://doi.org/10.1046/j.1365-263x.2003.00439.x.

80. Erasmus CE, van Hulst K, Rotteveel JJ, Willemsen MA, Jongerius PH. Clinical practice: swallowing problems in cerebral palsy. Eur J Pediatr. 2012;171(3):409–14. https://doi.org/10.1007/s00431-011-1570-y.

81. Silvestre-Rangil J, Silvestre FJ, Puente-Sandoval A, Requeni-Bernal J, Simó-Ruiz JM. Clinical-therapeutic management of drooling: review and update. Med Oral Patol Oral Cir Bucal. 2011;16(6):e763–6. https://doi.org/10.4317/medoral.17260.

82. Marpole R, Blackmore AM, Gibson N, Cooper MS, Langdon K, Wilson AC. Evaluation and management of respiratory illness in children with cerebral palsy. Front Pediatr. 2020;8:333. https://doi.org/10.3389/fped.2020.00333.

83. Crary MA, Carnaby GD, Mathijs L, et al. Spontaneous swallowing frequency, dysphagia, and drooling in children with cerebral palsy. Arch Phys Med Rehabil. 2022;103(3):451–8. https://doi.org/10.1016/j.apmr.2021.09.014.

84. Lorca Larrosa M, Ruiz Roca JA, Ruiz Roca MI, López-Jornet P. Effects of the neuromuscular bandage as rehabilitative treatment of patients with drooling and intellectual disability: an interventional study. J Intellect Disabil Res. 2019;63(6):558–63. https://doi.org/10.1111/jir.12593.

85. Shea SE. Intellectual disability (mental retardation). Pediatr Rev. 2012;33(3):110–21. https://doi.org/10.1542/pir.33-3-110.

86. Glycopyrronium for severe drooling in children. Drug Ther Bull. 2017;55(8):93–6. https://doi.org/10.1136/dtb.2017.8.0517.

87. Sjögreen L, Mogren Å, Andersson-Norinder J, Bratel J. Speech, eating and saliva control in rare diseases—a database study. J Oral Rehabil. 2015;42(11):819–27. https://doi.org/10.1111/joor.12317.

88. Morales Chávez MC, Nualart Grollmus ZC, Silvestre-Donat FJ. Clinical prevalence of drooling in infant cerebral palsy. Med Oral Patol Oral Cir Bucal. 2008;13(1):E22–6.

89. Blasco PA, Allaire JH. Drooling in the developmentally disabled: management practices and recommendations. Consortium on drooling. Dev Med Child Neurol. 1992;34(10):849–62.

90. Macknin ML, Piedmonte M, Jacobs J, Skibinski C. Symptoms associated with infant teething: a prospective study. Pediatrics. 2000;105(4 Pt 1):747–52. https://doi.org/10.1542/peds.105.4.747.

91. Villa A, Connell CL, Abati S. Diagnosis and management of xerostomia and hyposalivation. Ther Clin Risk Manag. 2014;11:45–51. https://doi.org/10.2147/TCRM.S76282.
92. Choi JH, Kim MJ, Kho HS. Oral health-related quality of life and associated factors in patients with xerostomia. Int J Dent Hyg. 2021;19(3):313–22. https://doi.org/10.1111/idh.12528.
93. Talha B, Swarnkar SA. Xerostomia. In: StatPearls. Treasure Island (FL): StatPearls Publishing; 2022.
94. Turner MD. Hyposalivation and xerostomia: etiology, complications, and medical management. Dent Clin N Am. 2016;60(2):435–43. https://doi.org/10.1016/j.cden.2015.11.003.
95. Närhi TO, Meurman JH, Ainamo A, et al. Association between salivary flow rate and the use of systemic medication among 76-, 81-, and 86-year-old inhabitants in Helsinki, Finland. J Dent Res. 1992;71(12):1875–80. https://doi.org/10.1177/00220345920710120401.
96. Orellana MF, Lagravère MO, Boychuk DG, Major PW, Flores-Mir C. Prevalence of xerostomia in population-based samples: a systematic review. J Public Health Dent. 2006;66(2):152–8. https://doi.org/10.1111/j.1752-7325.2006.tb02572.x.
97. Jamieson LM, Thomson WM. Xerostomia: its prevalence and associations in the adult Australian population. Aust Dent J. 2020;65(Suppl 1):S67–70. https://doi.org/10.1111/adj.12767.
98. Johansson AK, Johansson A, Unell L, Ekbäck G, Ordell S, Carlsson GE. Self-reported dry mouth in Swedish population samples aged 50, 65 and 75 years. Gerodontology. 2012;29(2):e107–15. https://doi.org/10.1111/j.1741-2358.2010.00420.x.
99. Osailan S, Pramanik R, Shirodaria S, Challacombe SJ, Proctor GB. Investigating the relationship between hyposalivation and mucosal wetness. Oral Dis. 2011;17(1):109–14. https://doi.org/10.1111/j.1601-0825.2010.01715.x.
100. Suresh KV, Ganiger CC, Ahammed YA, et al. Psychosocial characteristics of oromucosal diseases in psychiatric patients: observational study from Indian dental college. N Am J Med Sci. 2014;6(11):570–4. https://doi.org/10.4103/1947-2714.145471.
101. Suresh KV, Shenai P, Chatra L, et al. Oral mucosal diseases in anxiety and depression patients: hospital based observational study from South India. J Clin Exp Dent. 2015;7(1):e95–9. https://doi.org/10.4317/jced.51764.
102. Veerabhadrappa SK, Chandrappa PR, Patil S, Roodmal SY, Kumarswamy A, Chappi MK. Evaluation of xerostomia in different psychological disorders: an observational study. J Clin Diagn Res. 2016;10(9):ZC24–7. https://doi.org/10.7860/JCDR/2016/19020.8437.
103. Takiguchi T, Yoshihara A, Takano N, Miyazaki H. Oral health and depression in older Japanese people. Gerodontology. 2016;33(4):439–46. https://doi.org/10.1111/ger.12177.
104. Bulthuis MS, Jan Jager DH, Brand HS. Relationship among perceived stress, xerostomia, and salivary flow rate in patients visiting a saliva clinic. Clin Oral Investig. 2018;22(9):3121–7. https://doi.org/10.1007/s00784-018-2393-2.
105. Pires ALPV, Simoura JADS, Cerqueira JDM, et al. Relationship of psychological factors with salivary flow rate and cortisol levels in individuals with oral lichen planus: a case-control study. Oral Surg Oral Med Oral Pathol Oral Radiol. 2020;130(6):675–80. https://doi.org/10.1016/j.oooo.2020.10.004.
106. Thase ME. When are psychotherapy and pharmacotherapy combinations the treatment of choice for major depressive disorder? Psychiatry Q. 1999;70(4):333–46. https://doi.org/10.1023/a:1022042316895.
107. Gillman PK. Tricyclic antidepressant pharmacology and therapeutic drug interactions updated. Br J Pharmacol. 2007;151(6):737–48. https://doi.org/10.1038/sj.bjp.0707253.
108. Howland RH. The antidepressant effects of anticholinergic drugs. J Psychosoc Nurs Ment Health Serv. 2009;47(6):17–20. https://doi.org/10.3928/02793695-20090508-01.
109. Friedlander AH, Friedlander IK, Marder SR. Bipolar I disorder: psychopathology, medical management and dental implications. J Am Dent Assoc. 2002;133(9):1209–17. https://doi.org/10.14219/jada.archive.2002.0362.

110. Ben-Aryeh H, Naon H, Horovitz G, Szargel R, Gutman D. Salivary and lacrimal secretions in patients on lithium therapy. J Psychiatr Res. 1984;18(3):299–306. https://doi.org/10.1016/0022-3956(84)90020-7.
111. Markitziu A, Shani J, Avni J. Salivary gland function in patients on chronic lithium treatment. Oral Surg Oral Med Oral Pathol. 1988;66(5):551–7. https://doi.org/10.1016/0030-4220(88)90374-x.
112. Veiga FF, Johann ACBR, da Kagy VS, et al. Action of lithium carbonate on parotid acini. Dent Oral Craniofac Res. 2016;2:287–91.
113. Gottlieb G, Paulson G. Salivation in depressed patients. Arch Gen Psychiatry. 1961;5:468–71. https://doi.org/10.1001/archpsyc.1961.01710170046005.
114. Palmai G, Blackwell B. The diurnal pattern of salivary flow in normal and depressed patients. Br J Psychiatry. 1965;111:334–8. https://doi.org/10.1192/bjp.111.473.334.
115. Tanaka H, Ogata S, Ikebe K, et al. Association between salivary flow rate and depressive symptoms with adjustment for genetic and family environmental factors in Japanese twin study. Clin Oral Investig. 2017;21(4):1291–7. https://doi.org/10.1007/s00784-016-1883-3.
116. Javitt DC. Balancing therapeutic safety and efficacy to improve clinical and economic outcomes in schizophrenia: a clinical overview. Am J Manag Care. 2014;20(8 Suppl):S160–5.
117. Scully C, Bagan JV. Adverse drug reactions in the orofacial region. Crit Rev Oral Biol Med. 2004;15(4):221–39. https://doi.org/10.1177/154411130401500405.
118. Ben-Aryeh H, Jungerman T, Szargel R, Klein E, Laufer D. Salivary flow-rate and composition in schizophrenic patients on clozapine: subjective reports and laboratory data. Biol Psychiatry. 1996;39(11):946–9. https://doi.org/10.1016/0006-3223(95)00296-0.
119. Rabinowitz T, Frankenburg FR, Centorrino F, Kando J. The effect of clozapine on saliva flow rate: a pilot study. Biol Psychiatry. 1996;40(11):1132–4. https://doi.org/10.1016/S0006-3223(96)89255-9.
120. Takeuchi I, Hanya M, Uno J, Fujita K, Kamei H. Effectiveness of the repeated administration of scopolamine ointment on clozapine-induced hypersalivation in patients with treatment-resistant schizophrenia: a preliminary study. Asia Pac Psychiatry. 2017;9(4):12269. https://doi.org/10.1111/appy.12269.
121. Praharaj SK, Jana AK, Goswami K, Das PR, Goyal N, Sinha VK. Salivary flow rate in patients with schizophrenia on clozapine. Clin Neuropharmacol. 2010;33(4):176–8. https://doi.org/10.1097/WNF.0b013e3181e204e0.
122. Ekström J, Godoy T, Loy F, Riva A. Parasympathetic vasoactive intestinal peptide (VIP): a likely contributor to clozapine-induced sialorrhoea. Oral Dis. 2014;20(3):e90–6. https://doi.org/10.1111/odi.12139.
123. Ishikawa S, Kobayashi M, Hashimoto N, et al. Association between N-desmethylclozapine and clozapine-induced sialorrhea: involvement of increased nocturnal salivary secretion via muscarinic receptors by N-desmethylclozapine. J Pharmacol Exp Ther. 2020;375(2):376–84. https://doi.org/10.1124/jpet.120.000164.
124. Rajagopal V, Sundaresan L, Rajkumar AP, et al. Genetic association between the DRD4 promoter polymorphism and clozapine-induced sialorrhea. Psychiatr Genet. 2014;24(6):273–6. https://doi.org/10.1097/YPG.0000000000000058.
125. Ekström J, Godoy T, Riva A. Clozapine: agonistic and antagonistic salivary secretory actions. J Dent Res. 2010;89(3):276–80. https://doi.org/10.1177/0022034509356055.
126. Teoh L, Moses G, McCullough MJ. A review and guide to drug-associated oral adverse effects—dental, salivary and neurosensory reactions. Part 1. J Oral Pathol Med. 2019;48(7):626–36. https://doi.org/10.1111/jop.12911.
127. Lo YC, Chen HH, Huang SS. Panic disorder correlates with the risk for sexual dysfunction. J Psychiatr Pract. 2020;26(3):185–200. https://doi.org/10.1097/PRA.0000000000000460.
128. American Psychiatric Association. Diagnostic and statistical manual of mental disorders. 5th ed. Arlington: American Psychiatric Publishing; 2013. p. 214–7.
129. Nardi AE, Machado S, Almada LF, et al. Clonazepam for the treatment of panic disorder. Curr Drug Targets. 2013;14(3):353–64. https://doi.org/10.2174/1389450111314030007.

130. Mattioli TM, Alanis LR, da Sapelli SS, et al. Effects of benzodiazepines on acinar and myo-epithelial cells. Front Pharmacol. 2016;7:173. https://doi.org/10.3389/fphar.2016.00173.
131. Mummolo S, Nota A, Caruso S, Quinzi V, Marchetti E, Marzo G. Salivary markers and microbial flora in mouth breathing late adolescents. Biomed Res Int. 2018;2018:8687608. https://doi.org/10.1155/2018/8687608.
132. Weiler RM, Fisberg M, Barroso AS, Nicolau J, Simi R, Siqueira WL Jr. A study of the influence of mouth-breathing in some parameters of unstimulated and stimulated whole saliva of adolescents. Int J Pediatr Otorhinolaryngol. 2006;70(5):799–805. https://doi.org/10.1016/j.ijporl.2005.09.008.
133. Schneyer LH, Pigman W, Hanahan L, Gilmore RW. Rate of flow of human parotid, sublingual, and submaxillary secretions during sleep. J Dent Res. 1956;35(1):109–14. https://doi.org/10.1177/00220345560350010301.
134. Dawes C. Circadian rhythms in human salivary flow rate and composition. J Physiol. 1972;220(3):529–45. https://doi.org/10.1113/jphysiol.1972.sp009721.
135. Orr WC, Heading R, Johnson LF, Kryger M. Review article: Sleep and its relationship to gastro-oesophageal reflux. Aliment Pharmacol Ther. 2004;20(Suppl 9):39–46. https://doi.org/10.1111/j.1365-2036.2004.02239.x.

Chapter 3
Congenital/Developmental Defects

Louis Mandel

Abstract Congenital defects of organs and tissues are constant sources of concern. Manifestation of these defects may be apparent at birth, during young adulthood or in adults. The salivary glands (SG) are not immune to these developmental errors. Aplasia of the SG may be noted at birth. The parotid gland is most commonly affected, usually in association with another syndrome such as aplasia of the lacrimal gland and SG or with the lacrimo-auriculo-dento-digital (LADD) syndrome. The congenital incomplete hollowing out of the anterior submandibular duct and its orifice (atresia) results in salivary retention and proximal duct ballooning in the newborn that mimics a ranula. Dysgenetic polycystic disease is considered a congenital defect of the intercalated ducts that usually presents as spontaneous intermittent painless parotid gland swellings. Parotid duct dilations are congenital problems observed in all ages, but predominantly in adults. Unique horizontal tube-like buccal facial swellings, exacerbated during meals, that contain voluminous amounts of saliva are its hallmarks.

Congenital/Developmental Defects

Introduction

A variety of congenital/developmental salivary gland (SG) defects have been observed in patients examined in the Columbia University Salivary Gland Center (SGC). At times, a hereditary genetic background has been determined as the etiologic factor. Although intrinsic and extrinsic causes have been suggested, the specific causative process for many defects is not always satisfactorily confirmed. Intrinsic causes often have a genetic provenance and originate in the fetus during the prenatal period. Extrinsic causes encompass a variety of environmental factors that

L. Mandel, *Clinical Management of Salivary Gland Disorders*,
https://doi.org/10.1007/978-3-031-50012-1_3

include infection, nutritional problems, lifestyle, radiation, chemicals, etc. Inevitably, all body organs and tissues are subject to the vagaries of congenital/developmental abnormalities. The salivary glands are not immune from involvement in these aberrations. Consequently, the salivary gland proper and/or its ductal system may become victimized by these discrepancies. This chapter will review those congenital/developmental abnormalities that have been reported to involve the salivary glands.

Congenital/Developmental Defects

Congenital Parotid Duct Dilation

The major parotid duct (PD) or Stensen duct of the parotid gland (PG) is usually formed within the PG by the union of two or three smaller glandular interlobular ducts. The PD then emerges from the anterior border of the PG and traverses the lateral aspect of the masseter muscle on a path corresponding to a line from the lower border of the tragus of the ear to a point midway between the ala of the nose and the red margin of the upper lip [1]. At the anterior border of the masseter muscle, the duct turns medially and goes around or through the buccal fat pad, pierces the buccinator muscle, runs obliquely forward for a very short distance between the buccinator muscle and oral mucous membrane, and then exits intraorally on a papilla located on the buccal mucosa adjacent to the maxillary second molar. The PD is 4–6 cm in length and has a width that varies between 0.2 and 2.3 mm [2, 3] and an ostium that represents its narrowest portion. Histologically pseudostratified epithelium, two to four cells thick with interspersed goblet cells, lines the lumen. A thin smooth muscle layer, running longitudinally, surrounds the duct peripherally [4].

Gross dilation of the PD is not a rare entity. Wang et al. [5] reviewed 200 patients with non-neoplastic PG disease and found PG duct dilations in 3.5% of the patients, while Seifert et al. [6] found its presence in 1.5% of 360 patients. Etiologically, PD dilation is thought to result from a congenital defect of the duct with hereditary factors that play a key role [5, 7]. Obstruction or infection can intensify further dilations of the already existing congenitally defective duct wall.

Clinically, congenital duct dilation patients will present themselves with unique and peculiar horizontal facial swellings, somewhat tubular in configuration, corresponding to the course of the PD (Fig. 3.1). These duct distentions usually have a long-standing history with periods during which they became more prominent. Generally, the condition is painless, but pain and exacerbations of swelling associated with eating may develop with the onset of secondary obstruction and/or infection. Aggressive extraoral massage of the swelling will cause a voluminous intraoral salivary discharge visible at the intraoral orifice of the involved PD and a decrease in the extraoral size of the swelling.

The extraoral swellings become apparent at any age, and because initially they tend to be painless, patients delay treatment. Medical consultation is usually sought

Fig. 3.1 (**a**) Duct dilation. Patient A. Facial swelling (arrows) along the horizontal course of parotid duct. (Mandel L, J Oral Maxillofac Surg 2007;65:2089). (**b**) Duct dilation. Patient A. CT scan demonstrates a dilated parotid duct (arrows). (Mandel L, J Oral Maxillofac Surg 2007;65:2089)

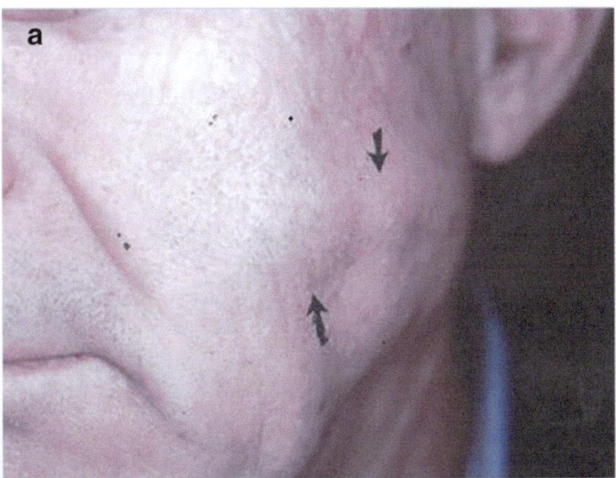

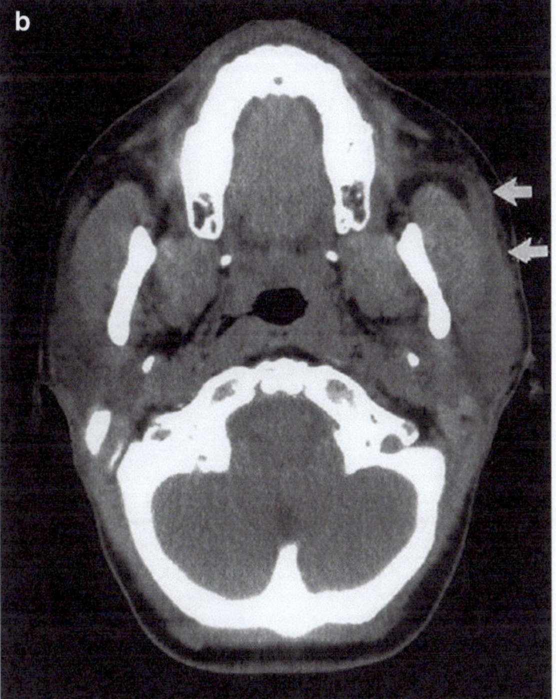

when pain and infection develop or because of a cosmetic issue. Clinically, a unilateral facial swelling will be present, but, on occasion, bilateral swellings from a bilateral duct defect may be seen. Palpation indicates that these swellings, caused by salivary accumulations within the distended ductal dilations, are painless, soft, compressible, and cyst-like. The swellings may become firmer and painful if infection enters the picture. The intraoral gush of saliva produced by extraoral pressure and massage of the PD dilation represents the evacuation of the retained and copious intraductal saliva that normally is clear in appearance. A cloudy salivary flow testifies to an infectious involvement of the PD and/or the PG.

Although the normal width of the PD has been stated to vary between 0.2 and 2.3 mm [2, 3], ultrasound in cases of congenital duct dilation has revealed that the duct's hypoechoic image width can measure as much as 15–20 mm [8]. Diagnosis of a widened PD with distinct borders may also be attained via sialography (Fig. 3.2a) or a CT scan (Figs. 3.1b and 3.2b). The distended duct with its contained trapped saliva will be clearly imaged by the CT scan as the duct traverses the lateral surface of the masseter muscle. With its availability, the MRI has become another popular unit in the imaging armamentarium. An MRI will enhance the contained saliva within the PD dilation and substantiate the increased luminal width of the PD (Fig. 3.3).

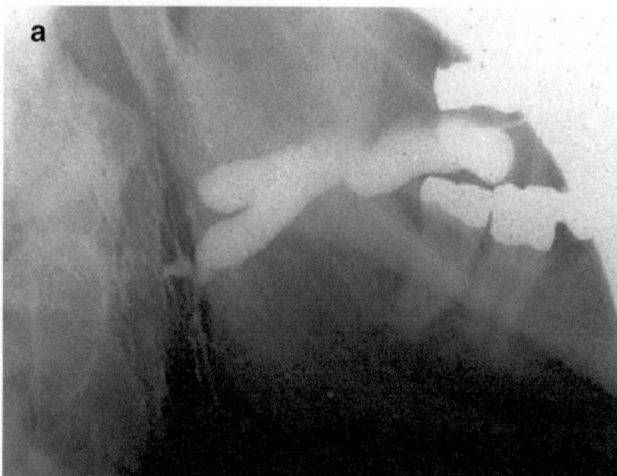
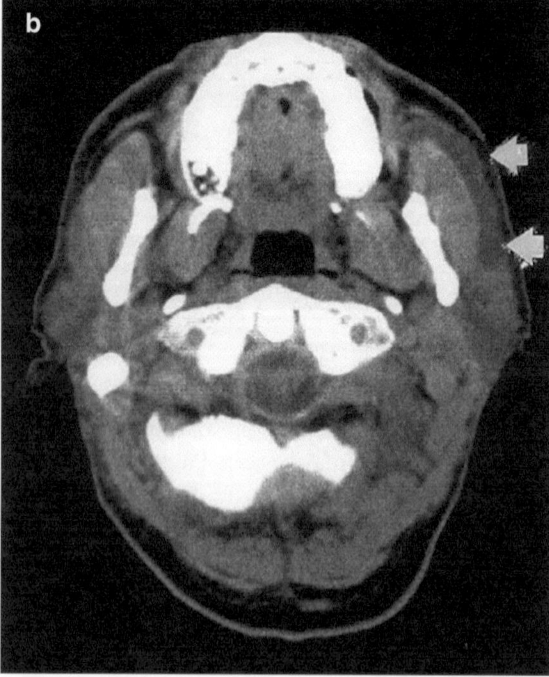

Fig. 3.2 (**a**) Duct dilation. Patient B. Sialogram reveals grossly dilated parotid duct. (Mandel L, J Oral Maxillofac Surg 2007;65:2089). (**b**) Duct dilation. Patient B. CT scan demonstrates dilated parotid duct (arrows). (Mandel L, J Oral Maxillofac Surg 2007;65:2089)

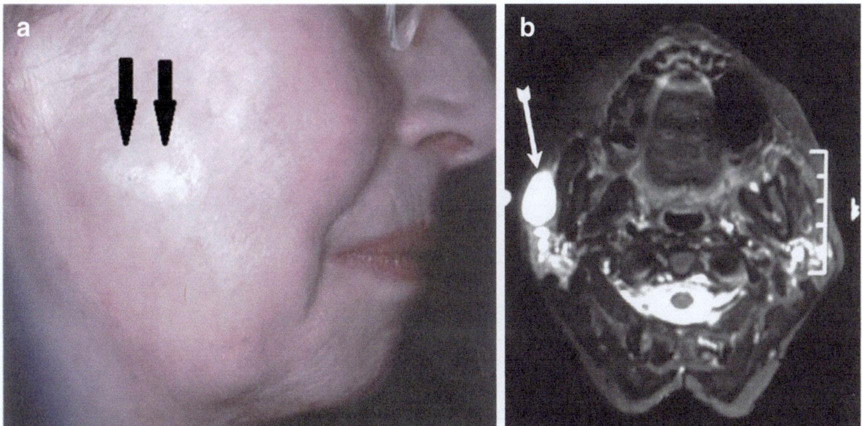

Fig. 3.3 (**a**) Duct dilation. Patient C. Facial swelling following path of parotid duct (arrows). (Mandel L, J Oral Maxillofac Surg 2007;65:2089). (**b**) Duct dilation. Patient C. MRI demonstrates dilated parotid duct (arrows). (Mandel L, J Oral Maxillofac Surg 2007;65:2089)

Some diagnostic confusion may arise from the fact that duct dilations can also develop from obstruction and lead to chronic parotitis. Stones, mucus plugs, and foreign bodies can act as obstructive agents that eventually cause a secondary duct dilation and an infectious process. Duct strictures, the end product of infection, form and lead to more obstruction. Regardless of the cause of the blockage, salivary retention and stagnation develop, thus enhancing the opportunity for repetitive ascending infections. Although duct dilations from the infection will occur, the PD dilation pattern from obstruction and infectious sequelae is readily recognized because the PD will appear segmented ("sausaged"). The segmentation, readily visible sialographically, is a consequence of a strictured duct's narrowing combined with a resulting salivary retention that favors ductal widening (Fig. 3.4). In contrast, the congenitally distended non-infected PD will have straight smooth walls devoid of strictures unless it becomes secondarily infected. With the onset of infection, the congenitally involved PD will mimic the sausage pattern associated with the infectious involvement of a normal PD. The difference rests in the fact that the sausaging in the congenitally dilated duct tends to be more gross. Nevertheless, differentiation demands clinical correlation.

In the early stages of a clinically apparent congenital PD dilation, conservative care is feasible. Frequent aggressive massage of the facial swelling and good oral hygiene must be practiced by the patient. Botulinum toxin A has been advocated as an alternative conservative therapeutic approach to decrease secretions [9]. If infection develops, symptomatic care (antibiotics, analgesics, etc.) can be instituted. Sialendoscopy may be of value therapeutically if stricturing from secondary infection has exacerbated salivary retention with retrograde PD dilation. Superficial parotidectomy may be necessary if an ascending secondary infection has compromised the PG. A definitive and permanent solution, wherein the dilated anterior segment of the PD is surgically dissected free and sutured to the buccal mucosa, has been suggested by Baurmash [10].

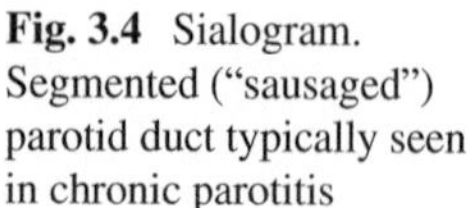

Fig. 3.4 Sialogram. Segmented ("sausaged") parotid duct typically seen in chronic parotitis

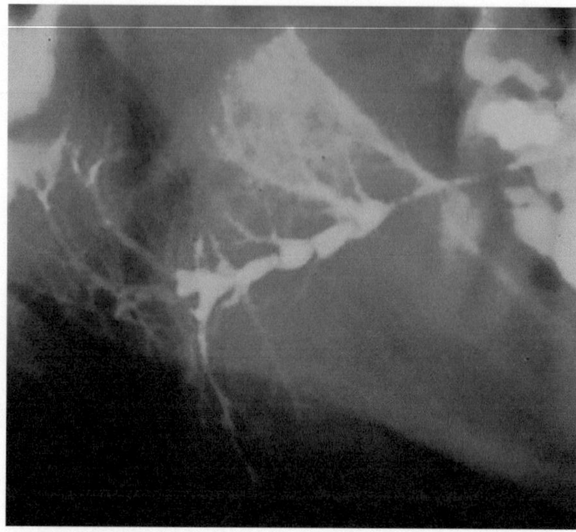

Congenital/Developmental Defects

Submandibular Duct Atresia

Submandibular duct (SMD) orifice atresia, first reported by Scher et al. [11], is a congenital anomaly observed in newborns and infants. The submandibular salivary gland (SMSG) develops during the sixth to eighth week of fetal life [12]. Its major duct arises as a solid cord from the ectoderm in the oral medial paralingual groove. At approximately 28 weeks of fetal life, a hollowing out of the cord, to form a patent duct lumen, occurs as one of the last acts in the development of the SMSG [13]. Anterior SMD atresia results when the duct hollowing process is incomplete and fails to incorporate the anterior orifice area. The resulting salivary retention, posterior to the blocked imperforate SMD, causes a visible cyst-like unilateral distention of the normal duct segment in the mouth floor (Fig. 3.5a). The swelling closely resembles the appearance of a ranula and has frequently been mistakenly referred to as a congenital ranula.

Males are more frequently involved than females. Bilateral involvement from bilateral atresia is not uncommon. Clinically, a bluish cyst-like swelling, oriented antero-posteriorly generally following the anatomic path of the SMD and containing a translucent fluid, can be observed. The overlying mucosa is not inflamed, and palpation indicates that the swelling is soft, cyst-like, painless, and compressible. Tongue displacement, caused by the swelling, may be present. Because the SMD is not patent, salivary flow from its orifice area is non-existent. An associated feeding problem may result in a fussy crying baby.

The sum of the lesion's clinical signs and symptoms often leads to the misdiagnosis of a ranula. Although SMD atresia can usually be diagnosed with an oral

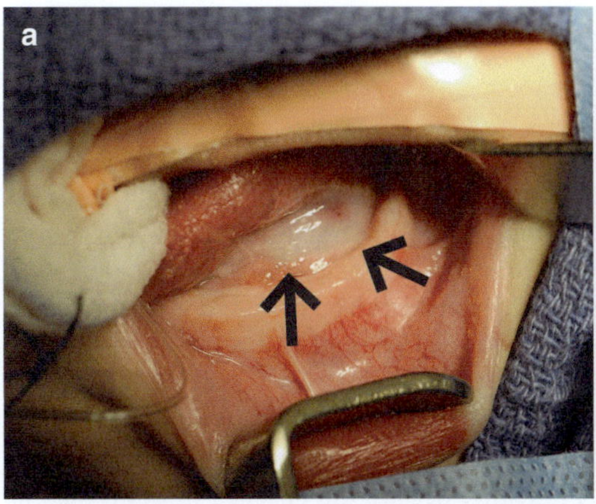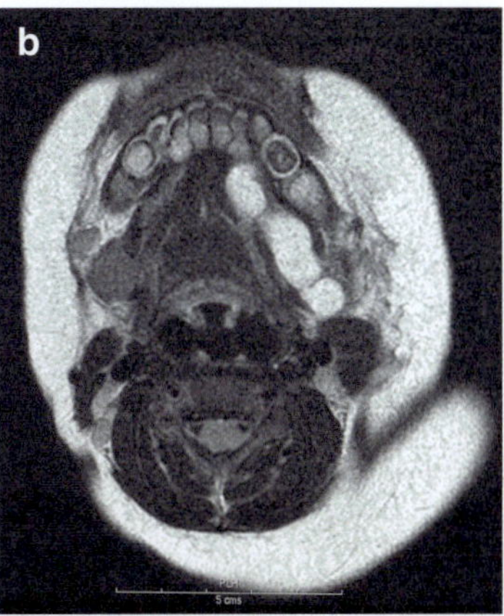

Fig. 3.5 (**a**) Atresia. Patient D. Swelling involving anterior mouth floor (arrows). (Mandel L, J Oral Maxillofac Surg 2012;70:2819). (**b**) Atresia. Patient D. MRI reveals segmentally lobed and dilated submandibular duct. (Mandel L, J Oral Maxillofac Surg 2012;70:2819)

examination, its existence and differentiation from a ranula are best established via imaging. An MRI will clearly show an elongated dilated tubular structure, segmentally lobed in the mouth floor, that is consistent with the anatomic course of an intact SMD (Fig. 3.5b). The normal SMD diameter does not exceed 3 mm, while duct atresia results in duct dilations that are well beyond 5 mm [14]. The MRI observed duct segmentation may be a result of the presence of resistant intraductal sphincters [15] or contraction of the SMD's surrounding smooth muscle fibers [16]. Besides a ranula, differential diagnosis must include dermal/epidermal inclusion cysts, thyroglossal cysts, branchial cysts, lymphatic and vascular lesions, and neoplasms.

Histologically, SMD atresia results in a cyst-like cavity lined by pseudostratified columnar epithelium consistent with a dilated duct [17]. Therein lies its difference from the misdiagnosed ranula which does not have an epithelial wall. The ranula's wall reflects the presence of the surrounding tissue's inflammatory response, manifested by granulation tissue, to extravasated secretions from a leaking sublingual salivary gland duct.

Because of the physical swelling, feeding of the infant and airway compromise may become issues. Sialadenitis and/or gland atrophy, secondary to salivary retention, can also develop and cause problems. Therefore, therapeutic intervention is indicated. Successful treatment can readily be achieved via simple surgery. A longitudinal antero-posterior incision is required along the anterior superior aspect of the distended SMD. The contained fluid immediately posterior to the atresia will be released and the swelling will collapse. The resulting filleted duct wall can now be sutured to the adjoining floor mucosa. A posteriorly placed and permanent patent orifice will evolve and prove to be functionally satisfactory. Although other surgical techniques have been advocated, the simplicity of this described surgical marsupialization of the SMD makes it the treatment of choice.

Congenital/Developmental Defects

Salivary Gland Aplasia

Aplasia of the major salivary glands, parotid (PG) and/or submandibular (SMSG), results from an ectodermal structural abnormality. The salivary gland aplasia may occur alone [18] or in association with other anomalies, particularly with defects in the lacrimal apparatus. Salivary gland (SG) aplasia can be partial or total and unilateral or bilateral. Patients with aplasia of the SG demonstrate a pattern of genetic inheritance which is autosomal dominant with a variable expressivity [19]. However, SG aplasia has also been reported to develop in the absence of a familial history [20].

SG aplasia, whether isolated or in association with other anomalies, most frequently involves the PG [21, 22]. Clinically, despite the absence of SG tissue, an anatomic defect in facial contour is not present because adipose tissue fills in the void created by the missing SG. Loss of the intraoral PG orifice and papilla is seen in all PG aplasias (Fig. 3.6a, b). With SG aplasia, the resulting hyposalivation may lead to increased dental caries if more than one SG is involved. Absence of the SG, most often seen in males, is usually partnered with the aplasia syndrome of lacrimal and salivary glands (ALSG) or with the lacrimo-auriculo-dento-digital (LADD) syndrome. Aplasia of the SG can also be observed in Down syndrome, mandibulo-facial dysostosis (Treacher-Collins), hemifacial microsomia, ectodermal dysplasia, Klinefelter syndrome, and cleft palate patients and as a feature in first and second branchial arch anomalies [23].

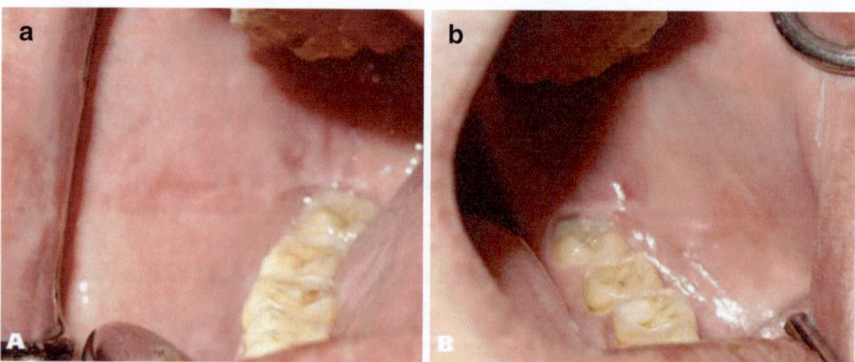

Fig. 3.6 (**a**) Aplasia. Patient E. Right buccal mucosa with the absence of Stensen papilla. (Mandel L, JADA 2006;137:984). (**b**) Aplasia. Patient E. Left buccal mucosa with the absence of Stensen papilla. (Mandel L, JADA 2006;137:984). (**c**) Aplasia. Patient E. Panoramic radiograph. Extensive occlusal enamel loss except in recently erupted third molars. (Mandel L, JADA 2006;137:984). (**d**) Aplasia. Patient E. Chipping of palatal dental surfaces right maxillary teeth. (Mandel L, JADA 2006;137:984). (**e**) Aplasia. Patient E. Chipping of palatal dental surfaces left maxillary teeth. (Mandel L, JADA 2006;137:984). (**f**) Aplasia. Patient E. Normal scintiscan demonstrates normal radioisotope pickup by both parotid and submandibular glands. (Mandel L, JADA 2006;137:984). (**g**) Aplasia. Patient E. Scintiscan reveals the absence of both parotids and both submandibular glands. (Mandel L, JADA 2006;137:984)

Fig. 3.6 (continued)

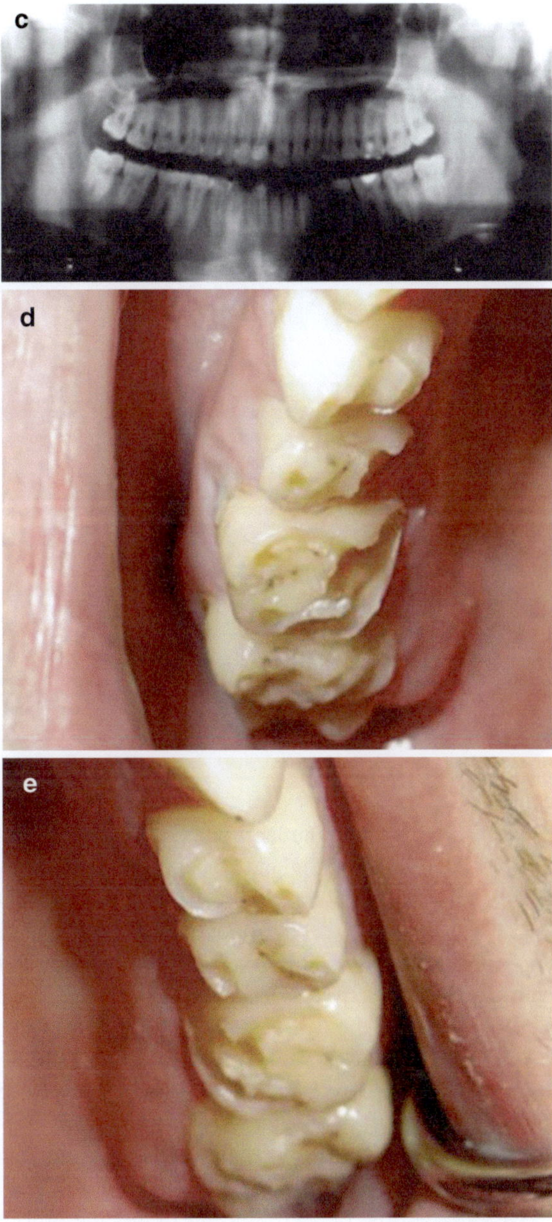

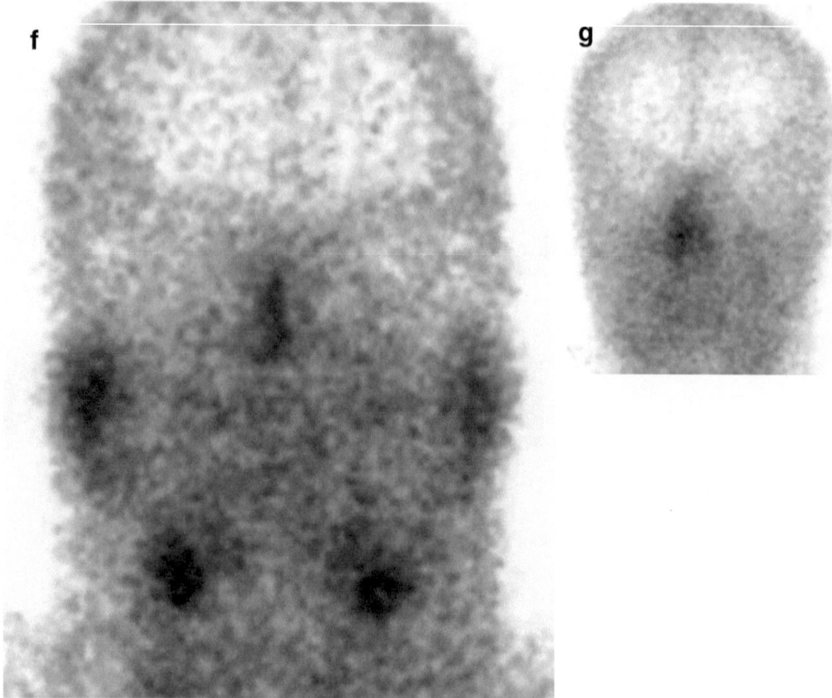

Fig. 3.6 (continued)

The disturbance in the lacrimal system seen in ALSG manifests itself as unilateral or bilateral lacrimal gland aplasia. The consequent loss of lacrimation results in eye irritations. Absence of the lacrimal puncta will also be evident. A mutation of the FGF-10 gene has been proposed as the cause of ALSG [19].

Aplasia of the SG is observed most commonly in LADD, where it is associated with abnormalities of the lacrimal gland similar to what is seen in ALSG. The possibility exists that the ALSG syndrome represents an incomplete form of LADD. In LADD, the SG aplasia, unilateral or bilateral, is usually accompanied by cup-shaped ears with hearing loss. There also is a decrease in eye lubrication caused by the lacrimal gland aplasia. Dentally, microdontia and hypodontia are present. Digitally, clinodactyly of the fifth digit and bony and soft-tissue tapering of the thumb are frequent findings in LADD [18].

Despite the loss of secreting SG tissue, the oral mucous membrane can remain lubricated, and widespread caries may be absent because of a compensatory increased salivary flow from the minor salivary glands and/or remaining uninvolved major glands [24, 25]. Nevertheless, dry mouth symptoms will usually develop in the presence of SG aplasia. The intensity of the hyposalivation will be in direct proportion to the extent of major/minor SG loss. The hyposalivation can be severe and result in rampant caries that may mimic the carious pattern seen in Sjögren's syndrome or following head and neck irradiation.

Saliva is a crucial factor in maintaining the integrity of the dental structures. However, the salivary volume in SG aplasia may be insufficient to totally buffer the oral acids. Dental demineralization can be expected to result from inadequate salivation. With demineralization, the enamel is softened and lost [26] (Fig. 3.6c), dentin is exposed, and the teeth become susceptible to episodes of chipping (Fig. 3.6d, e), a dental breakdown pattern different from hyposalivation-induced caries. The time frame and method in which the chipping develops depend on the extent of salivary reduction, the duration of exposure to the decreased saliva, masticatory stresses, dietary acids, and oral hygiene practices. A cupping pattern of the dental occlusal surface may also occur when the softer occlusal surface of any exposed dentin dissolves faster than the surrounding enamel. In addition, a peephole configuration can develop from point contact of an involved tooth with the cuspal height of an opposing tooth during mastication.

Diagnosis of SG aplasia and any associated syndrome is best accomplished via clinical observation of the patient's signs and symptoms. Confirmation of SG aplasia can be achieved from imaging (CT, MRI, ultrasound) techniques. A radioisotope study will serve as an accurate method to evaluate in real-time the presence and simultaneous functioning of all the salivary glands (Fig. 3.6f, g).

Sialogogic agents (pilocarpine or cevimeline) can be prescribed to increase salivation from any existing glandular tissues. Salivary flow can also be amplified with sugarless chewing gum or sour candy. Salivary substitutes, oral lubricants, and mouthwashes can be helpful as adjunctive aids. Fluoride use should be encouraged. Constant dental care is mandatory.

Congenital/Developmental Defects

Idiopathic Bone Cavity (Stafne)

Stafne in 1942 [27] was the first to describe the mandibular lingual ovoid concavities that are usually located in the Gonial angle area of the mandible (Fig. 3.7). The entity has been variously referred to as idiopathic bone cavity (IBC), static bone defect, or Stafne cavity. Because the defect is asymptomatic, it is identified only incidentally during routine radiographic examinations of the mandible. Most commonly found in males with a mean age of 52 years, it has a reported incidence of 0.08–0.48% [28]. A radiograph, usually a panoramic film, will image the IBC as a circular well-defined unilocular gonial angle area radiolucency, below the inferior alveolar canal and limited by a hyperostotic bony border and a thin connective tissue lining (Fig. 3.8). Although most commonly located in the mandibular angle, the ovoid IBC has been identified in all areas of the mandible including the ramus and anterior body [29]. It almost always occurs unilaterally, but bilateral cases have been reported [29]. No associated dento-alveolar pathology is present.

Examination of the IBC contents in the mandibular angle usually reveals the presence of normal submandibular salivary gland (SMSG) tissue. Evidence for this

Fig. 3.7 (**a**) Idiopathic bone cavity. Patient F. (**b**) Idiopathic bone cavity (IBC). Patient F. CT scan (axial view) bone window IBC defect (arrow). (**c**) Idiopathic bone cavity (IBC). Patient F. CT scan (coronal view) bone window IBC defect (arrow)

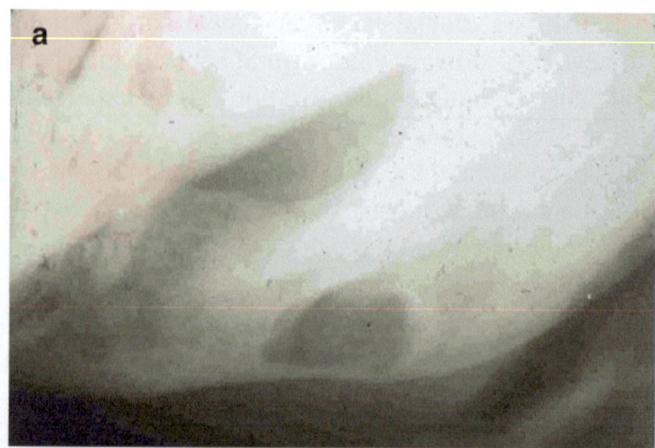

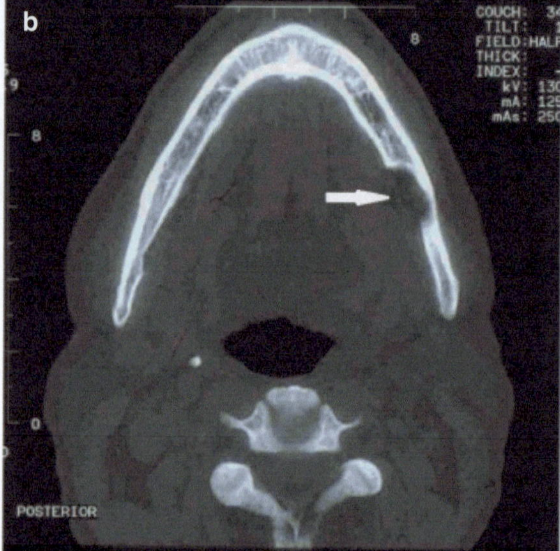

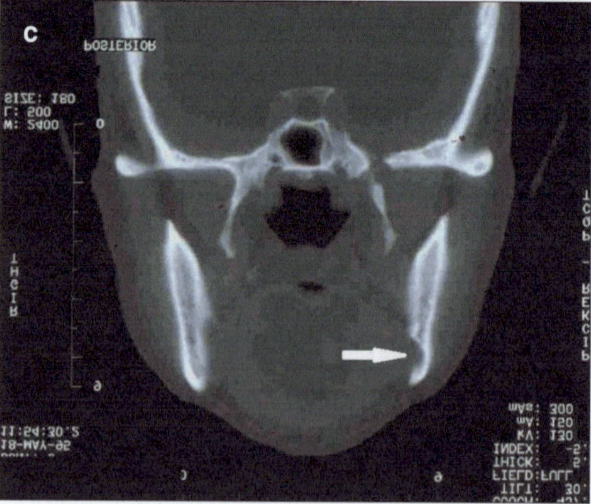

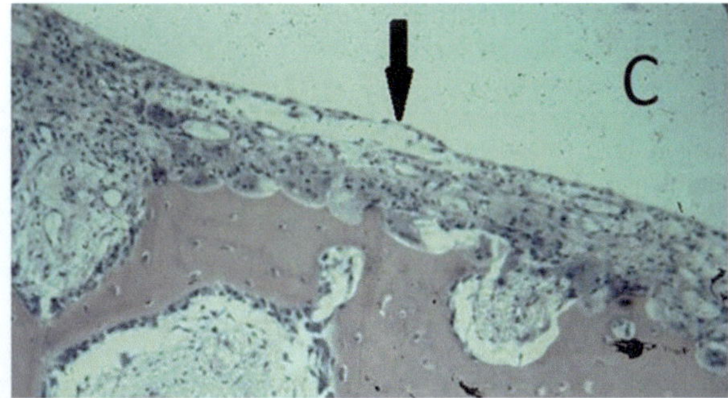

Fig. 3.8 Idiopathic bone cavity (IBC). Microscopic view. Bone cavity (C). Thin connective tissue lining (arrow)

SMSG extension into the IBC can also be obtained from MRI and CT scan imaging. Direct extension of the SMSG into the lingual concavity will be imaged. Confirmation of this SMSG prolapse is further substantiated by the fact that the signal intensity of the contained tissue in the IBC, imaged by the MRI or CT scan, corresponds to that of the SMSG [30]. It is also interesting and puzzling to note that a ramus located IBC concavity has been reported to contain parotid gland tissue [31], while sublingual salivary gland tissue was reported to inhabit a mandibular body lingual concavity [32].

The etiology of the IBC has not been determined. A developmental origin has frequently been advocated wherein there is the inclusion of a portion of the SMSG during mandibular development. However, the fact that the IBC is not seen in youngsters argues against this theory. More likely, there is an active chronic progressive pressure by juxtaposed glandular tissue against the mandible, and this brings about the concave bony resorption with contained glandular tissue that is seen in the mandibular IBC [28, 31].

Once a diagnosis has been made, no therapeutic intervention is indicated. If doubt regarding the diagnosis of the lucency is an issue, follow-up imaging studies are indicated to ascertain the existence of an on-going pathologic process that will be reflected by alterations in the lucent image. Active intervention may then be required.

Congenital/Developmental Defects

Dysgenetic Polycystic Disease

Dysgenetic polycystic disease (DPD) is a rare disorder, autosomal dominant primarily in females and hereditary in pattern, that usually involves portions of the parotid gland (PG) bilaterally but can occur unilaterally (Fig. 3.9). It has also been reported to develop in the submandibular [33] and minor [34] salivary glands. First described by Seifert et al. [6] in 1981, it is considered to be a congenital defect of the intercalated ducts of the salivary glands. DPD generally involves a PG lobule in young adult females whose median age at the time of examination is 31 years [34].

Fig. 3.9 (**a**) Dysgenetic polycystic disease (DPD). Patient G. Sialogram. Gross polycystic pattern seen in DPD. (Mandel L, J Oral Maxillofac Surg 1991;49:1228). (**b**) Dysgenetic polycystic disease. Patient G. Anterior–posterior sialogram demonstrates a polycystic pattern. (Mandel L, J Oral Maxillofac Surg 1991;49:1228)

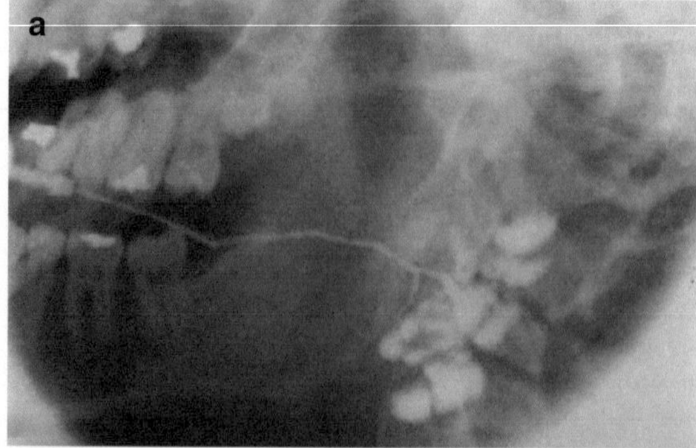

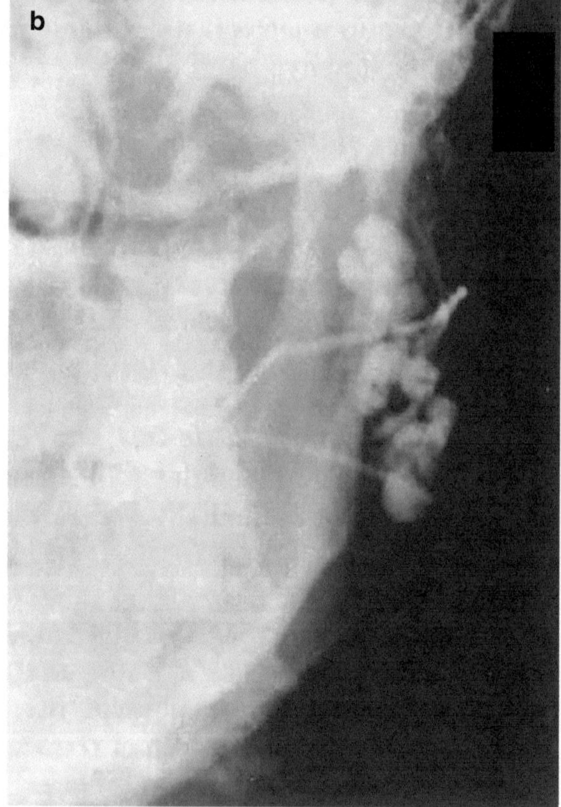

Patients present themselves with histories of intermittent painless PG swellings that often started in childhood and were not related to eating. A progression in the symptomatology and cosmetic concerns regarding the swellings serve to initiate a desire for medical attention.

An MRI will clearly demonstrate the presence in the PG of DPD's multiple varied-sized cysts. The hypoechoic areas seen with ultrasound, another useful

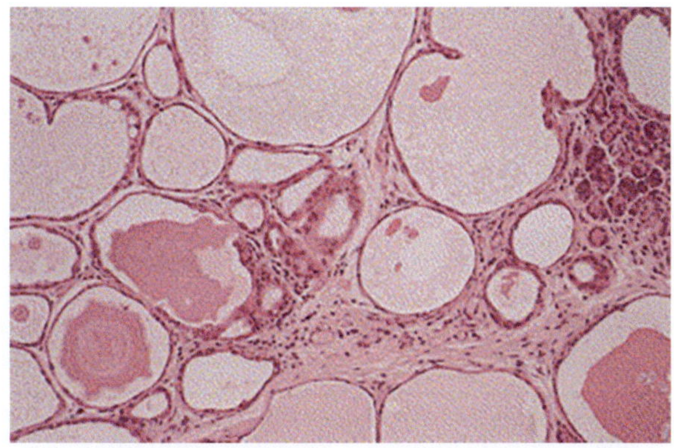

Fig. 3.10 Dysgenetic polycystic disease. Microscopic view. Multicystic spaces in connective tissue stroma. [Eveson JW, Current Diagnostic Pathology. 2006;12(1):22–30]

diagnostic imaging tool, also confirm the presence of these cystic lesions. Nevertheless, a definitive diagnosis demands the microscopic examination of a surgical specimen.

Microscopically, multiple cystic lesions, varying in size and surrounded by a loose connective tissue stroma, are present (Fig. 3.10). The lining of the cysts consists of one to three layers of flattened columnar/cuboidal epithelium [6, 34]. At times, small ducts can be seen opening directly into the cysts, thus suggesting DPD's origin from the intercalated duct system [34]. Inspissated proteinaceous secretions, in various stages of accretion, reside in the cystic spaces [35]. No inflammatory infiltrates surrounding the fluid-containing cysts are present. A scarcity of glandular acini exists between the cystic lesions [36]. Of interest is the fact that the described developmental and pathologic picture of DPD parallels the polycystic disease reported to occur in the pancreas, kidney, liver, and lung [34]. However, a common denominator uniting these disparate conditions has not been identified.

Because DPD is non-neoplastic and usually involves only lobules of the PG, a limited superficial lobectomy is an acceptable surgical approach. Total superficial lobe parotidectomy is only indicated when the pathology is extensive. Follow-up care is always necessary because recurrences can develop in any retained PG tissue or even develop in another salivary gland.

References

1. Williams PL, Warwick R, editors. Gray's anatomy. 36th ed. Philadelphia: Saunders; 1980. p. 1280.
2. Zenk J, Hosemann WG, Iro H. Diameters of the main excretory ducts of the adult human submandibular and parotid gland: a histologic study. Oral Surg Oral Med Oral Pathol Oral Radiol Endod. 1998;85(5):576–80. https://doi.org/10.1016/s1079-2104(98)90294-3.
3. Stringer MD, Mirjalili SA, Meredith SJ, Muirhead JC. Redefining the surface anatomy of the parotid duct: an in vivo ultrasound study. Plast Reconstr Surg. 2012;130(5):1032–7. https://doi.org/10.1097/PRS.0b013e318267d610.

4. Takeda Y. Histoarchitecture of the human parotid duct. Light-microscopic study. Acta Anat (Basel). 1987;128(4):291–4. https://doi.org/10.1159/000146356.

5. Wang Y, Yu GY, Huang MX, Mao C, Zhang L. Diagnosis and treatment of congenital dilatation of Stensen's duct. Laryngoscope. 2011;121(8):1682–6. https://doi.org/10.1002/lary.21854.

6. Seifert G, Thomsen S, Donath K. Bilateral dysgenetic polycystic parotid glands. Morphological analysis and differential diagnosis of a rare disease of the salivary glands. Virchows Arch A Pathol Anat Histol. 1981;390(3):273–88. https://doi.org/10.1007/BF00496559.

7. Lee DH, Yoon TM, Lee JK, Lim SC. Congenital dilatation of Stensen's duct in siblings. Int J Pediatr Otorhinolaryngol. 2015;79(11):1952–4. https://doi.org/10.1016/j.ijporl.2015.08.033.

8. Yoruk O, Kılıc K, Kantarcı M. "Mustache sign" due to Stensen duct dilation. Oral Surg Oral Med Oral Pathol Oral Radiol. 2013;116(6):e514–6. https://doi.org/10.1016/j.oooo.2013.08.002.

9. Le Roux MK, Graillon N, Hadj-Saïd M, Scemama U, Lutz JC, Chossegros C. Stensen duct dilation: case series of minimally invasive treatment. Oral Surg Oral Med Oral Pathol Oral Radiol. 2019;127(6):e114–7. https://doi.org/10.1016/j.oooo.2019.01.078.

10. Baurmash HD. Sialectasis of Stensen's duct with an extraoral swelling: a case report with surgical management. J Oral Maxillofac Surg. 2007;65(1):140–3. https://doi.org/10.1016/j.joms.2005.12.033.

11. Scher LB, Scher I. Case of imperforate submandibular ducts in an infant. Br Dent J. 1955;98:324–6.

12. Quirós-Terrón L, Arráez-Aybar LA, Murillo-González J, De-la-Cuadra-Blanco C, Martínez-Álvarez MC, Sanz-Casado JV, Mérida-Velasco JR. Initial stages of development of the submandibular gland (human embryos at 5.5–8 weeks of development). J Anat. 2019;234(5):700–8. https://doi.org/10.1111/joa.12955.

13. Ulualp SO, Rodriguez SC, Hernandez J, Hay M. Bilateral atresia of the submandibular duct orifices. Am J Otolaryngol. 2007;28(3):184–6. https://doi.org/10.1016/j.amjoto.2006.06.020.

14. Aasen S, Kolbenstvedt A. CT appearances of normal and obstructed submandibular duct. Acta Radiol. 1992;33(5):414–9.

15. Marchal F, Kurt AM, Dulguerov P, Lehmann W. Retrograde theory in sialolithiasis formation. Arch Otolaryngol Head Neck Surg. 2001;127(1):66–8. https://doi.org/10.1001/archotol.127.1.66.

16. Teymoortash A, Ramaswamy A, Werner JA. Is there evidence of a sphincter system in Wharton's duct? Etiological factors related to sialolith formation. J Oral Sci. 2003;45(4):233–5. https://doi.org/10.2334/josnusd.45.233.

17. Prosdócimo ML, Barreto Nogueira AP, de Albuquerque A, Cavalcante M, Agostini M, Benevenuto de Andrade BA, Romañach MJ. Congenital dilatation of the submandibular duct. Int J Pediatr Otorhinolaryngol. 2018;113:16–8. https://doi.org/10.1016/j.ijporl.2018.07.008.

18. Inan UU, Yilmaz MD, Demir Y, Degirmenci B, Ermis SS, Ozturk F. Characteristics of lacrimo-auriculo-dento-digital (LADD) syndrome: case report of a family and literature review. Int J Pediatr Otorhinolaryngol. 2006;70(7):1307–14. https://doi.org/10.1016/j.ijporl.2005.12.015.

19. Neagu D, Patiño-Seijas B, Luaces-Rey R, Collado-López J, García-Rozado-González Á, López-Cedrún-Cembranos JL. Aplasia of the lacrimal and major salivary glands (ALSG). First case report in Spanish population and review of the literature. J Clin Exp Dent. 2018;10(12):e1238–41. https://doi.org/10.4317/jced.55350.

20. Daniel SJ, Blaser S, Forte V. Unilateral agenesis of the parotid gland: an unusual entity. Int J Pediatr Otorhinolaryngol. 2003;67(4):395–7. https://doi.org/10.1016/s0165-5876(02)00375-0.

21. Al-Talabani N, Gataa IS, Latteef SA. Bilateral agenesis of parotid salivary glands, an extremely rare condition: report of a case and review of literature. Oral Surg Oral Med Oral Pathol Oral Radiol Endod. 2008;105(3):e73–5. https://doi.org/10.1016/j.tripleo.2007.10.013.

22. Yilmaz MD, Yücel A, Dereköy S, Altuntaş A. Unilateral aplasia of the submandibular gland. Eur Arch Otorrinolaringol. 2002;259(10):554–6. https://doi.org/10.1007/s00405-002-0492-8.

23. Taji SS, Savage N, Holcombe T, Khan F, Seow WK. Congenital aplasia of the major salivary glands: literature review and case report. Pediatr Dent. 2011;33(2):113–8.

24. Günbey HP, Günbey E, Tayfun F, Kaytez SK. A rare cause of unilateral parotid gland swelling: compensatory hypertrophy due to the aplasia of the contralateral parotid gland. J Craniofac Surg. 2014;25(3):e265–7. https://doi.org/10.1097/SCS.0000000000000629.
25. Yerli H. Dynamic sonography and CT findings of unilateral submandibular gland agenesis associated with herniated hypertrophic sublingual gland. J Clin Ultrasound. 2014;42(3):176–9. https://doi.org/10.1002/jcu.22072.
26. Fracaro MS, Linnett VM, Hallett KB, Savage NW. Submandibular gland aplasia and progressive dental caries: a case report. Aust Dent J. 2002;47(4):347–50. https://doi.org/10.1111/j.1834-7819.2002.tb00550.x.
27. Stafne EC. Bone cavities situated near the angle of the mandible. J Am Dent Assoc. 1942;29:1969–72.
28. He J, Wang J, Hu Y, Liu W. Diagnosis and management of Stafne bone cavity with emphasis on unusual contents and location. J Dent Sci. 2019;14(4):435–9. https://doi.org/10.1016/j.jds.2019.06.001.
29. Aps JKM, Koelmeyer N, Yaqub C. Stafne's bone cyst revisited and renamed: the benign mandibular concavity. Dentomaxillofac Radiol. 2020;49(4):20190475. https://doi.org/10.1259/dmfr.20190475.
30. Mauprivez C, Sahli Amor M, Khonsari RH. Magnetic resonance sialography of bilateral Stafne bone cavities. J Oral Maxillofac Surg. 2015;73(5):934.e1–934.e9347. https://doi.org/10.1016/j.joms.2015.01.034.
31. Kaya M, Ugur KS, Dagli E, Kurtaran H, Gunduz M. Stafne bone cavity containing ectopic parotid gland. Braz J Otorhinolaryngol. 2018;84(5):669–72. https://doi.org/10.1016/j.bjorl.2016.02.004.
32. Hayashi K, Onda T, Iwasaki T, et al. A case of a Stafne bone defect associated with sublingual glands in the lingual side of the mandible. Case Rep Dent. 2020;2020:8851174. https://doi.org/10.1155/2020/8851174.
33. Koudounarakis E, Willems S, Karakullukcu B. Dysgenetic polycystic disease of the minor and submandibular salivary glands. Head Neck. 2016;38(6):E2437–9. https://doi.org/10.1002/hed.24401.
34. Srikant N, Yellapurkar S, Boaz K, et al. Dysgenetic polycystic disease of minor salivary gland: a rare case report and review of the literature. Case Rep Pathol. 2017;2017:5279025. https://doi.org/10.1155/2017/5279025.
35. Batsakis JG, Bruner JM, Luna MA. Polycystic (dysgenetic) disease of the parotid glands. Arch Otolaryngol Head Neck Surg. 1988;114(10):1146–8. https://doi.org/10.1001/archotol.1988.01860220080029.
36. Kumar KA, Mahadesh J, Setty S. Dysgenetic polycystic disease of the parotid gland: report of a case and review of the literature. J Oral Maxillofac Pathol. 2013;17(2):248–52. https://doi.org/10.4103/0973-029X.119744.

Chapter 4
Sialolithiasis

Louis Mandel

Abstract Sialolithiasis, or salivary stones is defined as the formation of calcific concretions within the ductal system of a salivary gland (SG). The submandibular salivary gland is most frequently involved. The presence of stones is less common in the parotid gland, while its occurrence in the sublingual and minor salivary glands is infrequent. Salivary stasis in the presence of a nidus favors salt precipitation and sialolith formation. The stone's obstruction to salivary flow favors the development of objective and subjective symptomatology, pain and swelling, primarily associated with periods of increased salivary demand. Inevitably in time, an acute suppurative sialadenitis will develop secondary to the occurrence of an ascending duct invasion by oral bacteria. Therapeutic intervention to remove the offending sialolith is required. Sialolithectomy is usually rewarded by salivary gland recovery.

Sialolithiasis

Introduction

Sialolithiasis, or salivary stones, is defined as the formation of calcific concretions within the ductal system of a major or minor salivary gland. It is not an uncommon occurrence, with a reported estimated annual incidence in the general population ranging from 1 per 10,000 to 30,000 individuals [1]. Sialoliths are the most frequent cause of salivary gland swelling. Patients, with males and females equally susceptible, between 30 and 60 years of age are most often affected [2, 3]. Only 3% of all sialolithiasis cases have been reported in children [4]. Approximately 83% of sialolithiasis cases involve the submandibular salivary gland (SMSG) while the parotid gland (PG) is involved 10% of the time and the sublingual and minor salivary glands represent the remainder [5]. Recurrences after removal are reported to be 8.9% [3].

L. Mandel, *Clinical Management of Salivary Gland Disorders*, https://doi.org/10.1007/978-3-031-50012-1_4

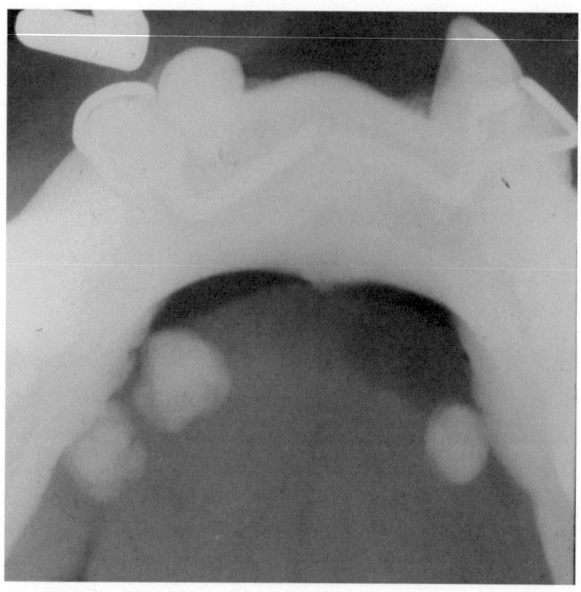

Fig. 4.1 Sialolithiasis. Occlusal radiograph. Bilateral submandibular duct stones

Single sialoliths are found 70–80% of the time with their size varying from 1 mm to 2–3 cm in diameter [3]. Two sialoliths are found in about 20% of the cases and three or more in about 5% of the patients [3] (Fig. 4.1). The sialoliths may develop unilaterally or even bilaterally and can be located extraglandularly in the major salivary duct or within an intraglandular duct. Generally, stones that form within a duct tend to be elongated (Fig. 4.2d), taking on the configuration dictated by the limiting confines defined by the duct wall, while those that develop within the hilus or gland proper tend to be oval in shape. Salivary stones are composed of organic (glycoproteins, cellular debris) and inorganic (mainly calcium carbonate and phosphate) substances [1].

The exact methodology of sialolith evolution has not been definitively determined. However, three physical prerequisites stand out as being identified with stone formation. Initially, a nidus is necessary and may result from a subclinical retrograde infection of a salivary duct that causes a change in the mucoid molecule within the saliva. A complex glycoprotein gel develops and serves as the nidus [6]. Alternatively, it has been suggested that the nidus can be a foreign body within the duct, desquamated inflammatory cellular debris, or clumps of microorganisms [4]. Regardless of its origin, the nidus creates a partial obstruction to salivary flow with a resulting salivary stasis, with salivary stasis being the second prerequisite needed for the formation of a sialolith. In turn, stasis favors precipitation of salivary salts into the glycoprotein matrix, the third process in the development of a stone [6, 7]. A clinically apparent sialolith becomes evident with continued mineral deposition. The exact reason for the growth of a sialolith has not been precisely determined, but a recent study indicates that an enhanced intraductal influx of neutrophils, brought about by inflammation, is an essential element [8]. Inevitably with the passage of time, the obstruction caused by the stone will produce subjective and objective

Fig. 4.2 (**a**) Sialolithiasis. Patient A. Mandibular dental radiographs. Incidental finding of submandibular sialoliths. (**b**) Sialolithiasis. Patient A. Extraoral view. No submandibular swelling. (**c**) Sialolithiasis. Patient A. Intraoral view. Bulging of non-inflamed sublingual tissue (right) caused by large underlying sialolith. (**d**) Sialolithiasis. Patient A. Occlusal radiograph. Ductal sialoliths. (Mandel L, Salivary Gland Disorders. Med Clin North Am 2014;98:1416)

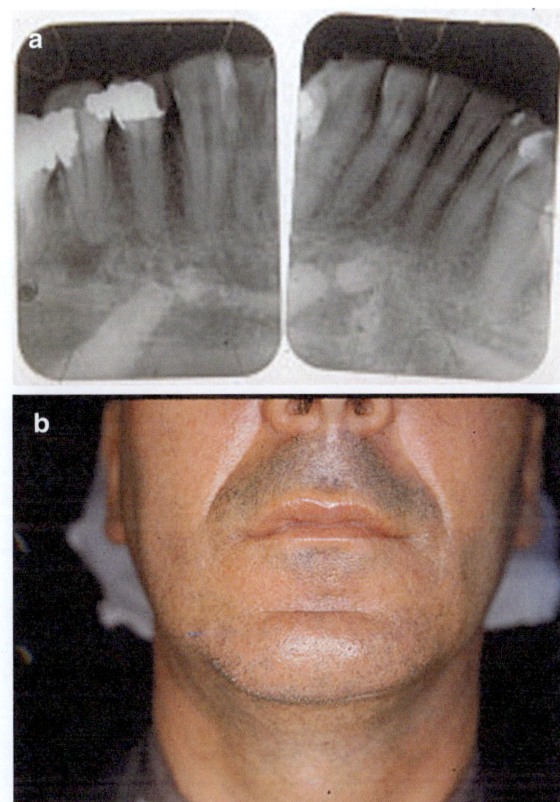

glandular symptomatology, most marked during periods of increased salivary demand such as while eating. Long-term obstruction of salivary flow inevitably leads to retrograde infection with degenerative glandular changes and decreases in salivary production.

Sialolithiasis

Submandibular Sialolithiasis

The increased frequency of sialoliths, or stones in the submandibular salivary gland (SMSG) duct system, as compared with its somewhat limited occurrence in the parotid gland (PG), has been attributed to several factors. The saliva from the SMSG normally contains greater concentrations of calcium and phosphate salts, fundamental stone ingredients, than the saliva secreted by the other salivary glands [6]. The SMSG saliva also has a higher pH than PG saliva, and this relative alkalinity, when compared with the more acidic PG saliva, favors salt precipitation [9]. The

Fig. 4.2 (continued)

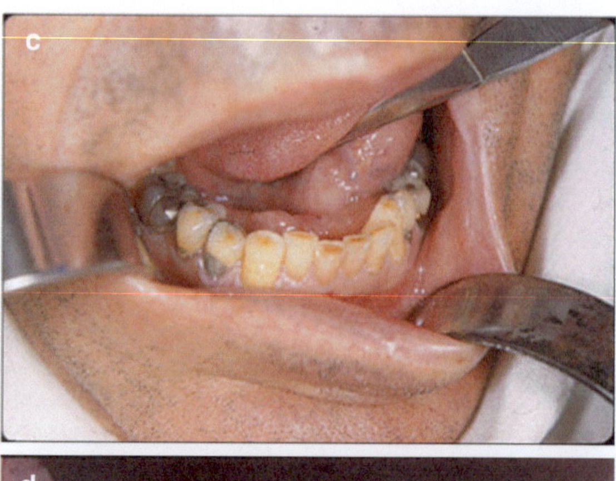

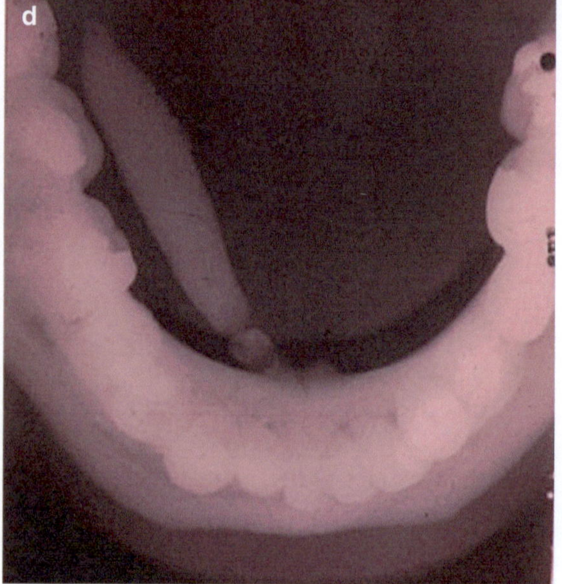

precipitation needed for stone formation is also facilitated by the fact that SMSG saliva runs an uphill anatomic trajectory that encourages stasis as the saliva moves through its major duct toward its orifice. Furthermore, SMSG saliva contains a significant element of viscous mucus, whereas the PG produces an aqueous serous secretion. The relative viscosity of the SMSG secretion when compared with the PG's aqueous secretion favors salivary stagnation with ensuing salt deposition.

The Columbia University Salivary Gland Center has noted that patients with stones in the SMSG duct system can be classified into three different clinical symptom groups. In the first group, there may be a total absence of symptoms (Fig. 4.2). The sialolith may have been present for varying periods of time and was identified incidentally only during a routine dental/medical imaging examination. It is also possible that a firm bulge in the mouth floor along the course of the Wharton duct,

Fig. 4.3 (**a**) Sialolithiasis. Patient B. Extraoral view. Left submandibular gland swelling. (**b**) Sialolithiasis. Patient B. Intraoral view. Modest mouth floor inflammation with edema

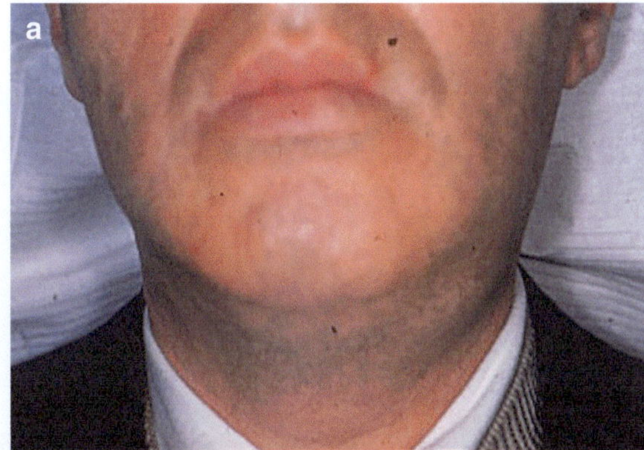

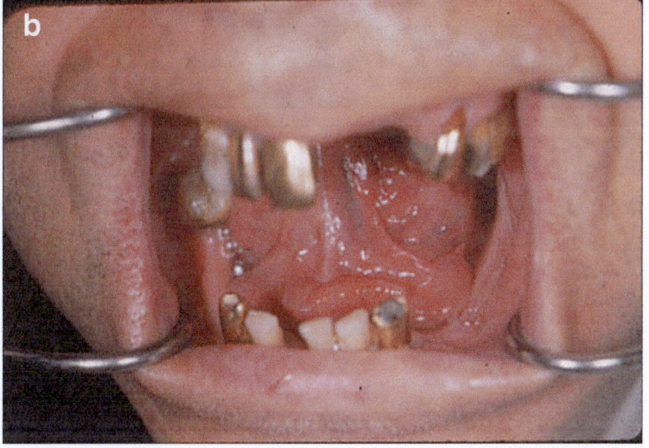

marking the position of the stone, is noted during an intraoral examination. The patients in this first category have no subjective symptomatology because the stone blockage of the duct is incomplete. Sufficient duct luminal patency is available to accommodate normal resting and stimulated salivary flow. Salivary retention, with its accompanying subjective and objective problems, is avoided.

More often a history of transient moderately painful gland swellings, initiated by eating, will be elicited from the second symptom group (Fig. 4.3). The swellings may last from a few minutes to several days and then subside only to develop again with a subsequent salivary stimulus. Such episodes may repeat themselves over a span of weeks or even months and be followed by varying periods of remission. The explanation may rest in the fact that the stone-narrowed residual duct lumen has now become additionally obstructed by a mucus plug that formed from stagnant saliva retained by the stone. It is also possible that inflammatory debris, resulting from oral bacteria whose retrograde ductal invasion is facilitated by the sialolith, further impeded salivary flow and contributed to the obstruction. The increased salivary production during meals cannot totally negotiate the narrowed patent lumen and salivary retention with SMSG swelling becomes evident. When eating with its increased salivary production ceases, the retained saliva gradually seeps past the

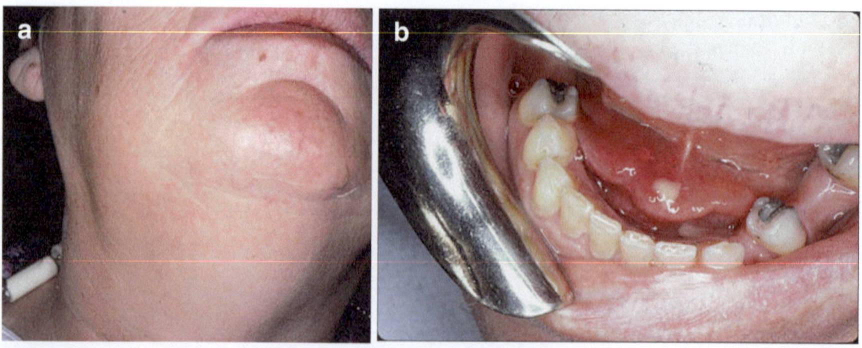

Fig. 4.4 (**a**) Sialolithiasis. Patient C. Extraoral view. Acute suppurative sialadenitis right submandibular gland secondary to sialolith. (Mandel L, Salivary Gland Disorders. Med Clin North Am 2014;98:1416). (**b**) Sialolithiasis. Patient C. Intraoral view. Acute suppurative sialadenitis. Pus exiting submandibular duct orifice. (Mandel L, Salivary Gland Disorders. Med Clin North Am 2014;98:1416)

thinned duct lumen and gland swelling subsides. Eventually, the soft gel-like mucus plug is eliminated, possibly by the hydrostatic pressure of salivary flow, and varying periods of remission occur. Unfortunately, recurrences that seem to progressively increase in intensity can be anticipated and will result in the third presenting clinical symptom picture, an acute suppurative sialadenitis (Fig. 4.4). This acute infectious process develops when an ascending bacterial ductal infection, presumably originating from the oral cavity and facilitated by salivary stasis, localizes in the gland proper. The SMSG becomes swollen and quite painful and the swelling does not subside between meals. The pain in the distended SMSG increases in intensity when eating because salivary retention exacerbates SMSG symptomatology. Usually, the patient relates a history of previous transient episodes of SMSG swelling that were associated with only mild discomfort.

The examination of a patient with acute infection will reveal a febrile patient who is in obvious distress. Extraorally, the SMSG is visibly swollen, firm, and very painful when palpated and the overlying skin is erythematous. Intraorally, the mouth floor along the course of the involved Wharton duct is markedly inflamed and the inflammation may even extend to the opposite side. Palpation of the involved mouth floor will indicate that the tissues are indurated and painful. Gentle extraoral milking of the involved gland and its duct in the mouth floor will produce a tell-tale sign, pus will be seen exiting from the duct orifice located adjacent to the lingual frenum.

There are numerous modalities that are available to diagnose the presence of an SMSG sialolith. Obviously, the history and clinical picture are essential elements in diagnosis. Close visual scrutiny of the mucosa in the mouth floor along the duct's path may reveal a yellow discoloration caused by the intraductal stone, provided that the stone is close to the surface. Stretching and making the soft tissues of the mouth floor taut serve to thin the overlying mucosa and may make the stone's yellow color visible. Furthermore, palpation of the mouth floor along the course of the duct, while simultaneously exerting extraoral pressure upon the SMSG, may be

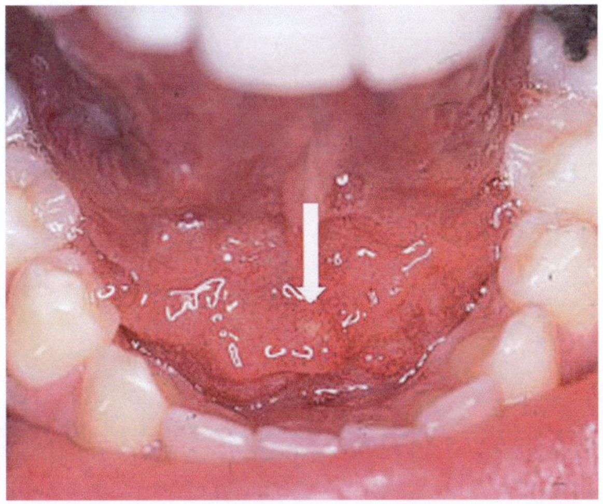

Fig. 4.5 Sialolithiasis. Small stone at orifice left submandibular duct (arrow). Close inspection reveals yellow discoloration

successful in locating the hard sialolith. The depth of the duct in the oral soft tissues and stone size are the determining factors as to whether the stone's position is palpable and/or visible. Diagnostic aid may also be obtained with a metallic probe that is gently inserted into the duct. The probe can serve as a marker of a sialolith's precise presence when metal contact with the calcified sialolith causes a grating sensation. It is also important to remember that the Wharton duct makes a right-angle bend at the posterior border of the mylohyoid muscle and then runs horizontally forward in the mouth floor. This genu area of the duct demands attention. The slowing and stasis of salivary flow, caused by the anatomic bend at the genu, encourage salt precipitation and are thought to be the cause of the increased occurrence of stones in this proximal portion of the duct. The duct's orifice on the caruncle adjoining the lingual frenum also requires meticulous inspection. Small stones, superficially located, locked in position by the narrow SMSG duct orifice often can be identified by their yellow coloration (Fig. 4.5). They can be made more visible via a manually stretched tightly drawn mucosa.

Patients with sialolithiasis seen in an office-based setting can be diagnosed via various radiographic techniques. Stones in the anterior two-thirds of the Wharton duct are best visualized with an occlusal radiograph of the mouth floor, provided that there is sufficient calcification. The soft tissues of the anterior mouth floor and its contained submandibular duct are distinctly pictured without any obliteration from adjacent calcified bony structures. However, with this technique, it is difficult to image posteriorly positioned stones that are located in the duct's genu or hilar region. An oblique angulated occlusal radiographic view, using an occlusal film, can successfully reveal such stones by radiographically displacing these stones into a more anterior position (Fig. 4.6). Problems also arise when using an occlusal film to view a stone in the orifice area of the duct. Care must be taken to avoid superimposing the sialolith on the opacity of the mandible's lingual cortical plate and making the sialolith visually difficult to identify (Fig. 4.7).

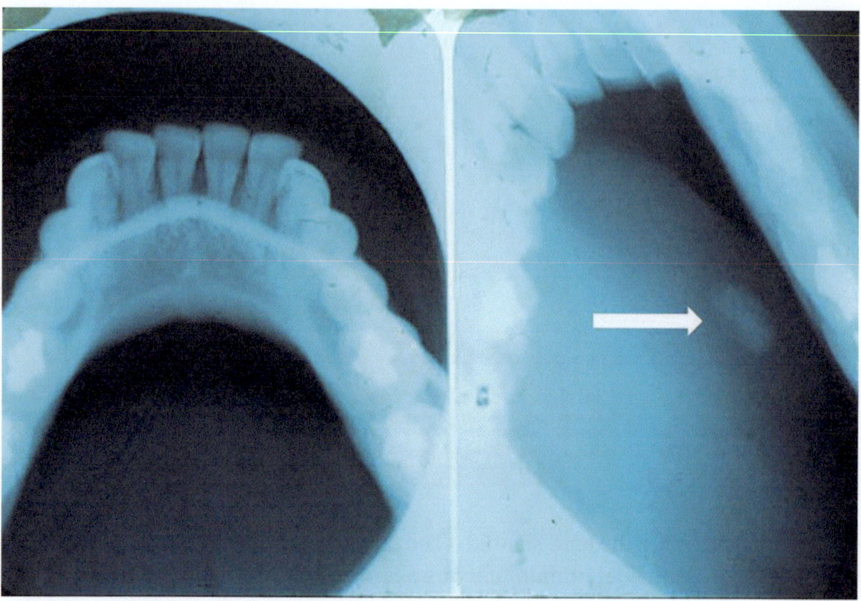

Fig. 4.6 Sialolithiasis. Occlusal radiographs. Posteriorly positioned sialolith not visible with a standard occlusal view (left film). Sialolith clearly seen (arrow) when projected forward via occlusal oblique view

Fig. 4.7 (**a**) Sialolithiasis. Patient D. Occlusal view. Lingual cortical plate blots out the orifice area of the submandibular duct. (**b**) Sialolithiasis. Patient D. Occlusal view. X-ray cone at a right angle to the occlusal film reveals a small sialolith (arrow)

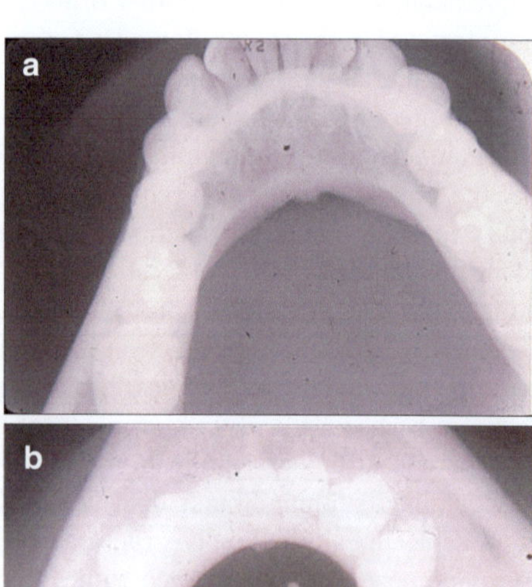

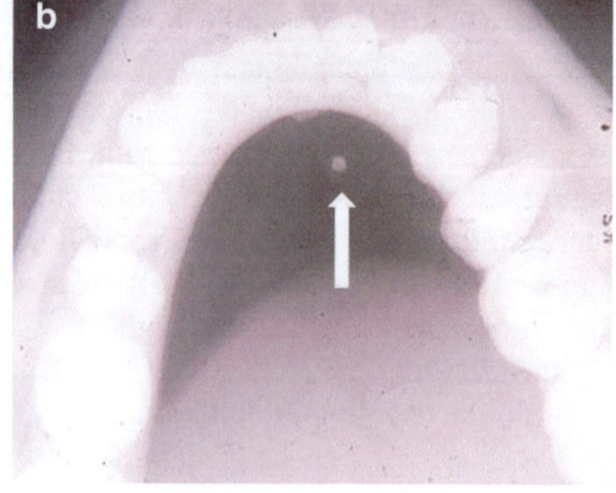

Fig. 4.8 Sialolithiasis. Lateral radiograph. Superimposition of mandibles. Sialolith present in the hilar area of the submandibular gland

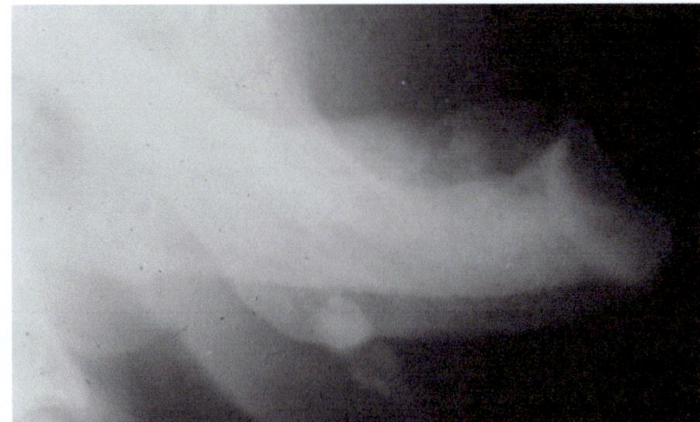

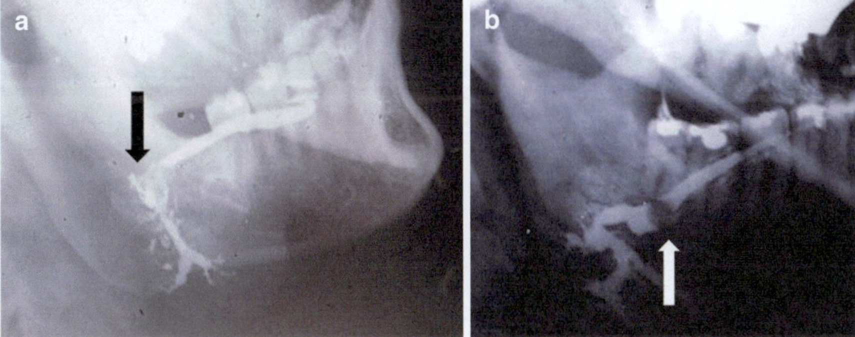

Fig. 4.9 (**a**) Sialolithiasis. Sialogram. Sialolith in the genu of submandibular duct (arrow). (**b**) Sialolithiasis. Sialogram. Sialolith in the posterior segment of the submandibular duct (arrow)

Lateral radiographic or panoramic views may be used as diagnostic supplemental aids. However, such views are hampered by the overlapping of the calcified stone upon the opaque mandible. The mandible will blot out a stone in the Wharton duct because the duct runs parallel to and at the horizontal level of the mandibular body. The value of these views rests in their ability to demonstrate stones within the duct hilus or gland proper because these sialoliths are positioned anatomically just below the inferior border of the mandible (Fig. 4.8).

Sialography, a not frequently used diagnostic procedure, has proven clinical value. The ductal introduction of a contrast solution serves to identify and localize radiopaque and relatively lucent sialoliths in the hilar area or body of the duct. Furthermore, the effect of the stone and the usual accompanying inflammation on the duct wall, intra- and/or extra-glandularly, will be portrayed (Fig. 4.9). However, the procedure should not be performed in the presence of active infection or in patients allergic to the contained iodine.

The CT scan has proven to be a very valuable aid in stone visualization (Fig. 4.10). Many sialoliths are small and only sparsely calcified. Consequently, standard radiography will fail to uncover their existence. The CT scan is exquisitely sensitive to

Fig. 4.10 (**a**)
Sialolithiasis. CT scan.
Sialolith in the body of the
submandibular gland
(arrow). (**b**) Sialolithiasis.
CT scan. Posteriorly
positioned submandibular
sialolith in the duct
(arrow). (Courtesy of Dr.
Daria Vasilyeva). (**c**)
Sialolithiasis. CT scan.
Anteriorly positioned
submandibular sialolith in
the duct (arrow)

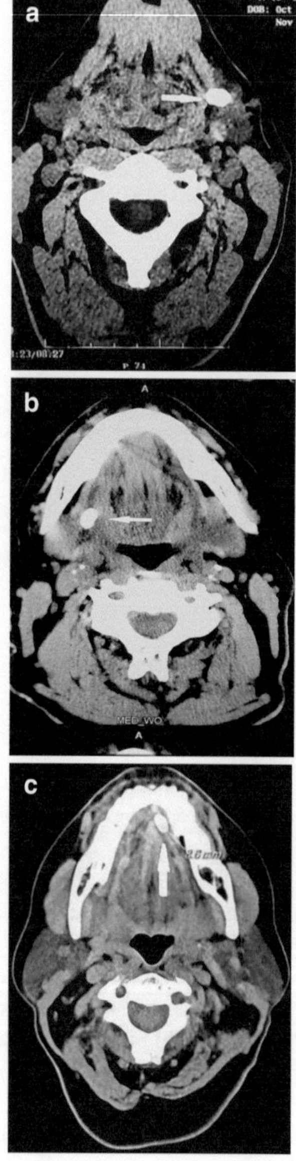

minute amounts of calcium salts and will clearly reveal stones that are relatively
radiolucent and small. Additionally, the CT scan can function to establish the exact
position of the stone within the duct while simultaneously assessing the status of the
gland. CT scanning is most effective without the use of contrast because the opacity
of contrast in a vessel can simulate the presence of a sialolith.

Ultrasonography has also proven to be a useful tool for the diagnosis of SMSG
sialoliths. Besides avoiding radiation, ultrasonography offers real-time image

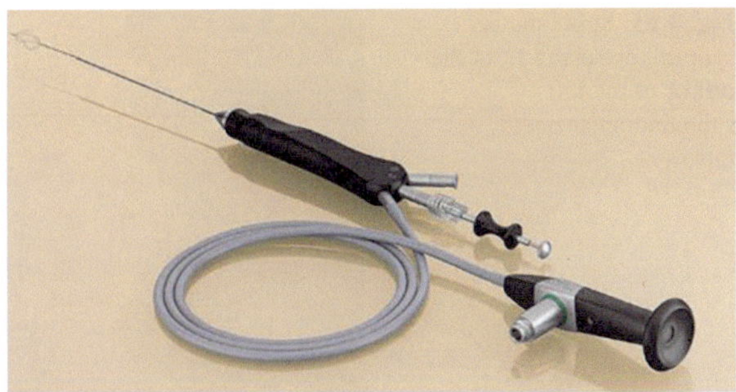

Fig. 4.11 Sialendoscope (Karl Storz Mfg.)

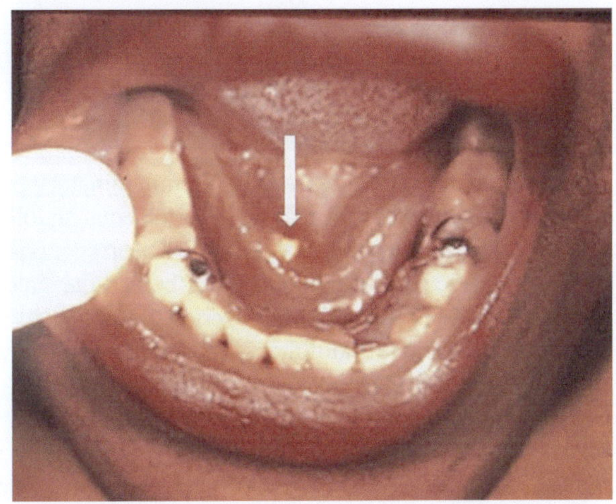

Fig. 4.12 Spontaneous sialolith extrusion from the body of the right submandibular duct (arrow)

interpretation, widespread availability, and rapid diagnostic information [10]. Ultrasonography for stone diagnosis has a reported sensitivity and specificity of 90% and 95%, respectively [11]. Stones are hyperechoic and will cast a posteriorly placed acoustic shadow. A major drawback of the procedure is that smaller stones are difficult to detect [4].

The introduction of the sialendoscope has added a new dimension to the armamentarium used in the diagnosis of salivary stones (Fig. 4.11). With upgradings of its design, the sialendoscope can be introduced directly into a major duct. The semi-rigid sialendoscope, designed to traverse duct curvatures, is available in a variety of diameters that facilitate its ability to negotiate the orifice and lumen of the SMSG duct. Visualization of the stone and ductal contents can be obtained because the sialendoscope has a miniaturized imaging system for optical viewing by the operator. Not only will the stone be seen, but any existing deleterious effect of the stone on the duct wall will also be visualized.

Although a variety of therapeutic techniques for sialolithectomy have been suggested, spontaneous exfoliation can occur and negate the need for intervention. A sialolith located close to the oral surface and surrounded by an acute inflammatory process can on occasion be spontaneously extruded into the mouth (Fig. 4.12). The

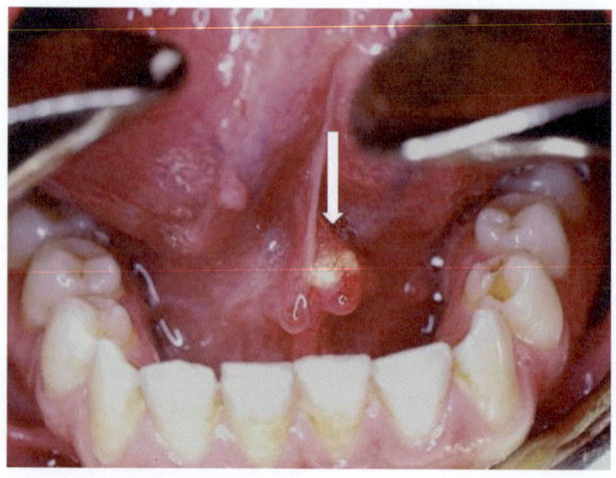

Fig. 4.13 Spontaneous sialolith extrusion from the orifice of the left submandibular duct (arrow)

sequestration aided by the surrounding inflammatory process represents the body's attempt to rid itself of an irritant. Spontaneous sialolith removal may also occur when small stones escape through the duct orifice, possibly facilitated by the salivary hydrostatic pressure that develops behind the sialolith (Fig. 4.13). Patients do relate histories of such natural deliveries.

Before a definitive sialolithectomy is performed, any existing manifestations of an acute suppurative sialadenitis should be controlled. Antibiotics, analgesics, antipyretics, and good oral hygiene are to be therapeutically deployed. The duct system acts as an excellent natural drainage mechanism with pus often observed exiting from the orifice, thus serving to mitigate symptoms. Once the acute symptoms subside, definitive therapy can be initiated.

Besides its diagnostic value, sialendoscopy can also be used therapeutically for stone removal. Sialendoscopy for SMSG sialolithectomy has a reported success rate of 86–93% [7]. Therefore, it has become a treatment of choice, particularly when the patient desires to avoid surgery [12]. The advantages of this minimally invasive technique are derived from its ability to directly visualize, assess, and remove an obstructing sialolith, thus avoiding open surgery and its associated complications [13]. The available commercial integrated sialendoscope is composed of a visualization channel and two operating channels. The scope's two operating channels include an irrigation channel to flush out debris and dilate the duct, and a working channel designed to accommodate a variety of auxiliary devices that can be used to remove sialoliths and eradicate strictures. Sialoliths <5 mm in the SMSG's major duct are amenable to sialendoscopic removal. The operator should be aware that problems develop when the sialendoscope attempts to negotiate the duct's posterior right angle bend in the genu area. The actual stone removal is made possible with the use of the instrument's supplemental tools, a wire basket or grasping forceps, introduced through the working channel. Laser appliances can also be introduced through the working channel to fracture larger stones into smaller segments that can be removed via standard sialendoscopic procedures. Transoral surgery is indicated if sialendoscopy fails or only partially succeeds in removing all the remnants of the fragmented stone [12]. Encasement of the sialolith by scar tissue also limits the effectiveness of sialendoscopy.

Unfortunately, sialendoscopy for stone removal has some disadvantages [12]. A learning curve by the operator is necessary to develop the skills to successfully manipulate the scope through the duct. Often the small SMSG duct orifice located on the movable caruncle is difficult to identify and enter. Narrowed, stenosed, and strictured ducts, as well as the posteriorly positioned anatomic bend of the SMSG duct, also present impediments in the passage of the sialendoscope. Surgical papillotomy as a means of entering the duct has been abandoned because of postoperative orifice stricture formation. It has been replaced by slow and deliberate serial duct dilatations by calibrated probes [14]. Surgical exposure of a distal luminal segment of the SMSG duct represents another means for the scope to enter the duct. Stones that are fixed in position or >5 mm in diameter often cannot be delivered. Such situations require transoral surgery or the use of ancillary procedures (lasers, lithotripsy) aimed at stone fragmentation.

Transoral surgical removal of SMSG duct stones is recommended for those stones that are not amenable because of location to sialendoscopic procedures or are large or fixed in position by scar tissue [15–17]. Some practitioners even prefer it as the therapeutic approach for nearly all SMSG stones [2, 18]. Intraoral surgical SMSG stone removal can be performed in an office setting, provided that the sialolith is located in an accessible portion of the duct. The key to success lies in the isolation and visualization of the duct. No matter where the stone is located, the duct is dissected free in the anterior mouth floor where it is superficially placed and accessible as it approaches its orifice (Fig. 4.14). A 2–3 cm anteroposterior incision is made superficially through the mouth floor mucosa, in the mandibular cuspid–bicuspid area, just medial and parallel to the sublingual fold (Fig. 4.15b). Blunt dissection will readily locate the duct lying in a bed of soft tissue in close relation to

Fig. 4.14 Submandibular duct dissected free

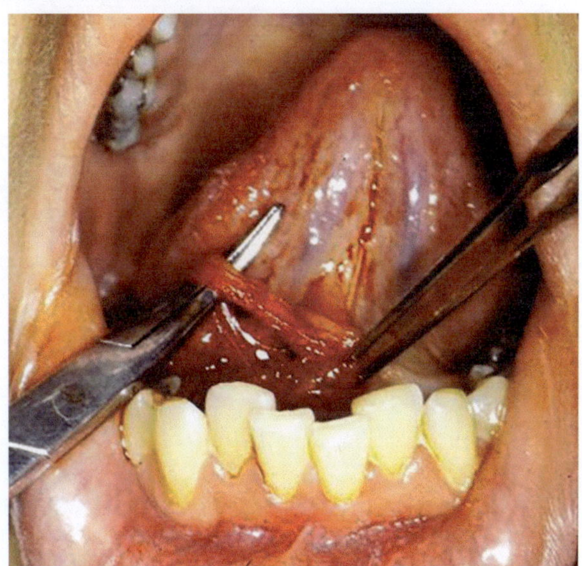

Fig. 4.15 (**a**) Sialolithiasis. Patient E. Transoral surgery. Probe entering the orifice of the left submandibular duct. (**b**) Sialolithiasis. Patient E. Transoral surgery. Incision made parallel and medial to sublingual fold. (**c**) Sialolithiasis. Patient E. Transoral surgery. Dilation of the submandibular duct by sialolith (arrow 9)

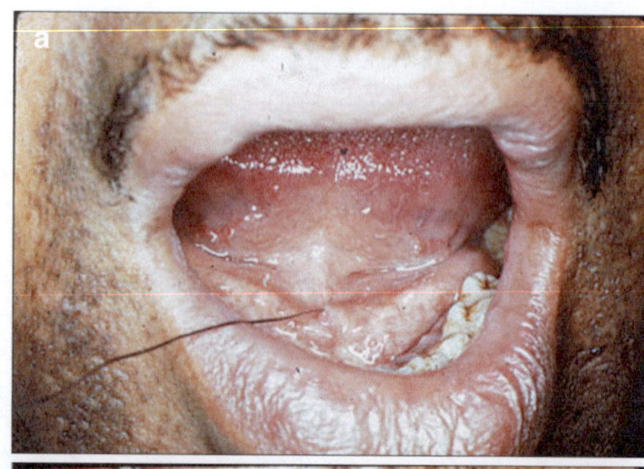

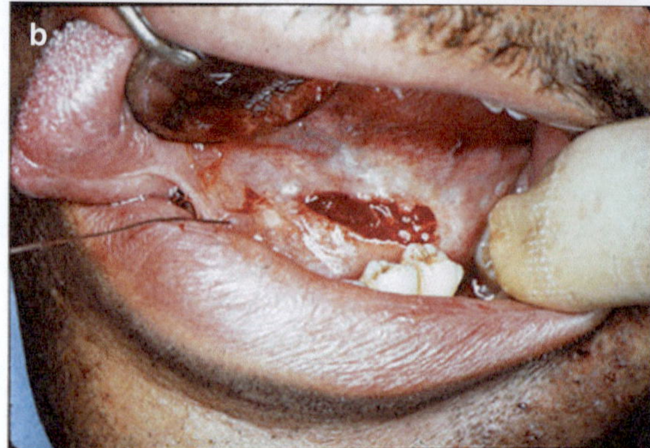

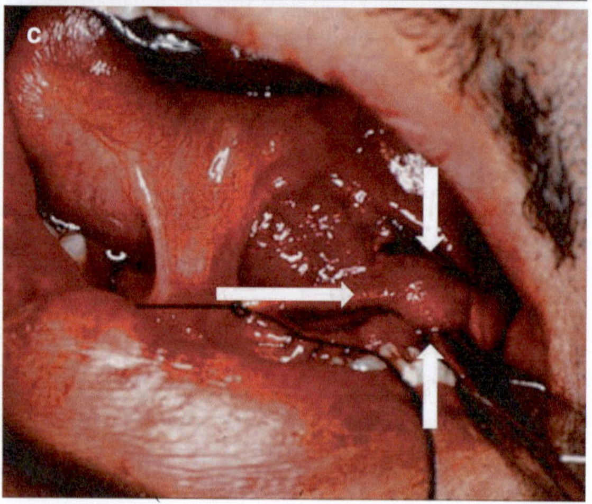

the sublingual salivary gland. Preoperative insertion of a metallic probe into the SMSG duct aids in duct identification during surgery (Fig. 4.15a). Once the duct is dissected free, it can be circumscribed with ¼ inch umbilical tape. With imaging having previously identified the sialolith's position, the dissection is extended, while the duct is gently retracted superiorly and anteriorly by tension on the umbilical tape and surgically followed to the anterior or posterior location of the stone. Surgically dissecting in the proximal area of the duct requires caution to avoid the inferiorly traversing lingual nerve. Removal of proximally placed stones demands that the surgical assistant use extraoral pressure to displace the SMSG superiorly such that the proximal areas of the duct take a more oral, accessible and visible position. Success demands this key maneuver. No matter where the stone is located, it is recognized by its yellow color visualized through the thin dilated duct wall (Fig. 4.15c). A widening of the duct, induced by the physical presence of the stone, is another distinguishing feature identifying the stone location. A linear anteroposterior incision is made in the superior duct wall immediately above the stone which is then curetted free from its ductal crypt. The overlying mucosa is sutured, but no attempt needs to be made to suture the duct which rapidly heals without any further intervention. Surprisingly, within 7–10 days postoperatively, the salivary flow will be observed at the duct orifice. The postoperative course includes moderate mouth floor swelling and discomfort. The operator should also be aware of the possibility of ranula formation resulting from trauma to the ducts of the surrounding sublingual gland during the dissection of the SMSG duct.

Stones in the genu or hilar area of the Wharton duct often are large and offer an opportunity for a different and simpler approach for their surgical removal. Those sialoliths that approach diameters of 1 cm or more can be brought into a more oral position by extraoral pressure on the SMSG. Intraoral palpation will then readily reveal the large stone's position. A shallow incision through the overlying oral mucosa followed by a blunt dissection to the palpable stone's location and an incision into the duct will successfully deliver larger proximally positioned sialoliths. Remember that surgery in this duct area demands caution to avoid the lingual nerve as it inferiorly crosses the duct on its way to the tongue.

No matter what technique is used for stone removal, clinical recovery of the resilient SMSG can be anticipated. Generally, a need for the simultaneous removal of the inflamed SMSG does not exist. Admittedly, some inflammatory gland destruction caused by sialolithiasis is present. Nevertheless, the gland will mostly recover and return to clinical function, albeit at a slightly decreased level resulting from some acinar destruction. Occasionally, advanced parenchymal destruction, from a prolonged or aggressive sialadenitis secondary to the sialolith, mandates the removal of the SMSG. The presence of large or multiple stones within the body of the SMSG represents another reason for sialoadenectomy.

Sialolithiasis

Parotid Gland Sialolithiasis

Statistically, parotid gland (PG) sialolithiasis occurs less frequently (10%) than SMSG sialolithiasis (83%) [5]. The aqueous aspect of PG saliva derived from its serous content, the horizontal path rather than an uphill course of PG saliva, PG saliva's lessened calcium salt content, and its relative acidity when compared with SMSG saliva all decrease the incidence of PG sialolithiasis. Sialoliths in the PG usually evolve in the same manner as SMSG duct stones. Nidus formation, salivary stagnation, and chemical salt precipitation are the factors that lead to the creation of the PG stone. However, PG sialolithiasis presents many more challenges in relation to diagnosis and therapy. Gland degeneration and surgical removal with serious consequences can be anticipated if treatment is delayed.

PG stones can form at any age, but the peak incidence occurs in patients who are in their 30s and 40s. The majority (64%) of PG stones are located within the major secreting duct (Stensen duct), while 23% are located in the intraglandular duct system, and 13% are in the hilus [15, 19]. Parotid duct stones tend to be small in size, single, and unilateral. Regardless of size, obstructive symptomatology can be expected. Parotid swellings with discomfort develop when an increased salivary volume, stimulated by eating, meets the obstruction caused by the sialolith. Saliva is retained and backs up, and PG swelling with discomfort results. Because luminal blockage by the stone is not total, the swelling and discomfort subside as retained saliva seeps past the partial obstruction. However, the failure of adequate salivary lavage, along with salivary stagnation from obstruction, can eventually pave the way for an ascending bacterial infection from the oral cavity. Unilateral parotitis will develop, and with recurrent intermittent exacerbations, a persistent diffuse PG swelling evolves and is usually moderately present even during remissions. Extraoral manual pressure on the PG will produce a suppurative discharge at the PG duct's orifice when infection has become an issue. Apparently, the three symptom groups seen in SMSG sialolithiasis are also observed when the PG is involved. The absence of symptoms, the occasional flare-ups of moderate glandular pain and swelling, and an acute infectious process have all been reviewed in the section on SMSG sialolithiasis.

In summary, the scenario of PG sialolithiasis involves the formation of a stone with a clinical PG infection developing secondarily to the obstructive stone. However, it is not unusual for this sequence to be reversed. Chronic parotitis (CP) (reviewed in Chap. 5) is a common pathologic condition whose etiology develops from a retrograde ductal infection originating from the oral cavity. The ensuing ductal infection provides the essential prerequisites for secondary stone development: nidus, salivary stagnation, and salt precipitation. Therefore, imaging of patients with recurrent exacerbations of CP will occasionally reveal a ductal stone whose obstructive presence will add to and exacerbate the symptomatology associated with CP. It should be emphasized that, in these situations, the PG sialolith represents a secondary complication resulting from the presence of a CP.

Although the history and physical examination are key elements in diagnosing the existence of a PG sialolith, imaging is required to clearly reveal its location and its effect on the gland. Parotid stones often are not amenable to conventional radiographic study because they tend to be small, poorly calcified, and obscured by adjacent bony structures. Intraoral radiography, with a periapical film placed in the mucobuccal fold adjacent to the duct orifice, can only demonstrate stones in the anterior parotid duct. Extraoral radiography will not be successful because visualization is limited by the superimposition of the calcified mandibular ramus upon the sialolith's opacity.

Sialography has proven to be an excellent method for detecting parotid stones (Fig. 4.16). Many PG stones can be diagnosed by a sialographic filling defect that marks their location. In addition, the stone's position can be determined by its pathological effect on the adjacent portion of the duct. Ductal dilation, immediately

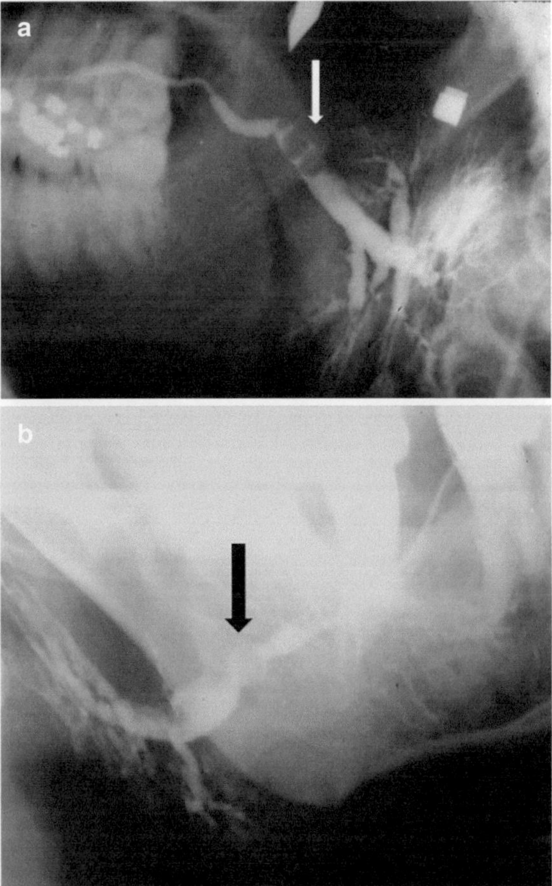

Fig. 4.16 (a) Sialolithiasis. Parotid sialogram. Sialoliths in the parotid duct (arrow) cause salivary retention and duct dilation. (b) Sialolithiasis. Parotid sialogram. Parotid duct sialolith (arrow). Incomplete contrast filling of dilated duct proximal to sialolith

proximal to the obstruction caused by the stone, testifies to the dilating effect of salivary retention upon the duct. Luminal stricturing, representing inflammatory changes caused by salivary retention with or without bacterial infection, may also be observed. Unfortunately, problems with sialography arise because the procedure requires a modicum of technical ability. Furthermore, small stones and their filling defect can be obliterated by the opaque dye used in sialography. Additionally, sialography is contraindicated during the acute manifestations of a parotitis and in patients who are allergic to the dye.

Ultrasonography is a rapid non-invasive procedure that images stones as hyperechoic nodules with posterior acoustical shadows. However small stones, which are common in the PG duct system, are difficult to identify and locate precisely. Imaging via a CT scan offers significant advantages in the diagnosis of PG stones (Fig. 4.17).

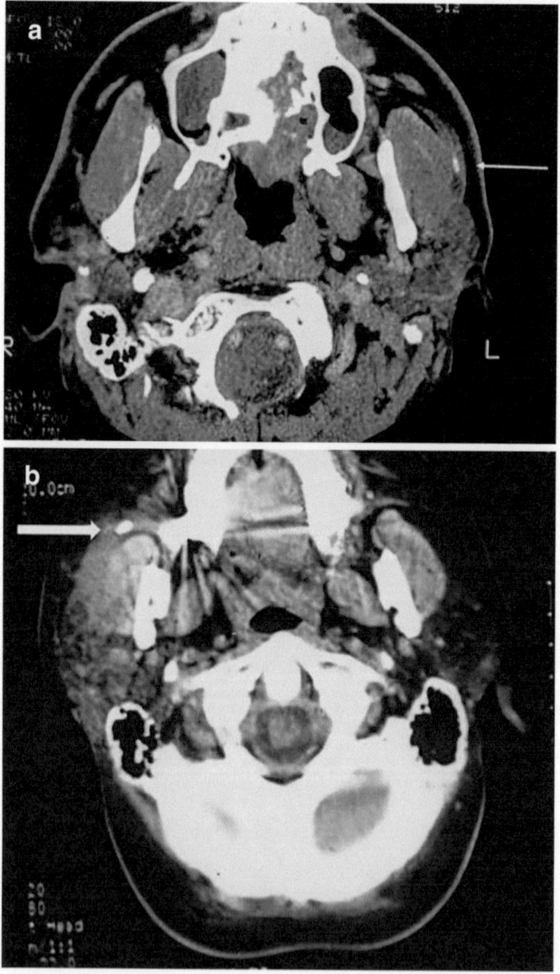

Fig. 4.17 (**a**) Sialolithiasis. CT scan. Sialolith in the body of the left parotid duct (arrow). (**b**) Sialolithiasis. CT scan. Sialolith in the orifice area of the right parotid duct (arrow)

Stones lucent to standard radiography contain minimal amounts of calcific materials. The CT scan has a heightened ability to clearly image minute amounts of calcium even in small stones that measure ≤1 mm. The extent of the PG sialadenitis, secondary to the stone, will also be seen and aid in determining a need for additional glandular care. Contrast should be avoided because the dye's presence in a blood vessel will mirror the appearance of a sialolith.

The advent of the sialendoscope has made available another procedure that can be utilized for the diagnosis of a PG stone. The thin semi-flexible scope with an optical lens can be introduced into the parotid duct orifice and advanced to visualize any existing stone and its effect on the duct wall. A more detailed review of sialendoscopy instrumentation and its use in the diagnosis and therapy of sialoliths can be found in this chapter under the section on SMSG sialolithiasis.

Besides its diagnostic abilities, the sialendoscope has taken a primary role in the removal of PG stones that occur along the entire extraglandular length of the parotid duct. Sialoliths (<5 mm) are engaged by the working tools of the sialendoscope and can be successfully delivered. Problems occur when the stone is larger than 5 mm or fixed in position by scar tissue. Therefore, various adjunctive instruments (lithotripsy, lasers, burs) have been integrated into the sialendoscope. They serve to fragment the sialolith into small manageable pieces that usually can be removed by the scope or lavaged out. In a review of 1285 patients with PG stones, successful treatment with sialendoscopy, with and without fragmentation, was reported to range from 71 to 100% [5]. The successful extraction of parotid sialoliths has made it possible to avoid transfacial surgical sialolithectomy or superficial lobe parotidectomy and their associated morbidities.

Occasionally, small PG duct stones are spontaneously delivered through the duct orifice (Fig. 4.18). However, intraoral surgery is usually required as a backup procedure, provided that the stone is positioned within 1.5 cm of the duct orifice. Surgery involves a 2 cm intraoral vertical semilunar incision, placed in the buccal mucosa approximately 1.0 cm anterior to the PG duct orifice (Fig. 4.19). The concavity of the incision should face in the posterior direction while the convexity faces anteriorly. A buccal flap, containing the Stensen papilla, is surgically mobilized and

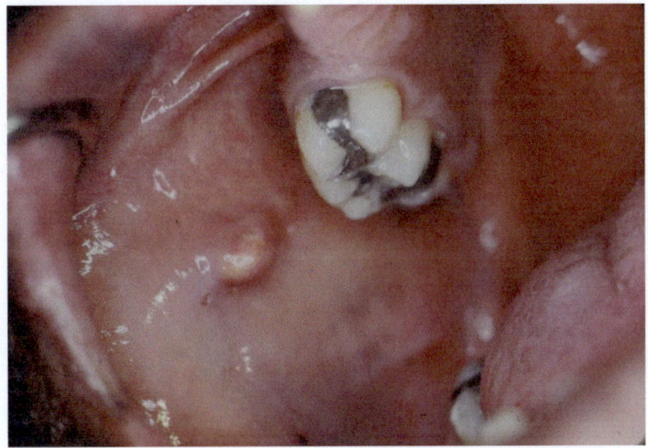

Fig. 4.18 Sialolithiasis. Spontaneous sialolith extrusion at the orifice of the parotid duct

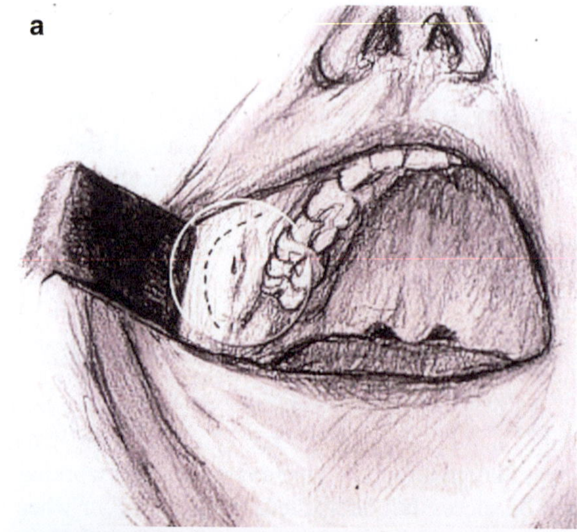

Fig. 4.19 (a) Sialolithiasis. Sketch demonstrates incision for sialolith removal in the anterior segment of the parotid duct. (b) Sialolithiasis. The retracted flap reveals the parotid duct on the undersurface of the retracted surgical flap

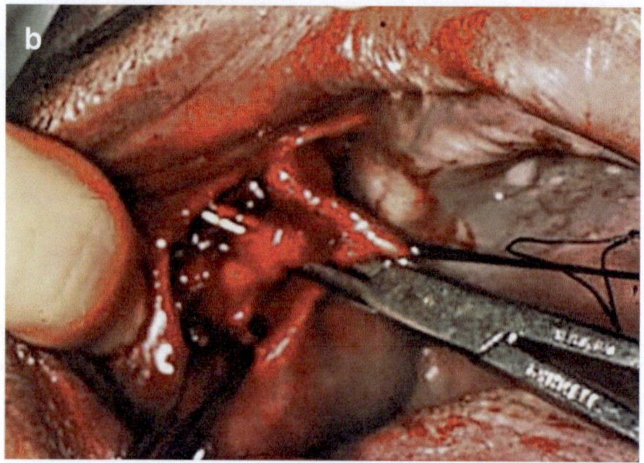

retracted posteriorly. Blunt dissection will reveal the parotid duct on the under surface of the flap as it approaches its orifice. With retraction of the duct and its posterior dissection, stones within 1.5 cm of the duct orifice can be identified and delivered. Surgical accessibility and visibility are severely compromised by adjacent anatomic structures when the stone is positioned more than 1.5 cm away from the duct orifice.

Chronic parotitis (CP) is the end result of a failure to retrieve an obstructing PG stone via sialendoscopy or intraoral/extraoral surgical sialolithectomy. Unfortunately, because of the refractory nature of CP, the usual therapeutic approach is a superficial lobe parotidectomy. Because of the possible associated complications (facial nerve damage, facial scarring, auriculotemporal syndrome), this surgical option has become a therapeutic procedure of last resort.

Sialolithiasis

Sublingual Gland Sialolithiasis

Sialolithiasis development in the sublingual salivary gland (SLSG) is considered an uncommon occurrence. Stones in the SLSG have been reported to represent only 1–6.5% of identified salivary stones [20]. This incidence is unexpectedly quite low despite the fact that SLSG saliva is six times more viscous than SMSG saliva and its upward trajectory of flow violates gravity and favors stasis [6]. Both conditions (viscosity and gravity) encourage stone formation. Conceivably, the very abbreviated length of each of the SLSG's ducts of Rivinus acts to discourage the intraductal development of stones.

When present, the duct of Bartholin (BD), the major SLSG duct, empties into the anterior segment of the SMSG duct or opens on the caruncle adjacent to the orifice of the SMSG duct. A high degree of suspicion should be held for the presence of SLSG stones at the junction of the SMSG duct and the BD. The tendency for sialolith occurrence at this ductal confluence demands a close examination of the area. Stones located at the junction of these ducts are not infrequent. Consequently, anterior SLSG stones often are misdiagnosed as the more common SMSG stones. A clue to differentiating an SMSG stone from an SLSG stone rests in the fact that a stone-incited SMSG swelling will be evident extraorally in the submandibular triangle, while an SLSG stone will cause SLSG swelling limited to the mouth floor.

Symptomatology associated with SLSG sialolith obstruction is not as severe as what occurs when the PG or SMSG are involved. An individual lobe, rather than the entire SLSG, is usually affected because there is no major secretory duct emptying the entire SLSG that can be obstructed and cause total gland symptomatology. Furthermore, because of the superficial location of the SLSG, as it rests on the mylohyoid muscle, swellings are limited intraorally to that section of the sublingual fold beneath which lies the responsible SLSG lobe.

The diagnosis of an SLSG stone is readily made when the history and physical examination are incorporated into the results of imaging. The occlusal film provides the best diagnostic radiographic view of the SLSG and adjacent soft tissues of the mouth floor. The anatomic locale of the SLSG and its duct system makes it possible to avoid interference from bone opacities when the gland is viewed radiographically with an occlusal film. Therefore, stones in the SLSG system are readily identified. A CT scan without contrast is advised if the SLSG sialolith is poorly calcified.

Successful removal of an SLSG stone is best accomplished via transoral surgery. Because the gland and its duct are accessible, superficially placed just beneath the oral mucosa, and because the stone has been located via imaging and palpation, surgical incision and delivery of the sialolith are simplified and successful. Moderate postoperative swelling and discomfort can be expected. The postoperative development of a ranula is always a possibility. If a stone is present in an existing BD and if the BD empties into the SMSG duct, sialolithectomy requires sectioning and ligation of the BD at its confluence with the SMSG duct. Otherwise, SMSG secretions will escape through a patent BD and accumulate in the anterior mouth floor.

Sialolithiasis

Minor Salivary Gland Sialolithiasis

Sialolithiasis involving a minor salivary gland (MSG) is a rare clinical finding. Patients are usually seen with circumscribed small firm painless persistent nodular swellings that involve the upper lip (Fig. 4.20a). Because these sialoliths are small and poorly calcified, imaging often is not successful in uncovering their presence. However, a soft tissue radiograph taken with a periapical film may demonstrate their existence (Fig. 4.20b). Excision of the presenting nodule is usually required for a definitive diagnosis. Histopathologically, the calcific mass will be identified in a dilated duct (Fig. 4.21). Periductal inflammation and acinar atrophy are also present and help to substantiate the diagnosis of MSG sialolithiasis.

The occurrence of sialoliths in the minor salivary glands has been previously reviewed. The details regarding the diagnosis and therapy of this pathologic entity are reviewed in Chap. 18 "Minor Salivary Glands."

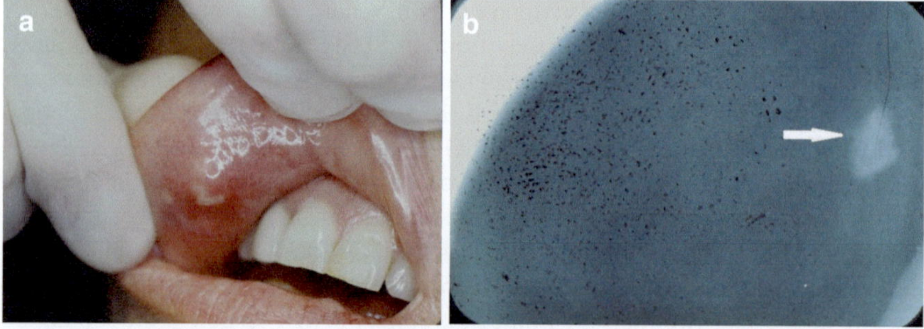

Fig. 4.20 (**a**) Sialolithiasis. Patient F. Upper lip. Nodular swelling of the minor salivary gland. (**b**) Sialolithiasis. Patient F. Soft tissue radiograph of the upper lip reveals sialolith (arrow)

Fig. 4.21 Sialolithiasis. Sialolith (S) in minor salivary gland duct. Excised with overlying mucosa (M)

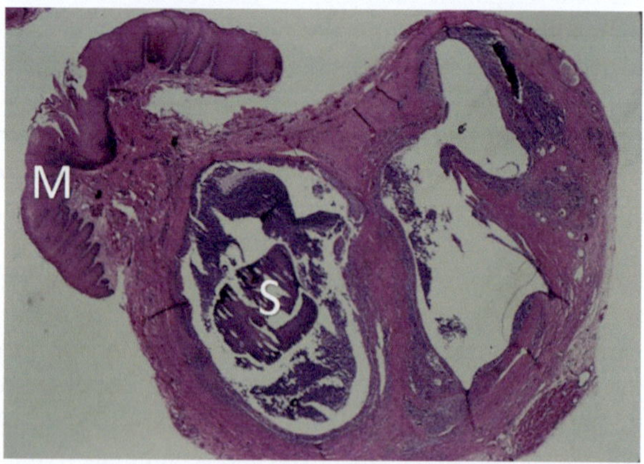

References

1. Huoh KC, Eisele DW. Etiologic factors in sialolithiasis. Otolaryngol Head Neck Surg. 2011;145(6):935–9. https://doi.org/10.1177/0194599811415489.
2. Kraaij S, Karagozoglu KH, Forouzanfar T, Veerman EC, Brand HS. Salivary stones: symptoms, aetiology, biochemical composition and treatment. Br Dent J. 2014;217(11):E23. https://doi.org/10.1038/sj.bdj.2014.1054.
3. Lustmann J, Regev E, Melamed Y. Sialolithiasis. A survey on 245 patients and a review of the literature. Int J Oral Maxillofac Surg. 1990;19(3):135–8. https://doi.org/10.1016/s0901-5027(05)80127-4.
4. Pachisia S, Mandal G, Sahu S, Ghosh S. Submandibular sialolithiasis: a series of three case reports with review of literature. Clin Pract. 2019;9(1):1119. https://doi.org/10.4081/cp.2019.1119.
5. Galdermans M, Gemels B. Success rate and complications of sialendoscopy and sialolithotripsy in patients with parotid sialolithiasis: a systematic review. Oral Maxillofac Surg. 2020;24(2):145–50. https://doi.org/10.1007/s10006-020-00834-x.
6. Mandel ID. Sialochemistry in diseases and clinical situations affecting salivary glands. Crit Rev Clin Lab Sci. 1980;12(4):321–66. https://doi.org/10.3109/10408368009108733.
7. Quiz J, Gillespie MB. Transoral sialolithotomy without endoscopes: an alternative approach to salivary stones. Otolaryngol Clin N Am. 2021;54(3):553–65. https://doi.org/10.1016/j.otc.2021.01.006.
8. Schapher M, Koch M, Weidner D, et al. Neutrophil extracellular traps promote the development and growth of human salivary stones. Cell. 2020;9(9):2139. https://doi.org/10.3390/cells9092139.
9. Suddick RP, Hyde RJ, Feller RL. Salivary water and electrolytes and oral health. In: Menaker L, editor. The biologic basis of dental caries. New York: Harper and Row; 1980.
10. Hammett JT, Walker C. Sialolithiasis. In: StatPearls. Treasure Island (FL): StatPearls Publishing; 2021.
11. Katz P, Hartl DM, Guerre A. Clinical ultrasound of the salivary glands. Otolaryngol Clin N Am. 2009;42(6):973. https://doi.org/10.1016/j.otc.2009.08.009.
12. Gallo A, Benazzo M, Capaccio P, et al. Sialoendoscopy: state of the art, challenges and further perspectives. Round table, 101(st) SIO National Congress, Catania 2014. Acta Otorhinolaryngol Ital. 2015;35(4):217–33.
13. Fabie JE, Kompelli AR, Naylor TM, Nguyen SA, Lentsch EJ, Gillespie MB. Gland-preserving surgery for salivary stones and the utility of sialendoscopes. Head Neck. 2019;41(5):1320–7. https://doi.org/10.1002/hed.25560.
14. Moorthy A, Bachalli PS, Krishna S, Murthy S. Sialendoscopic management of obstructive salivary gland pathology: a retrospective analysis of 236 cases. J Oral Maxillofac Surg. 2021;79(7):1474–81. https://doi.org/10.1016/j.joms.2020.11.032.
15. Zenk J, Constantinidis J, Kydles S, Hornung J, Iro H. Klinische und diagnostische Befunde bei der Sialolithiasis [clinical and diagnostic findings of sialolithiasis]. HNO. 1999;47(11):963–9. https://doi.org/10.1007/s001060050476.
16. Zenk J, Constantinidis J, Al-Kadah B, Iro H. Transoral removal of submandibular stones. Arch Otolaryngol Head Neck Surg. 2001;127(4):432–6. https://doi.org/10.1001/archotol.127.4.432.
17. Juul ML, Wagner N. Objective and subjective outcome in 42 patients after treatment of sialolithiasis by transoral incision of Wharton's duct: a retrospective middle-term follow-up study. Eur Arch Otorrinolaringol. 2014;271(11):3059–66. https://doi.org/10.1007/s00405-014-2905-x.
18. McGurk M, Escudier MP, Brown JE. Modern management of salivary calculi. Br J Surg. 2005;92(1):107–12. https://doi.org/10.1002/bjs.4789.
19. Ottaviani F, Galli A, Lucia MB, Ventura G. Bilateral parotid sialolithiasis in a patient with acquired immunodeficiency syndrome and immunoglobulin G multiple myeloma. Oral Surg Oral Med Oral Pathol Oral Radiol Endod. 1997;83(5):552–4. https://doi.org/10.1016/s1079-2104(97)90119-0.
20. Liao LJ, Hsiao JK, Hsu WC, Wang CP. Sublingual gland sialolithiasis: a case report. Kaohsiung J Med Sci. 2007;23(11):590–3.

Chapter 5
Parotid Infection

Louis Mandel

Abstract Human tissue is subject to bacterial invasion and the symptomatic sequelae associated with infection. The salivary glands (SG) are not immune to bacterial insult, with the parotid gland (PG) being more susceptible than the other SG. Both the submandibular (SM) and sublingual salivary (SL) glands contain a mucin element in their secretions, while the PG produces a serous secretion. It is the anti-microbial properties of mucin that may be responsible for the elevated resistance to infection of the SM and SL glands. Acute suppurative infection of the glands usually involves the PG with dehydration and hyposalivation in a debilitated patient acting as predisposing factors. Chronic SG infection, usually in the form of a recurrent unilateral PG swelling, seems to originate during a period of decreased salivary flow that favors an orally ascending bacterial invasion of the duct system. Subsequent duct wall damage with scarring and stricturing set the stage for further bacterial incursions and the onset of recurrent glandular swellings.

Overview

Inflammation is a complex tissue reaction to an irritant. Bacterial infection, brought about by a wide range of pathogens, represents a common example of a tissue irritant. The organisms' successful tissue invasion incites the host's reaction in the form of an inflammatory process that produces the classic signs associated with infection. These signs may include combinations of swelling, pain, heat, erythema, and loss of function. Systemic manifestations may also develop and include fever, sweating, fatigue, weight loss, and generalized pain. All body organs and tissues are susceptible to these bacterial incursions.

As with other anatomic structures, the salivary glands are liable to bacterial infection with the parotid gland (PG) being most vulnerable when compared with the other major

L. Mandel, *Clinical Management of Salivary Gland Disorders*, https://doi.org/10.1007/978-3-031-50012-1_5

salivary glands. The PG is a serous secreting gland, while the secretions of the submandibular (SMSG) and sublingual salivary glands (SLSG) contain a significant mucus element. The anti-microbial properties of mucin, a glycoprotein, are probably responsible for the relatively increased resistance to infection displayed by the SMSG and SLSG.

Parotid Infection

Acute Parotitis

Acute parotitis (AP) is defined as a bacterial suppurative process that is sudden in onset and develops in a previously non-infected parotid gland (PG). The submandibular salivary gland is infrequently involved. The disease is most commonly seen in the elderly and debilitated patients, the immunocompromised, and hospitalized patients recovering from surgery, usually abdominal in nature (Figs. 5.1, 5.2 and 5.3). Hospital admissions for AP have been reported to be in the range of 0.01–0.02% [1]. Its reported prevalence in 2008 in post-surgical patients was only 0.0028% [2]. Some succumb to fatal outcomes from multisystem organ failure [3]. The advent of antibiotics and emphasis on electrolyte and fluid balance have brought about a precipitous drop in the incidence of AP. A recent resurgence in its occurrence has been noted and attributed to the inciting presence of methicillin-resistant *Staphylococcus aureus* (MRSA) [4, 5].

It seems that a primary cause of AP is dehydration, a condition often seen in debilitated patients following abdominal surgery [1, 6]. Consequently, AP has also been referred to as surgical parotitis. In patients who have undergone abdominal surgery, intake of oral fluids is discouraged. Dehydration with hyposalivation becomes an issue when the patients fail to receive appropriate intravenous fluid management. Debilitating medical conditions and poor oral hygiene play key supporting roles in the onset of AP. Loss of blood, diarrhea, emesis, and sweating combined with inadequate fluid replacement actively effectuate the dehydration. The resulting dehydration-encouraged hyposalivation is accentuated if the patient uses medications that inhibit salivation. These prerequisites to the evolution of AP occur not only in post-surgical patients but also in ambulatory elderly systemically compromised individuals. Hyposalivation causes a quantitative loss of saliva's protective anti-bacterial and lavaging properties [7]. In addition, because many patients are forbidden, unwilling, or unable to take oral nourishment, they will lose the increased salivary flow that results from the stimulatory effect of mastication on the salivary glands. Furthermore, because poor oral hygiene often co-exists, a precipitous increase in the oral bacterial content develops with many of the organisms having the ability to trigger an acute pathologic process. The stage is now set for the development of an ascending PG ductal infection with the bacteria originating from the oral cavity. The most frequent organism causing AP is *Staphylococcus aureus*, but anaerobics and MRSA have also been identified [2, 5].

Unilateral acute suppurative PG swelling is the prevailing manifestation of AP, but bilateral PG involvement can also occur. Pain, fever, leukocytosis, and an

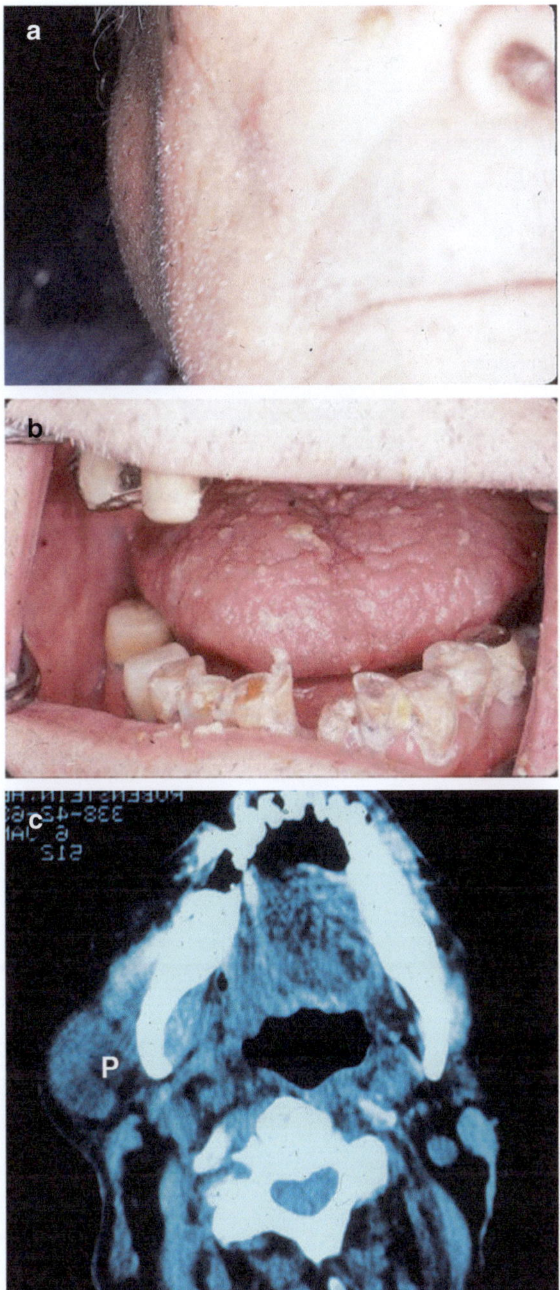

Fig. 5.1 (**a**) Acute parotitis. Patient A. Right parotid swelling in an elderly demented dehydrated patient. (**b**) Acute parotitis. Patient A. Dry mouth. Food debris adherent to the mucosa. (**c**) Acute parotitis. Patient A. CT scan. Parotid abscess (P)

Fig. 5.2 (**a**) Acute parotitis. Patient B. Right parotid abscess following abdominal surgery. (Mandel L, Salivary Gland Disorders. Med Clin North Am 2014;98:1411). (**b**) Acute parotitis. Patient B. Pus exiting parotid duct orifice (arrow) in dehydrated patient after abdominal surgery. (Mandel L, Salivary Gland Disorders. Med Clin North Am 2014;98:1411)

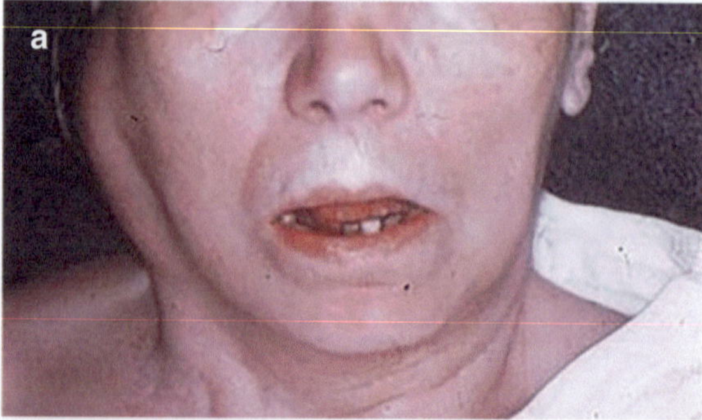

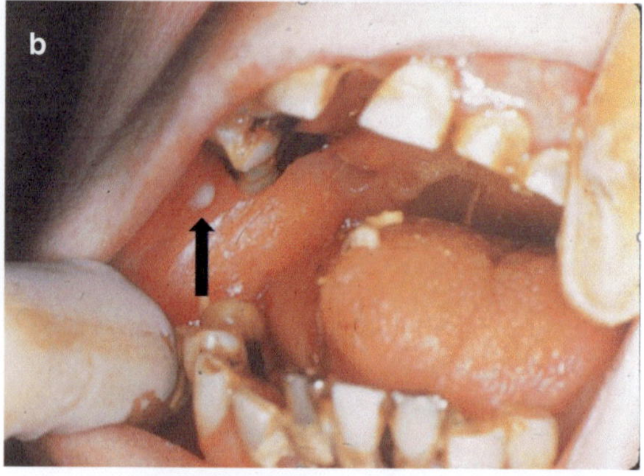

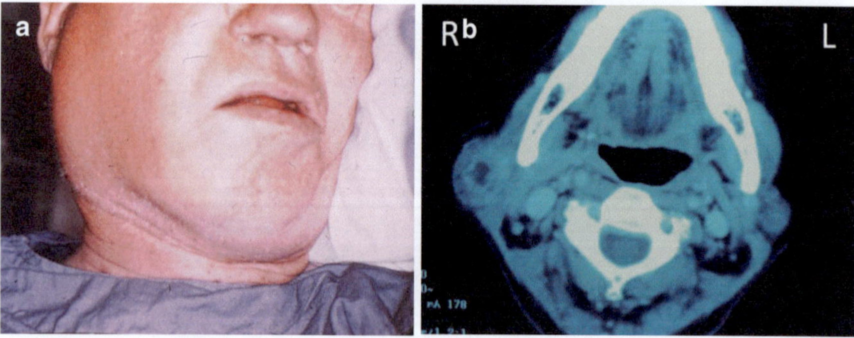

Fig. 5.3 (**a**) Acute parotitis. Patient C. Parotid abscess in a debilitated critically ill hospitalized patient. (**b**) Acute parotitis. Patient C. CT scan. Parotid abscess (right) in a debilitated critically ill hospitalized patient

elevated sedimentation rate are present. Extraorally, the PG area is erythematous and when palpated is found to be painful, warm, and firm. The firmness is caused by the intraglandular inflammatory infiltrate creating increased tension on the limiting surrounding fibrous PG capsule. A moderate trismus is usually present. Intraorally, the parotid duct orifice may be red and pouting. Additionally, because the parotid duct acts as a natural pathway for drainage (Fig. 5.4), an intraoral suppurative flow

Fig. 5.4 Acute parotitis. Microscopic view. Mucopurulent discharge in parotid duct lumen

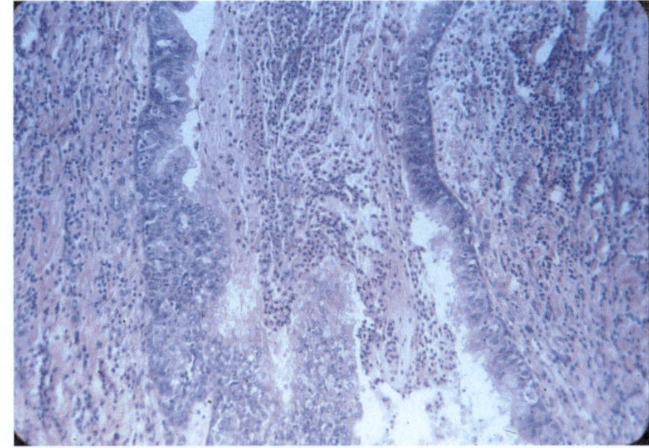

is usually observed exiting from the duct's orifice. Extraoral pressure upon the swollen PG will enhance this flow but will cause pain. The spread of the infectious process to adjoining tissues is infrequent because it is inhibited by the protection afforded by the surrounding dense fibrous PG capsule. Regardless, perforation of the capsule can occasionally occur and the infection may then spread to the adjacent tissues and cervical fascial planes [1, 2].

Imaging (CT, MRI) shows an increased PG density in direct proportion to the extent of the inflammatory infiltrate. Lucencies, depicting abscess formations that have peripheral contrast enhancements from the surrounding vascular inflammatory infiltrate will also be noted (Fig. 5.3b).

Treatment of AP can be conservative. Rehydration is the key, but it must be supported by appropriate antibiotic therapy. The immediate and initially prescribed antibiotic should be penicillin. Subsequent tailoring of the antibiotic may be required when the results of culture and sensitivity testing become available. Fluid and electrolyte replacement, treatment of any underlying medical condition, building the patient's resistance and good oral hygiene, and nursing care are also required. The duct serves as an excellent drainage mechanism, and with the inclusion of rehydration, antibiotics, and supportive therapy, a successful therapeutic outcome can be anticipated. Surgical incision and drainage are usually not necessary because the microabscesses that are present fail to form the macroabscess that would require such an approach [3, 8]. Therapeutic failure, after 5 days of hydration, antibiotics, and supportive therapy, signals the presence of a well-formed localized abscess. In such a situation, surgical intervention is mandated in order to achieve a successful outcome [1, 2, 8].

Parotid Infection

Chronic Parotitis

Chronic parotitis (CP) is the most common salivary gland pathologic entity seen in the Columbia University Salivary Gland Center. It is considered to be a non-specific sialadenitis characterized by recurrent unilateral, occasionally bilateral, parotid gland

(PG) swellings. Adults in the age range of 40–60 years, with a slight female dominance, represent the most susceptible patient group [9, 10]. The CP swellings are intermittent, often but not always associated with salivary retention caused by the stimulus of eating [11], and tend to be moderately painful. A single PG exacerbation may last from a few minutes to several days with the possibility of multiple exacerbations developing over a period of weeks. Subsidence of the individual swelling occurs when stimulation to salivary flow ceases, and the retained saliva seeps past an existing partial obstruction. The obstruction is initiated by a retrograde ascending ductal infection from the oral cavity and leads to the referral of CP as a chronic obstructive parotitis. These cycles of swelling alternate with intervals of remission in which the PG is clinically asymptomatic. The remission period may last for weeks, months, and even years, but symptom recurrences can be expected. The continued waxing and waning of the PG swellings serve to increase the extent of gland destruction [12].

Although the etiology of CP can be multifactorial, the generally accepted cause seems to be related to some previous period of decreased salivary production and flow [13]. The hyposalivation, which can be temporary, may be triggered by a systemic condition such as dehydration, result from the use of medically prescribed anti-sialogogic medications, or provoked idiopathically. With the decreased salivary flow, an inadequate lavage of the parotid duct ensues. Favorable conditions are now available for an ascending ductal infection caused by a variety of organisms originating from the oral cavity (Fig. 5.5). The bacterial invasion hones in on the duct wall. The ductal inflammatory response caused by these pathogens results in two significant factors that initiate the obstructive symptomatology of CP. Duct wall inflammation develops, and debris is produced and when shed serves to partially obstruct the duct lumen. Second, healing of the inflamed duct wall will result in its scarring and stricturing with luminal narrowing. The consequent luminal thinning from these two causes leads to two significant complicating clinical outcomes. Primarily, salivary stasis develops and favors repeated incursions of ascending infections from the oral cavity. Additional increased duct stricturing and parenchymal damage ensue (Figs. 5.6, 5.7 and 5.8). A revolving cycle of salivary stasis and ascending infection with ductal/parenchymal damage can be anticipated. Secondly, sialolith formation is encouraged because the requirements for stone evolution have been established. Bacterial and inflammatory debris act as a nidus while salivary stasis caused by the narrowed lumen presents the opportunity and environment for the precipitation of saliva's proteinaceous components and chemical salts that actively serve in the production of the calcified sialolith. In turn, the sialolith's physical presence accentuates the symptomatology associated with obstruction and infection (Fig. 5.9).

Generally, sialolithiasis in the PG system, as compared with the submandibular salivary gland, is somewhat unusual. The reported relatively high incidence of sialoliths in CP, varying from 6 to 43% [12, 14], probably emanates from the salivary stasis and the intraluminal conditions that exist in CP and serve to promote sialolithiasis. The presence of PG sialolithiasis further accentuates CP pathology because sialolith obstruction encourages salivary retention and the ascending infections that increase ductal and parenchymal injury (Fig. 5.9).

Sporadic meal-related PG swellings, intermingled with asymptomatic periods of remission, are classic features of CP. Patients usually seek attention because of their

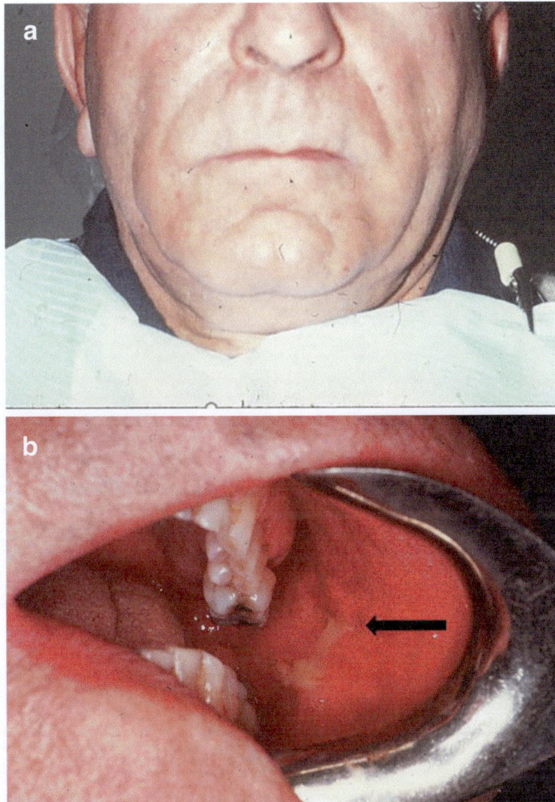

Fig. 5.5 (**a**) Chronic parotitis. Patient D. Left parotid swelling. (**b**) Chronic parotitis. Patient D (acute exacerbation). Suppurative discharge left parotid duct orifice (arrow)

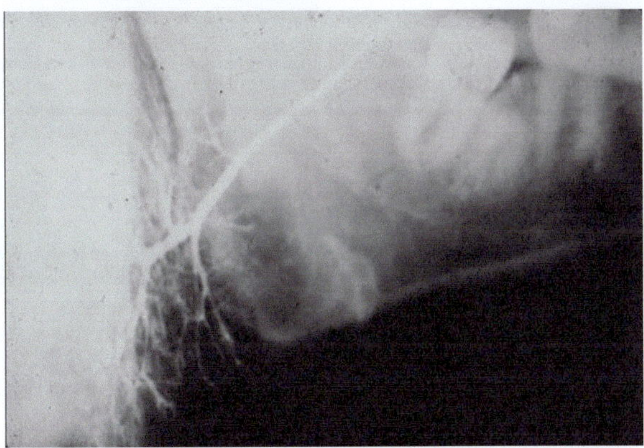

Fig. 5.6 Sialogram. Normal parotid duct arborization

long-standing histories of repeated undulating PG swellings that may have been accompanied by fever. Moderate discomfort is also part of the symptom complex. Upon extraoral examination during a remission period, a mild swelling following the anatomic contour of the PG will be noted. The PG is swollen from the chronic presence of inflammation and obstruction-incited salivary retention. The overlying skin

Fig. 5.7 Chronic parotitis. Sialogram. Early parotid duct inflammatory change

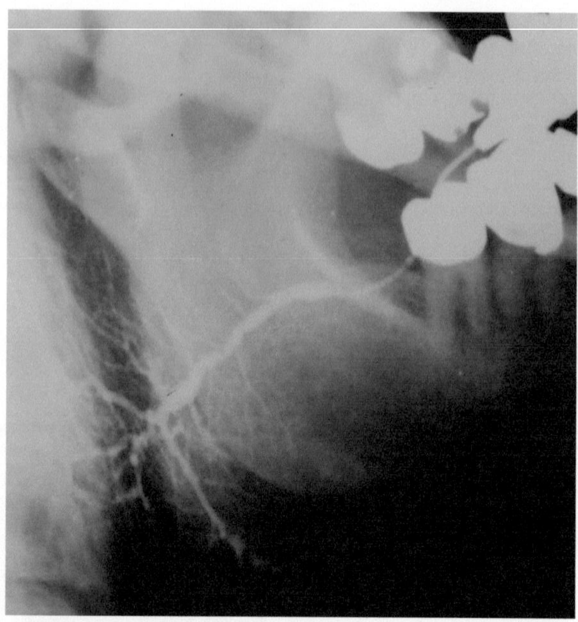

Fig. 5.8 Chronic parotitis. Sialogram. More advanced duct inflammation

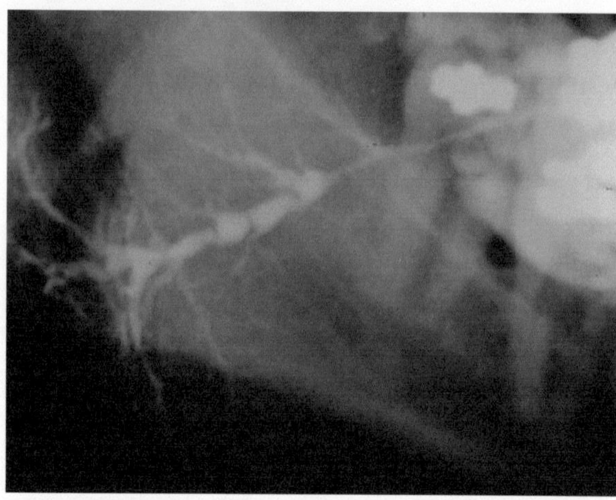

may be erythematous. Intraorally, a decrease in salivary flow will be observed exiting from the culpable PG duct's orifice. More importantly, the salivary quality is abnormal. Viscous flocculations in clear saliva, giving the return an "egg drop soup" appearance, may be present [15]. The flocculations consist mostly of albumin which has entered into the retained ductal saliva because of a breakdown of normal duct wall permeability barriers [15]. Alternatively, the salivary return may be cloudy from contained pus. The accumulation of viscous material adds to the duct obstruction and gland swelling by physically discouraging a free salivary flow. Any acute gland swelling is temporary because the soft clogging obstructive proteinaceous plug that

Fig. 5.9 Chronic parotitis. CT scan. Sialadenitis (arrow **b**) present in conjunction with sialolith (arrow **a**). Note dilated congested parotid duct

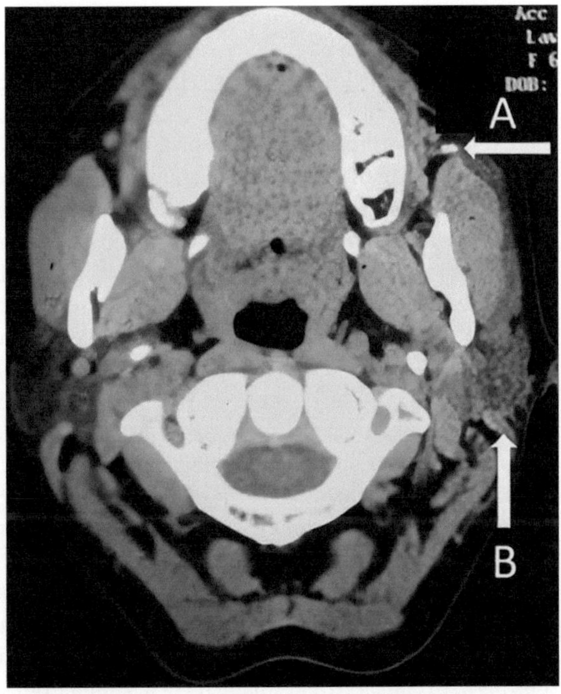

has formed will spontaneously clear itself and exit through the duct orifice. The clearance of the coagulum may have its origin in the hydrostatic pressure that builds up behind the plug or even from the compressing milking action of the facial musculature during mastication and speech. With the elimination of the proteinaceous plug, discomfort and swelling subside as normal luminal salivary flow resumes. A period of relative PG normality is now encountered. Mealtime swellings will no longer develop, and salivary quality will visually appear normal, but some measured decrease in salivary volume from glandular damage will be noted. However, the groundwork for recurrences from the presence of duct wall irregularities and strictures, and gland damage, is still in existence and serves as a platform for future incursions.

As stated, CP is often referred to as chronic obstructive parotitis. Certainly, obstruction is a major contributor to the symptomatology associated with CP. Obstruction from ductal scarring and stricturing, salivary plug formation, and sialolithiasis only adds fuel to the fire that originated from the orally ascending PG duct infection that is primarily responsible for CP. The essential etiologic cause of CP is the ascending infection with obstruction serving as an aggravating secondary complication.

Occasionally, a patient may develop symptoms of a debilitating acute suppurative infection of the PG superimposed on a pre-existing CP. Such a condition represents an acute exacerbation of the chronic infection seen in CP. The condition may occur because of a reduced patient resistance, and an increased virulence of the involved organisms complemented by a PG that has been weakened by multiple low-grade infectious episodes. With the descending spiral that results from the repeated bouts of glandular swelling, some patients develop very diseased glands that act as the basis for their predilection for acute exacerbation. These patients are in acute distress with pain, fever, and the presence of frank pus that can be observed intraorally at the PG duct ostium. This PG flare-up can mimic the symptomatology of an acute parotitis (AP). Because the therapeutic approaches to CP and AP are quite different, the presence of an underlying CP must be determined.

The evaluation of saliva, both quantity and quality, has proven to be an integral part of CP diagnosis. The constant insult to the PG parenchyma and ductal system by repeated glandular exacerbations leads to decreases in salivary volume. The investigation will also reveal alterations in salivary chemistry. Increased sodium and chloride content is evident in the saliva, a result of the decreased absorptive capacity of the injured duct wall [12, 15]. Elevations of albumin, lactoferrin, and IgA are also present because these elements can readily enter the saliva through damaged and porous duct walls [16].

Diagnosis of CP can be achieved via a variety of modalities. The history and clinical picture, buttressed by the salivary chemistry, are key features in diagnosis. Imaging has also proven to be a significant tool in diagnosis. Unfortunately, standard radiography is inadequate for visualizing duct structure or uncovering the possible complicating presence of a sialolith. Sialoliths are not an uncommon finding in conjunction with CP. Because parotid sialoliths associated with CP tend to be small and poorly calcified, they are not readily unmasked by radiography. Furthermore, PG sialoliths can be radiographically blotted out by their superimposition on surrounding well-calcified bony structures. Imaging via a CT scan has proven to be particularly useful in CP diagnosis (Fig. 5.9). An enhanced and enlarged PG resulting from salivary retention, inflammatory infiltrate, and fibrosis will be observed. The CT scan also serves to uncover the existence of small relatively radiographically lucent stones because the scan is exquisitely sensitive to minute amounts of calcification. The multiple planes used in CT scanning will also visually free a stone from surrounding obliterating calcified bony structures.

Sialography is extremely useful in revealing the status of a PG that has been subjected to repeated insults from CP. Degenerative duct changes will be seen and reflected as a "sausaged" pattern, primarily affecting the major duct and to a lesser degree the secondary ducts (Figs. 5.7 and 5.8). The pattern represents areas of duct stricturing alternating with duct dilations that result from obstruction and salivary retention, features that develop in direct proportion to CP's duration and severity [10, 17]. In addition, sialography can function as a therapeutic procedure by flushing out ductal debris and simultaneously cause some luminal widening during the injection process. The negativity for the use of sialography is derived from the need for a cooperative patient, a practitioner's skill set, and its radiation effect.

With the introduction of the sialendoscope, a new approach to diagnosing CP has been made available. The width of the sialendoscope has been designed such that it has the ability to enter the parotid duct through the duct's intraoral orifice. The scope contains optic fibers which make it possible to visualize the duct lumen as the scope is advanced along the length of the duct. The causes of the ductal obstruction can be visually identified. Besides the expected strictures, the lumen is usually compromised by debris. The debris represents inflammatory cell and tissue exfoliation plus coagulated salivary constituents. In addition, any sialolith that occupies the duct will readily be observed with the scope.

Histologically, manifestations of PG chronic parenchymal inflammation are evident [12, 18]. A periductal inflammatory infiltrate and duct epithelial metaplasia are seen. Lymphocytic infiltration in the gland parenchyma with fibrosis is also present. If an acute infectious process has been superimposed upon the CP, an abundance of neutrophils will be present. Eventually, with a prolonged history, the PG parenchyma will be replaced by a fibroadipose tissue and a mononuclear infiltrate [19, 20].

Initially, in the early mild self-limiting phase of CP, a conservative approach to treatment is acceptable. Antibiotics as indicated, analgesics, sialogogues, duct probing, duct irrigations, and massage of the gland have been reported to lead to symptom resolution in 50% of the cases [13]. Retrograde infusion of 1% methyl violet, a chemical irritant, has been used with success to cause duct sclerosis and glandular atrophy [21]. In the past, surgical parotidectomy was recommended when conservative therapy failed [13, 18]. Tympanectomy [13] and surgical duct ligation [21] have also been advocated. Failures and the morbidity associated with these surgical approaches may be negated with the therapeutic use of the sialendoscope. The advances in optical technology and the development of thin semi-rigid sialendoscopes have made salivary duct endoscopy possible [13]. The interventional sialendoscope contains an irrigation port that produces a pressured flush of fluid that may incorporate steroids and antibiotics and serve to wash out debris, overwhelm strictures, and even promote duct dilation. Working parts in the sialendoscope contain additional therapeutic components that function to balloon dilate the duct, grasp a stone, or cut a stricture. Sialendoscopy has been reported to be effective in 76–81% of patients treated for CP [22, 23]. In addition, botulinum toxin injections have been suggested for those CP cases that are refractory to the various therapeutic procedures [9].

Parotid Infection

Neonatal Acute Suppurative Parotitis

Neonatal acute suppurative parotitis (NASP) has features that are essentially identical to acute parotitis. There is one difference, and it rests in the fact that NASP uniquely occurs in the newborn. Because it is limited to the newborn, NASP has been listed and fully reviewed in Chap. 12 "Salivary Gland Disease in Children."

References

1. Fattahi TT, Lyu PE, Van Sickels JE. Management of acute suppurative parotitis. J Oral Maxillofac Surg. 2002;60(4):446–8. https://doi.org/10.1053/joms.2002.31234.
2. Belczak SQ, Cleva RD, Utiyama EM, Cecconello I, Rasslan S, Parreira JG. Acute postsurgical suppurative parotitis: current prevalence at Hospital das Clínicas, São Paulo University Medical School. Rev Inst Med Trop Sao Paulo. 2008;50(5):303–5. https://doi.org/10.1590/s0036-46652008000500010.

3. Sheppard DC, Chambers HF. Suppurative parotitis. West J Med. 1998;169(2):116–7.
4. Speirs CF, Mason DK. Acute septic parotitis: incidence, aetiology and management. Scott Med J. 1972;17(2):62–6. https://doi.org/10.1177/003693307201700204.
5. Brook I. Diagnosis and management of parotitis. Arch Otolaryngol Head Neck Surg. 1992;118(5):469–71. https://doi.org/10.1001/archotol.1992.01880050015002.
6. Berker M, Sahin A, Aypar U, Ozgen T. Acute parotitis following sitting position neurosurgical procedures: review of five cases. J Neurosurg Anesthesiol. 2004;16(1):29–31. https://doi.org/10.1097/00008506-200401000-00007.
7. Alaya S, Mofredj A, Tassaioust K, Bahloul H, Mrabet A. Acute parotitis as a complication of noninvasive ventilation. J Intensive Care Med. 2016;31(8):561–3. https://doi.org/10.1177/0885066616636021.
8. Brook I. Acute bacterial suppurative parotitis: microbiology and management. J Craniofac Surg. 2003;14(1):37–40. https://doi.org/10.1097/00001665-200301000-00006.
9. Ardekian L, Shamir D, Trabelsi M, Peled M. Chronic obstructive parotitis due to strictures of Stenson's duct—our treatment experience with sialoendoscopy. J Oral Maxillofac Surg. 2010;68(1):83–7. https://doi.org/10.1016/j.joms.2009.08.019.
10. Harbison JM, Liess BD, Templer JW, Zitsch RP 3rd, Wieberg JA. Chronic parotitis: a challenging disease entity. Ear Nose Throat J. 2011;90(3):E13–6. https://doi.org/10.1177/014556131109000317.
11. Strohl MP, Chang CF, Ryan WR, Chang JL. Botulinum toxin for chronic parotid sialadenitis: a case series and systematic review. Laryngosc Investig Otolaryngol. 2021;6(3):404–13. https://doi.org/10.1002/lio2.558.
12. Bhatty MA, Piggot TA, Soames JV, McLean NR. Chronic non-specific parotid sialadenitis. Br J Plast Surg. 1998;51(7):517–21. https://doi.org/10.1054/bjps.1997.0135.
13. Motamed M, Laugharne D, Bradley PJ. Management of chronic parotitis: a review. J Laryngol Otol. 2003;117(7):521–6. https://doi.org/10.1258/002221503322112923.
14. Moody AB, Avery CM, Walsh S, Sneddon K, Langdon JD. Surgical management of chronic parotid disease. Br J Oral Maxillofac Surg. 2000;38(6):620–2. https://doi.org/10.1054/bjom.2000.0478.
15. Baurmash HD. Chronic recurrent parotitis: a closer look at its origin, diagnosis, and management. J Oral Maxillofac Surg. 2004;62(8):1010–8. https://doi.org/10.1016/j.joms.2003.08.041.
16. Mandel ID, Baurmash H. Sialochemistry in chronic recurrent parotitis: electrolytes and glucose. J Oral Pathol. 1980;9(2):92–8. https://doi.org/10.1111/j.1600-0714.1980.tb01391.x.
17. Wang SL, Zou ZJ, Wu QG, Sun KH. Sialographic changes related to clinical and pathologic findings in chronic obstructive parotitis. Int J Oral Maxillofac Surg. 1992;21(6):364–8. https://doi.org/10.1016/s0901-5027(05)80764-7.
18. van der Lans RJL, Lohuis PJFM, van Gorp JMHH, Quak JJ. Surgical treatment of chronic parotitis. Int Arch Otorhinolaryngol. 2019;23(1):83–7. https://doi.org/10.1055/s-0038-1667006.
19. Bowling DM, Ferry G, Rauch SD, Goodman ML. Intraductal tetracycline therapy for the treatment of chronic recurrent parotitis. Ear Nose Throat J. 1994;73(4):262–74.
20. Nahlieli O, Bar T, Shacham R, Eliav E, Hecht-Nakar L. Management of chronic recurrent parotitis: current therapy. J Oral Maxillofac Surg. 2004;62(9):1150–5. https://doi.org/10.1016/j.joms.2004.05.116.
21. Wang S, Marchal F, Zou Z, Zhou J, Qi S. Classification and management of chronic sialadenitis of the parotid gland. J Oral Rehabil. 2009;36(1):2–8. https://doi.org/10.1111/j.1365-2842.2008.01896.x.
22. Nahlieli O, Shacham R, Yoffe B, Eliav E. Diagnosis and treatment of strictures and kinks in salivary gland ducts. J Oral Maxillofac Surg. 2001;59(5):484–92. https://doi.org/10.1053/joms.2001.22667.
23. Koch M, Iro H, Zenk J. Role of sialoscopy in the treatment of Stensen's duct strictures. Ann Otol Rhinol Laryngol. 2008;117(4):271–8. https://doi.org/10.1177/000348940811700406.

Chapter 6
Viral Disease and the Salivary Glands

Louis Mandel

Abstract Viruses are tiny microscopic germs consisting of genetic material surrounded by a coating of protein. They replicate by using the machinery and metabolism of a host cell, and form thousands of copies that lead to cell death with lysis of the cell membrane. The lysis allows for viral release and the ability to infect other cells. Numerous diseases have viral origins, two of which involve the salivary glands, mumps (epidemic parotitis) and HIV/AIDS. Mumps can occur systemically in all age groups, but is usually seen in the 5–9 year age category when painful bilateral parotid gland swellings develop. A subgroup of HIV/AIDS, patients with the diffuse infiltrative lymphocytosis syndrome, can demonstrate salivary gland involvement with the onset of lymphoepithelial cysts that involve the parotid gland, usually bilaterally.

Overview

Viruses are tiny microscopic germs, much smaller than bacteria, that are found wherever there is life. They consist of genetic material surrounded by a protein coating. Because they are acellular, they do not multiply through cell division. Rather, they replicate by infecting a host cell. By using the machinery and metabolism of the host cell, they rapidly form thousands of copies of themselves. Inevitably, they cause host cell death and lysis of the cell membrane. With membrane destruction, the viral copies are released to infect other body cells.

Viruses spread throughout a societal population via a variety of pathways. They can affect individuals who breathe in diseased aerosol droplets that are discharged into the air when an infected person sneezes or coughs. Sexual contact, exposure to infected blood or even saliva, and fecal contamination represent other modes for viral spread.

L. Mandel, *Clinical Management of Salivary Gland Disorders*,
https://doi.org/10.1007/978-3-031-50012-1_6

Numerous diseases originate from viral dissemination. Included are pathologic entities such as influenza, the common cold, smallpox, measles, herpes, human immunodeficiency virus (HIV)/acquired immune deficiency syndrome (AIDS), and mumps. Two of these viral conditions, namely, mumps and HIV/AIDS, are known to involve the salivary glands. The salivary gland symptomatology associated with these two viral diseases is the subject of this chapter.

Mumps

Mumps is a viral disease caused by a paramyxovirus. This highly contagious disease affects all age groups, but individuals in the 5–9-year age category are the primary prey. Although it has widespread systemic manifestations (orchitis, oophoritis, mastitis, encephalitis, pancreatitis), the most frequent and recognizable mumps symptom is painful bilateral parotid gland (PG) swellings (Fig. 6.1), with the other major salivary glands implicated to a lesser extent. Exposure to the very contagious mumps virus confers immunity upon the patient. With the development of the MMR (mumps, measles, rubella) vaccine, a striking drop in the incidence of this viral disease has occurred.

Because mumps primarily affects children, a full discussion of this pathologic entity can be found in Chap. 9 (Pediatric Salivary Gland Disease).

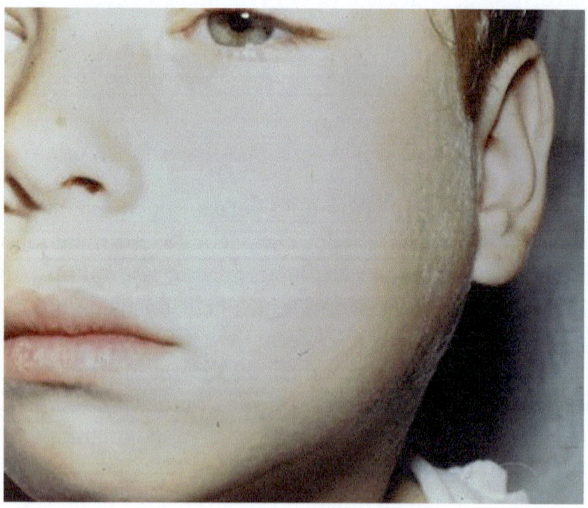

Fig. 6.1 Mumps. Left parotid gland (PG). Swelling. Right PG was also swollen

Human Immunodeficiency Virus Disease (HIV/AIDS)

As of 2016, reports indicate that 36.7 million people worldwide are infected with the human immunodeficiency virus (HIV) [1]. Head and neck HIV lesions are manifested in 41–50% of these patients (Fig. 6.2). Parotid gland (PG) swellings are present in 1–10% of this affected head and neck group (Fig. 6.3) [1–6]. In this cohort of patients with PG swellings, the most common cause of the swelling is the pathologic

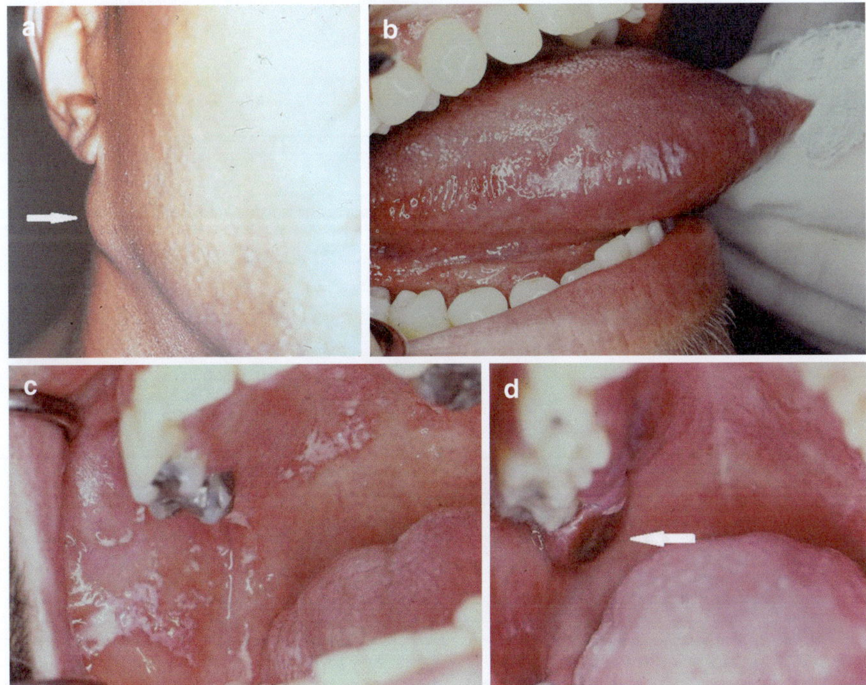

Fig. 6.2 (**a**) HIV. Lymphadenopathy (arrow). (**b**) HIV. Hairy leukoplakia tongue. (**c**) HIV. Candidiasis (buccal mucosa, palate). (**d**) HIV. Kaposi sarcoma (arrow)

Fig. 6.3 HIV. Bilateral parotid gland swelling

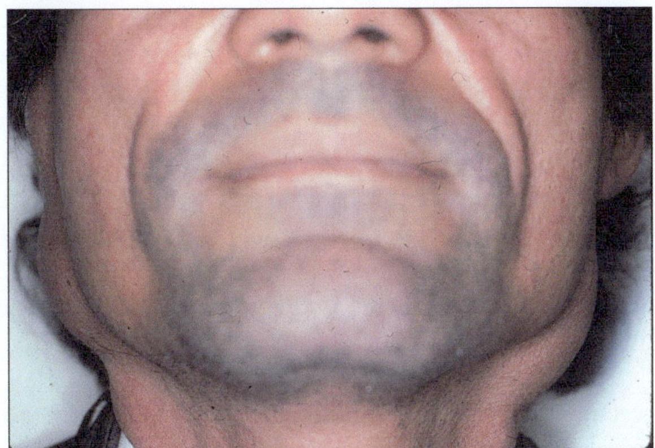

Fig. 6.4 (**a**) HIV. Patient
A. Bilateral parotid
swelling. (**b**) HIV. Patient
A. CT scan. Bilateral
parotid cysts

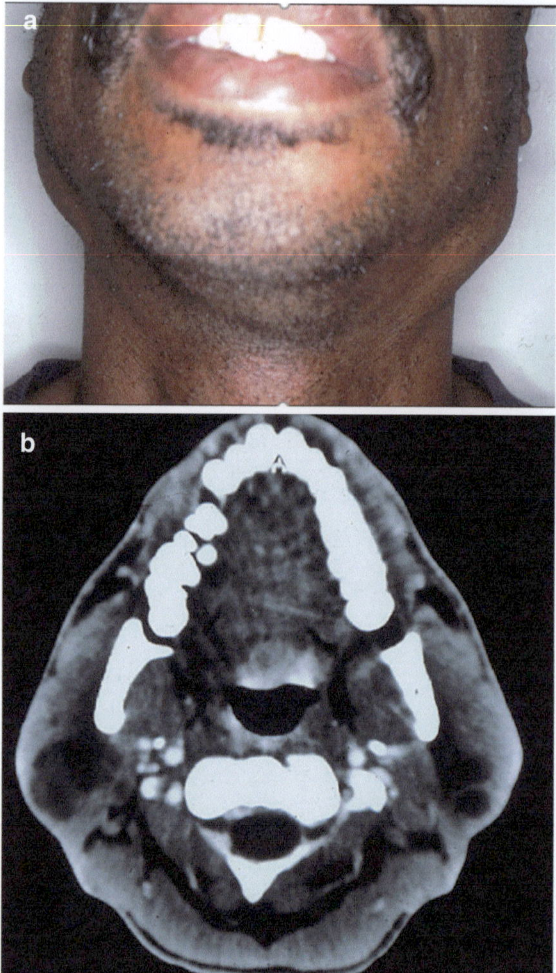

presence of a benign lymphoepithelial cyst (BLEC), which is usually observed bilaterally. The BLEC was first described by Hildebrandt in 1895 [7], and up to 1981, only 21 cases were identified [8]. The incidence of BLEC significantly increased with the onset of the HIV/acquired immune deficiency syndrome (HIV/AIDS). The Hildebrandt lesions differed from the now more commonly observed BLEC in that they occurred rarely, were unilateral, and developed in HIV-negative patients [1, 2, 9]. The recognition of a relationship between BLEC and HIV/AIDS was first appreciated by Ryan et al. in 1985 [10]. The PG swellings in these HIV patients result from either the onset of a florid glandular lymphoproliferation (Fig. 6.5) or more commonly the development of an intraglandular BLEC (Fig. 6.4) that is present in about 5% of HIV patients [5]. These pathologic changes may only involve and be limited to the PG but can also serve as indications of the presence of diffuse infiltrative lymphocytosis syndrome (DILS), a subset of HIV disease. DILS develops in certain immunogenetically distinct (HLA-DR5) adults and children [11–13].

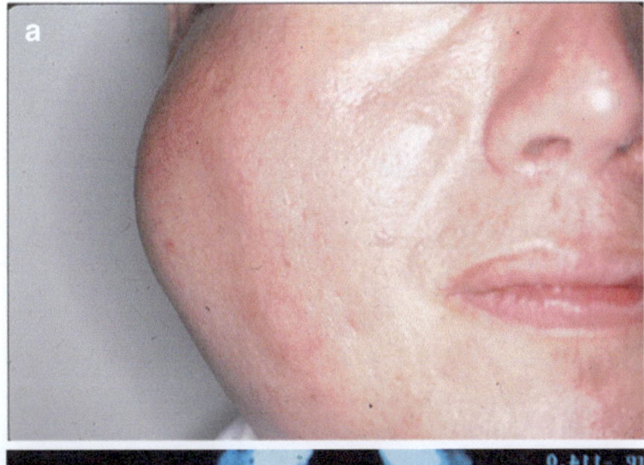

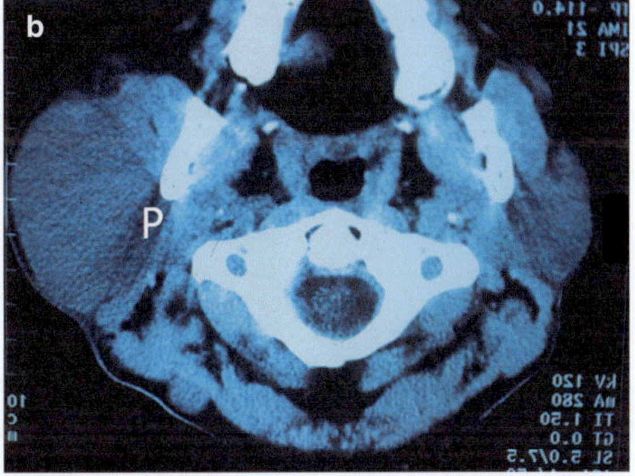

Fig. 6.5 (**a**) HIV. Patient B. Right parotid gland swelling. (Mandel L. Oral Surg Oral Med Oral Pathol Oral Radiol Endod 1998;85:565). (**b**) HIV. Patient B. CT scan. Right parotid swelling (P) caused by lymphoproliferation. (Mandel L. Oral Surg Oral Med Oral Pathol Oral Radiol Endod 1998;85:565)

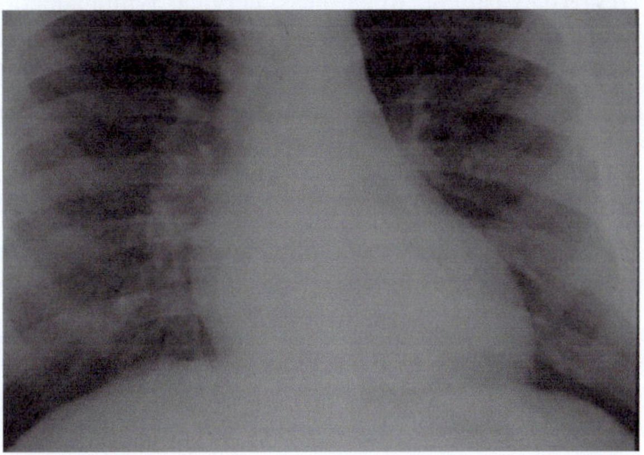

Fig. 6.6 HIV. Pulmonary involvement

The DILS subset of patients is characterized by a multisystem (salivary glands, lung, liver, kidney) visceral CD8 cell infiltration (Fig. 6.6) [11, 12]. Serologically, there is a CD8 increase accompanied by a decrease in circulating CD4 lymphocytes. The syndrome follows a less aggressive course than that observed in the standard

Fig. 6.7 (**a**) HIV. Patient
C. Bilateral parotid
swelling. (**b**) HIV. Patient
C. CT scan. Bilateral
parotid cysts. (Mandel
L. Chapter Salivary Gland
Disorders. Med Clin North
Am 2014;98:1407)

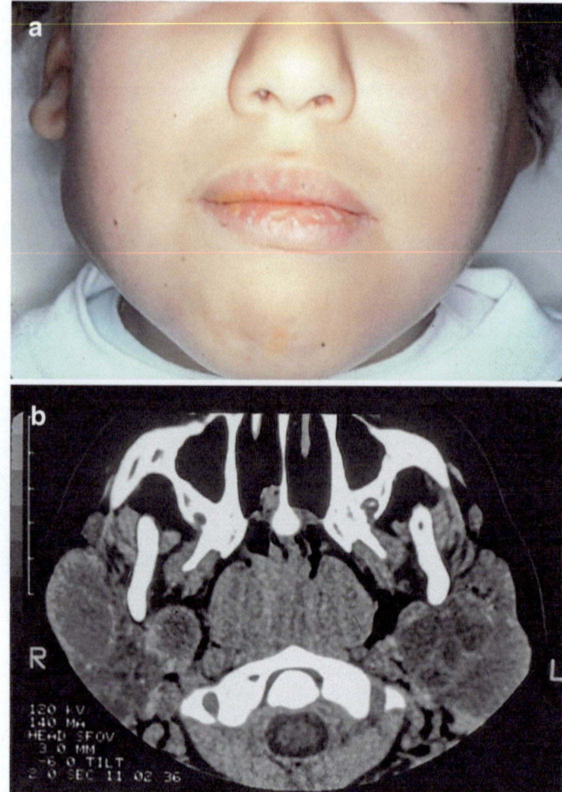

HIV/AIDS patient. Regardless, cervical lymphadenopathy is often present along with a fourfold increase in the onset of a non-Hodgkin lymphoma [14, 15].

The lymphoproliferation that is the other cause of PG swelling is reactive and originates from viral stimulation of the PG lymph nodes or an exuberant response of normally present intraglandular lymphocytes. It is also possible that the extraglandular CD8 lymphocytosis that develops can infiltrate into the PG and lead to glandular swelling [10].

The more frequent cause of the PG swelling is the presence of a BLEC (Figs. 6.5, 6.7 and 6.8). The pathogenesis for its evolution has not been clearly established, but two theories have been suggested [5, 7, 16–18]. During fetal life, elements of PG epithelium can become trapped within developing intraglandular PG lymph nodes. An average of 2–22 nodes are usually dispersed throughout the superficial lobe of the PG [19], mostly in the lobe's tail [5]. Viral stimulation leads to lymph node lymphoproliferation which in some way induces the trapped intranodal glandular epithelium to proliferate and form a cyst. A second hypothesis involves HIV-infected cells migrating into the PG. The migration can trigger a lymphoid proliferation and duct cell metaplasia that causes ductal obstruction and ductal dilation that is responsible for the cyst-like appearance.

Fig. 6.8 (**a**) HIV. Patient D. Parotid swelling on the left side. (**b**) HIV. Patient D. CT scan. Left parotid cyst

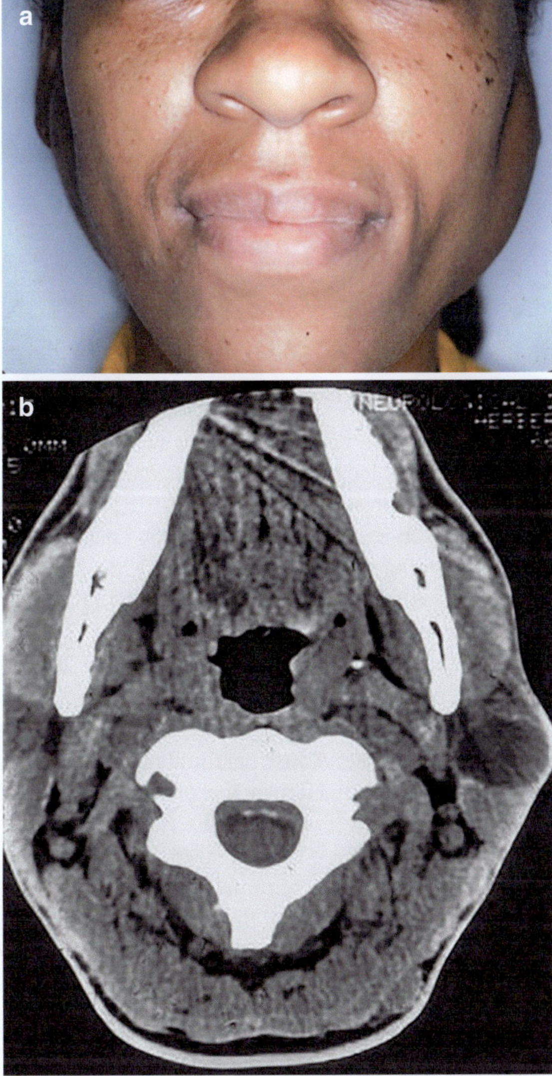

Clinically, the BLEC almost exclusively involves the PG, with the submandibular salivary gland (SMSG) rarely affected [5, 20, 21], maybe because of the absence of SMSG intraglandular lymph nodes. The BLEC is seen equally in males and females who are in their fifth decade of life [21]. Bilateral PG cystic involvement is the norm in HIV-positive patients with unilateral BLEC more commonly seen in HIV-negative individuals [17]. Occasionally, the cysts have been described in the other major salivary glands and even the minor salivary glands [1]. The cysts can be simple or multiple, multiloculated, circumscribed, and often become very large. They are painless with a history of slow growth that eventually becomes a cosmetic

Fig. 6.9 HIV patient with lymphoma involving salivary glands

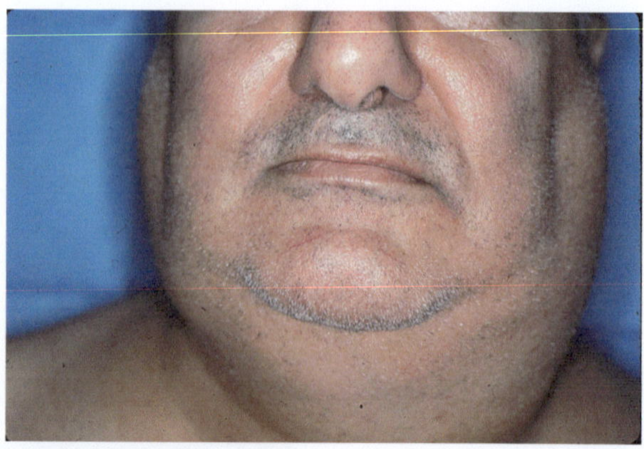

problem. Palpation indicates that the swellings are soft, compressible, painless, and cyst-like and are located in the PG's superficial lobe.

The clinical presence of a bilateral BLEC should serve to alert the practitioner to the probable co-existence of HIV/AIDS. These unique swellings frequently serve as an early harbinger of HIV disease [17, 20]. Although the PG swelling associated with BLEC is considered benign, monitoring is indicated because the transformation into a malignant lymphoma, originating from the florid glandular lymphoproliferation, is a known possibility (Fig. 6.9) [5, 20, 22]. Sudden increases in PG size herald the possibility of such a transformation.

Less objective data are available regarding the effect of HIV-related PG disease on salivary flow rate. A low unstimulated whole saliva flow rate has been reported [23–25]. The role of HIV in the pathogenesis of hyposalivation is unclear. This hyposalivation may result from the lymphoproliferation or BLEC acting to cause acinar atrophy [1, 26]. The decreased salivation may also represent the effect of the prescribed highly active antiretroviral therapy (HAART) on salivary secretion [27, 28]. However, objective oral dryness is not a common occurrence.

Imaging has a significant role in the diagnosis of BLEC. A CT scan will clearly delineate the BLEC's presence in the PG and the extent of the cyst which is usually multicentric rather than unicentric. The scan will also testify to the presence of any subclinical PG BLEC in the absence of a clinical PG swelling as well as its anatomical relationship to adjoining structures. Peripheral enhancement of the cystic lesions will be observed. If lymphoproliferation alone has initiated the PG enlargement, a diffuse glandular density, caused by the lymphocytic proliferation displacing normal gland parenchyma and fat, will be observed. Any associated cervical lymphadenopathy will also be visualized by a scan. An MRI (T2) will show multiple circumscribed cystic lesions, with high T2 signal intensity, within the PG [29]. Ultrasound offers a rapid simple imaging procedure for BLEC diagnosis (Fig. 6.10). Most commonly, small to large sonolucent areas, with well-defined borders and containing echogenic debris, are imaged [30]. A heterogeneous echotexture background will also be observed [5].

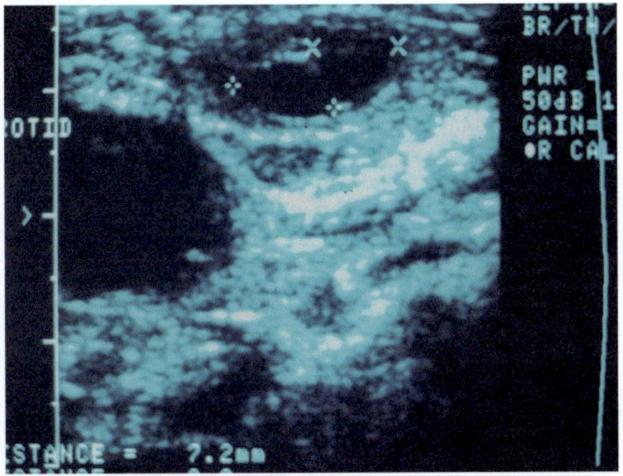

Fig. 6.10 HIV. Ultrasound reveals hypoechoic areas in heterogeneous stroma

Fine-needle aspiration biopsy is a simple and safe examination procedure that is helpful in achieving a diagnosis. Aspiration will deliver a straw-colored fluid that contains a mixture of squamous epithelial and lymphoid cells [18]. Histologically, multiple epithelial cysts accompanied by dense lymphoid tissue are present. Stratified squamous epithelium is the usual epithelial lining of the cyst. Lymphoid tissue will be seen to replace PG parenchyma. Existing lymphocytic follicles are larger and more irregularly shaped than those seen in a normal lymph node [17]. Labial salivary gland biopsy usually confirms the presence of a periductal CD8 T-lymphocytic infiltration with acinar atrophy, fibrosis, and ductal dilation [1, 31].

When BLEC was first recognized during the early HIV/AIDS era, its occurrence called attention to a need for an effective therapeutic solution. Parotidectomy became the treatment of choice (Fig. 6.11), but, because of the surgical morbidity (facial nerve paresis, sialoceles, fistulas), the surgical option was re-evaluated. Alternate therapeutic solutions (irradiation, repeated aspirations, sclerotherapy) were tried. Fortunately, the advent of HAART has succeeded as an effective therapeutic agent. As a consequence of HAART therapy for HIV/AIDS patients, a remarkable decrease in the incidence of HIV-related PG swelling has taken place. HAART's effectiveness in the elimination of PG swellings (Figs. 6.12 and 6.13) results from termination of viral replication, viral load reduction, and a CD4/CD8 cell count stabilization [1]. HAART results in elimination or a marked decrease in the size of the BLEC and should be used as the initial line of defense before considering a more aggressive approach [32]. Patients refractory to HAART can be treated with radiation (24 Gy) [33], a dosage low enough to avoid the threat of radiation-induced malignancy. Sclerotherapy is advocated for BLEC HIV-negative patients. Surgery for all BLEC conditions is considered a last resort because of the morbidities involved in the removal of the PG superficial lobe. Regardless of successful HAART treatment, patients must be monitored because of the possible evolution of a lymphocytic malignancy.

Fig. 6.11 (**a**) HIV. Patient E. Unilateral parotid swelling (left). (**b**) HIV. Patient E. CT scan. Left parotid cystic swelling. Right parotid was surgically removed previously because of cystic involvement

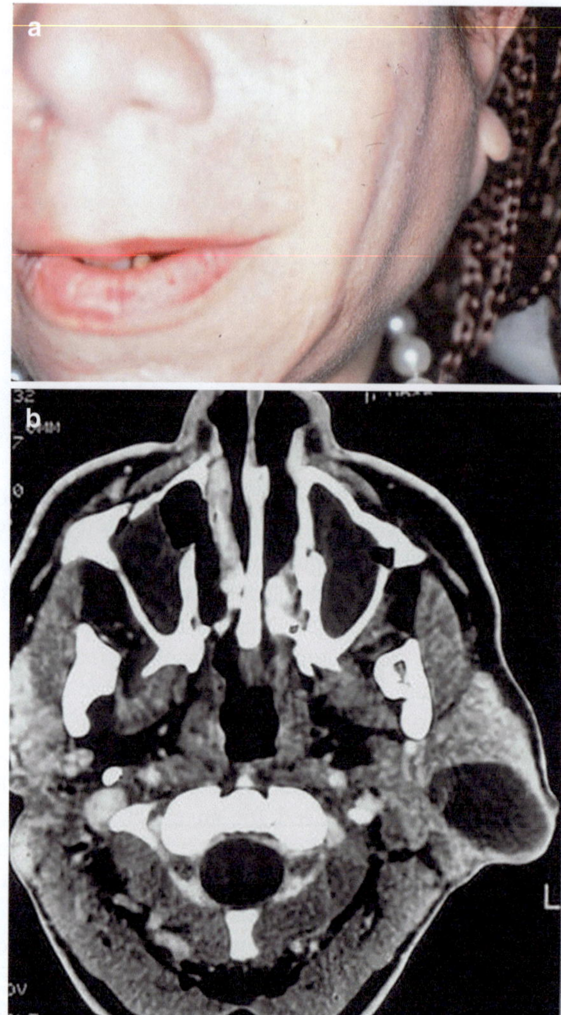

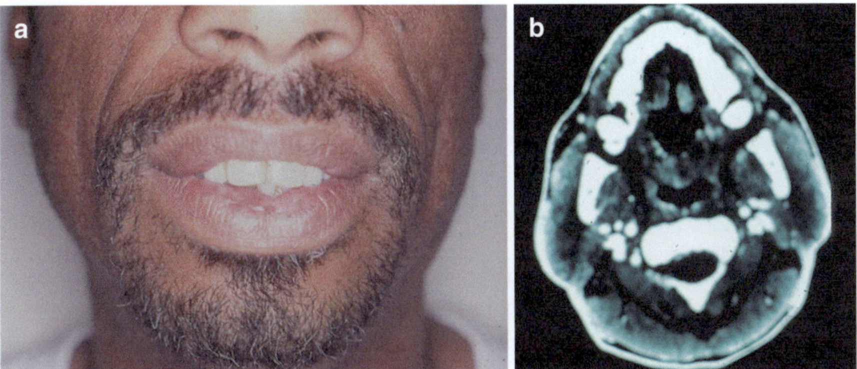

Fig. 6.12 (**a**) HIV. Patient A (seen in Fig. 6.4) following treatment with HAART. (**b**) HIV. Patient A (seen in Fig. 6.4). CT scan following treatment with HAART

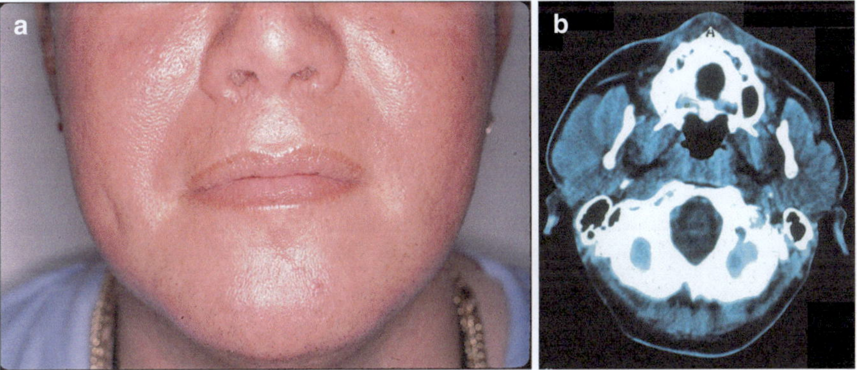

Fig. 6.13 (**a**) HIV. Patient B (seen in Fig. 6.5) following treatment with HAART. (**b**) HIV. Patient B (seen in Fig. 6.5). CT scan following treatment with HAART

References

1. Meer S. Human immunodeficiency virus and salivary gland pathology: an update. Oral Surg Oral Med Oral Pathol Oral Radiol. 2019;128(1):52–9.
2. Schiødt M, Greenspan D, Daniels TE, et al. Parotid gland enlargement and xerostomia associated with labial sialadenitis in HIV-infected patients. J Autoimmun. 1989;2(4):415–25.
3. Mandel L, Hong J. HIV-associated parotid lymphoepithelial cysts. J Am Dent Assoc. 1999;130(4):528–32.
4. Soberman N, Leonidas JC, Berdon WE, et al. Parotid enlargement in children seropositive for human immunodeficiency virus: imaging findings. AJR Am J Roentgenol. 1991;157(3):553–6.
5. Shivhare P, Shankarnarayan L, Jambunath U, Basavaraju SM. Benign lymphoepithelial cysts of parotid and submandibular glands in a HIV-positive patient. J Oral Maxillofac Pathol. 2015;19(1):107.
6. Iro S, Hmoura E, Slimani F. Parotid lymphoepithelial cysts revealing HIV infection in a 12-year-old girl: a case report. Ann Med Surg (Lond). 2021;67:102338.
7. Sujatha D, Babitha K, Prasad RS, Pai A. Parotid lymphoepithelial cysts in human immunodeficiency virus: a review. J Laryngol Otol. 2013;127(11):1046–9.

8. Dave SP, Pernas FG, Roy S. The benign lymphoepithelial cyst and a classification system for lymphocytic parotid gland enlargement in the pediatric HIV population. Laryngoscope. 2007;117(1):106–13.

9. Zanelli M, Zizzo M, Sanguedolce F, Annessi V, Ascani S. Benign lymphoepithelial cyst of the parotid gland: mind the underlying cause. Int J Surg Pathol. 2021;29(1):78–9.

10. Ryan JR, Ioachim HL, Marmer J, Loubeau JM. Acquired immune deficiency syndrome—related lymphadenopathies presenting in the salivary gland lymph nodes. Arch Otolaryngol. 1985;111(8):554–6.

11. Itescu S, Brancato LJ, Buxbaum J, et al. A diffuse infiltrative CD8 lymphocytosis syndrome in human immunodeficiency virus (HIV) infection: a host immune response associated with HLA-DR5. Ann Intern Med. 1990;112(1):3–10.

12. Itescu S, Winchester R. Diffuse infiltrative lymphocytosis syndrome: a disorder occurring in human immunodeficiency virus-1 infection that may present as a sicca syndrome. Rheum Dis Clin N Am. 1992;18(3):683–97.

13. Kazi S, Cohen PR, Williams F, Schempp R, Reveille JD. The diffuse infiltrative lymphocytosis syndrome. Clinical and immunogenetic features in 35 patients. AIDS. 1996;10(4):385–91.

14. Pillai S, Agarwal AC, Mangalore AB, Ramaswamy B, Shetty S. Benign lymphoepithelial cyst of the parotid in HIV negative patient. J Clin Diagn Res. 2016;10(4):MD05–MD6.

15. Islam NM, Bhattacharyya I, Cohen DM. Salivary gland pathology in HIV patients. Diagn Histopathol. 2012;18:366–72.

16. Shanti RM, Aziz SR. HIV-associated salivary gland disease. Oral Maxillofac Surg Clin N Am. 2009;21(3):339–43.

17. Sekikawa Y, Hongo I. HIV-associated benign lymphoepithelial cysts of the parotid glands confirmed by HIV-1 p24 antigen immunostaining. BMJ Case Rep. 2017;2017:bcr2017221869. https://doi.org/10.1136/bcr-2017-221869.

18. Steehler MK, Steehler MW, Davison SP. Benign lymphoepithelial cysts of the parotid: long-term surgical results. HIV AIDS (Auckl). 2012;4:81–6. https://doi.org/10.2147/HIV.S27755.

19. McKean ME, Lee K, McGregor IA. The distribution of lymph nodes in and around the parotid gland: an anatomical study. Br J Plast Surg. 1985;38(1):1–5. https://doi.org/10.1016/0007-1226(85)90078-5.

20. Ahamed AS, Kannan VS, Velaven K, Sathyanarayanan GR, Roshni J, Elavarasi E. Lymphoepithelial cyst of the submandibular gland. J Pharm Bioallied Sci. 2014;6(Suppl 1):S185–7. https://doi.org/10.4103/0975-7406.137464.

21. Joshi J, Shah S, Agarwal D, Khasgiwal A. Benign lymphoepithelial cyst of parotid gland: review and case report. J Oral Maxillofac Pathol. 2018;22(Suppl 1):S91–7. https://doi.org/10.4103/jomfp.JOMFP_252_17.

22. Corr P, Vaithilingum M, Thejpal R, Jeena P. Parotid MALT lymphoma in HIV infected children [published correction appears in J Ultrasound Med 1998;17(4):204]. J Ultrasound Med. 1997;16(9):615–7. https://doi.org/10.7863/jum.1997.16.9.615.

23. Flaitz CM, Hicks MJ, Carter AB, et al. Saliva collection technique for cytologic, microbiologic and viral evaluation in pediatric HIV infection. ASDC J Dent Child. 1998;65(5):318–55.

24. Nittayananta W, Chanowanna N, Pruphetkaew N, Nauntofte B. Relationship between xerostomia and salivary flow rates in HIV-infected individuals. J Investig Clin Dent. 2013;4(3):164–71. https://doi.org/10.1111/jicd.12052.

25. da Silva Rath IB, Beltrame AP, Carvalho AP, Schaeffer MB, Almeida IC. HIV-associated salivary gland disease—clinical or imaging diagnosis? Int J Paediatr Dent. 2015;25(4):233–8. https://doi.org/10.1111/ipd.12133.

26. Patton LL, van der Horst C. Oral infections and other manifestations of HIV disease. Infect Dis Clin N Am. 1999;13(4):879–900. https://doi.org/10.1016/s0891-5520(05)70114-8.

27. López-Verdín S, Andrade-Villanueva J, Zamora-Perez AL, Bologna-Molina R, Cervantes-Cabrera JJ, Molina-Frechero N. Differences in salivary flow level, xerostomia, and flavor alteration in Mexican HIV patients who did or did not receive antiretroviral therapy. AIDS Res Treat. 2013;2013:613278.

28. Kumar JV, Baghirath PV, Naishadham PP, Suneetha S, Suneetha L, Sreedevi P. Relationship of long-term highly active antiretroviral therapy on salivary flow rate and CD4 count among HIV-infected patients. J Oral Maxillofac Pathol. 2015;19(1):58–63. https://doi.org/10.4103/0973-029X.157203.
29. Loulergue P, Guerre A. Parotid gland swelling leading to human immunodeficiency virus infection diagnosis. Am J Med. 2015;128(12):e5–6.
30. Mandel L. Ultrasound findings in HIV-positive patients with parotid gland swellings. J Oral Maxillofac Surg. 2001;59(3):283–6.
31. Ghrenassia E, Martis N, Boyer J, Burel-Vandenbos F, Mekinian A, Coppo P. The diffuse infiltrative lymphocytosis syndrome (DILS). A comprehensive review. J Autoimmun. 2015;59:19–25. https://doi.org/10.1016/j.jaut.2015.01.010.
32. Naik AN, Clinkscales WB, Kato MG, Nguyen SA, Gillespie MB. Nonsurgical management of human immunodeficiency virus-associated parotid cysts: a systematic review and meta-analysis. Head Neck. 2018;40(5):1073–81.
33. Mourad WF, Young R, Kabarriti R, et al. 25-Year follow-up of HIV-positive patients with benign lymphoepithelial cysts of the parotid glands: a retrospective review. Anticancer Res. 2013;33(11):4927–32.

Chapter 7
Autoimmune Disease

Louis Mandel

Abstract In autoimmune disease (AID), the body's immune system produces antibodies that attack the body's own tissues. The attack can be against a single organ or be systemic in nature. There is evidence that indicates that over 100 varieties of AID exist, some of which have salivary gland implications. Sjögren syndrome (SS) is the AID that most frequently hones in on the salivary glands. Primary SS is marked by the presence of hyposalivation and xerophthalmia, while secondary SS occurs in the presence of another systemic AID such as rheumatoid arthritis or lupus erythematosus. In addition to SS, AIDs such as IgG4 related disease, primary biliary cholangitis, graft vs host disease, diabetes, autoimmune thyroid disease and myasthenia gravis are known to have salivary gland ramifications.

Overview

In autoimmune disease (AID), the body's immune system produces antibodies that do not perform their normal function. Instead of fighting infection, these antibodies attack the body's own tissues. The attack may be directed toward a single cell type or a single organ or be systemic in nature and affect multiple organs. The symptomatology that evolves is dependent on what organ or tissue has become the target and damaged.

There is evidence to indicate that over 100 varieties of AID can be identified [1]. Celiac disease, rheumatoid arthritis, multiple sclerosis, psoriasis, thyroid disease, type 1 diabetes, and lupus erythematosus are the more common AIDs that affect patients. It is estimated that about 4.5% of the population of the United States have an AID [2] with women being more susceptible than men. Some patients have more than one AID. Because AID runs in families, a genetic background is suspected. Although the etiology of AID has not been established, infection is thought to play a significant role in its onset. Environmental factors including infections,

L. Mandel, *Clinical Management of Salivary Gland Disorders,*
https://doi.org/10.1007/978-3-031-50012-1_7

antibiotics, anti-hypertensives, smoking, chemicals, and diet may also serve as adjunctive causes for the occurrence of AID.

Diagnosing AID is difficult because symptoms are often very similar to those seen in common illnesses. These symptoms tend to wax and wane and include fatigue, low-grade fevers, myalgia, arthralgia, and rashes. Some help in the diagnosis of an AID may be derived from the serologic presence of antinuclear antibodies in many of the AIDs. Most frequently, the structures involved include the blood vessels, underlying connective tissue, joints, muscles, skin, pancreas, and thyroid.

As stated, AID can impact a variety of organs. The salivary gland (SG) complex represents one such organ system that can be disrupted by an AID. Therefore, a review of those salivary gland conditions affected by AID serves as the subject of this chapter.

Sjögren Syndrome

The eponym Sjögren syndrome (SS) originated as a tribute to the Swedish ophthalmologist, Henrik Sjögren. In 1933, he presented a paper that linked together a disparate triad of symptoms (keratoconjunctivitis sicca, dry mouth, polyarthritis) into one disease entity that is now known as SS [3]. SS is defined as a chronic autoimmune disease characterized by a lymphocytic infiltration into the exocrine glands. Because of the particular involvement of the lacrimal and salivary glands, dry eyes and a dry mouth result. Systemic multiorgan manifestations may also be present and can involve the liver, respiratory tract, nervous system, gastrointestinal system, joints, and kidney. Fatigue is a key feature.

Two clinical forms of SS exist and are referred to as primary SS and secondary SS. Primary SS is recognized as an autoimmune disease that is limited to the salivary and lacrimal glands. In secondary SS, another autoimmune disease (rheumatoid arthritis (Fig. 7.1), lupus erythematosus (Fig. 7.2), systemic sclerosis (Fig. 7.3), and dermatomyositis) will be present along with an existing primary SS. Rheumatoid arthritis and lupus erythematosus are the more common SS-associated systemic

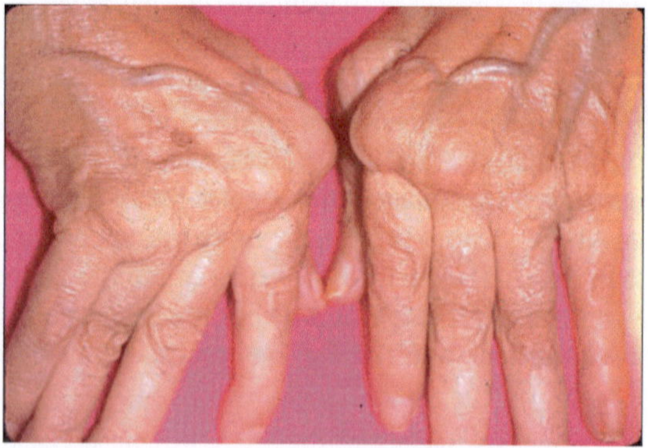

Fig. 7.1 Sjögren syndrome. Rheumatoid arthritis

Fig. 7.2 Sjögren syndrome. Facial erythema seen in lupus erythematosus

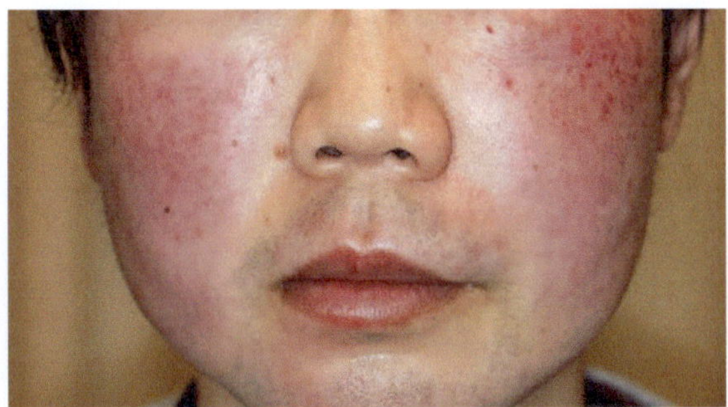

Fig. 7.3 Sjögren syndrome. Systemic sclerosis

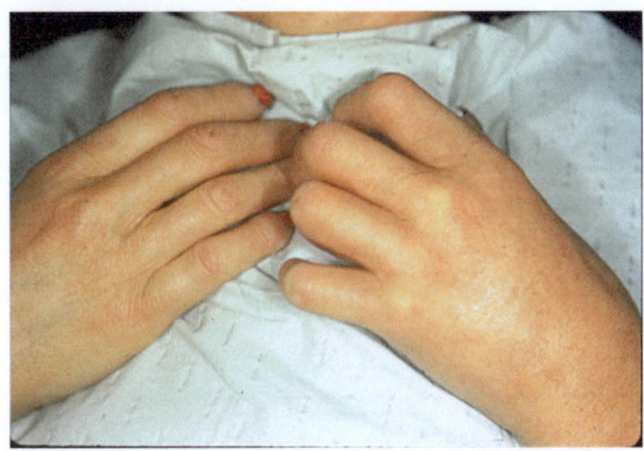

autoimmune diseases. Rheumatoid arthritis has been found in 53% of patients with SS, while lupus erythematosus has been identified in 22% [4]. Mikulicz disease, characterized by bilateral painless persistent salivary and lacrimal gland swellings, was previously included in the diagnostic confines of primary SS, but is now considered a manifestation of immunoglobulin G4-related disease.

SS predominantly involves females over males in a ratio of 9:1 [5–7] with the mean age at the time of diagnosis of 50 years [6, 7]. However, the Asian and Afro-American female-to-male ratios have been recognized as 27:1 and 7:1, respectively [8]. A systematic literature search reported an overall SS prevalence rate of 61 cases per 100,000 people [9].

The etiology of SS is unknown. However, exposure to environmental factors such as viral infections is considered a potential cause in a genetically predisposed individual [10]. The role of genetics is buttressed by the fact that one-third of SS patients have a relative with an autoimmune connective tissue disease [10, 11]. An appreciation has recently developed for the part that epithelial cells may play in SS pathogenesis [10]. These cells are targets of the autoimmune process, but they can also activate an immune reaction [10, 12]. B cell activation plays a major role in SS pathogenesis, while T cells serve as significant contributors in milder lesions [7].

The most frequent complaint of SS patients centers around their ocular (Fig. 7.4) and/or oral (Fig. 7.5) dryness, with 98% of the patients reporting at least one sicca

Fig. 7.4 Sjögren
syndrome. Patient
complained of dry eyes

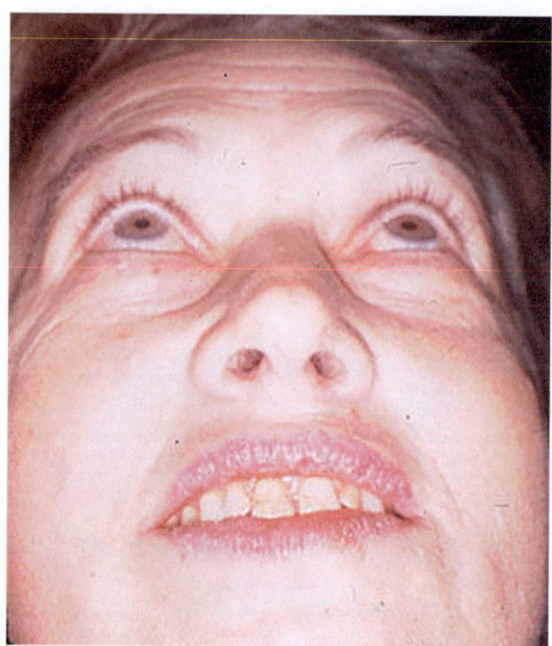

Fig. 7.5 Sjögren
syndrome. Dry mouth,
cobblestone tongue, and
dental caries

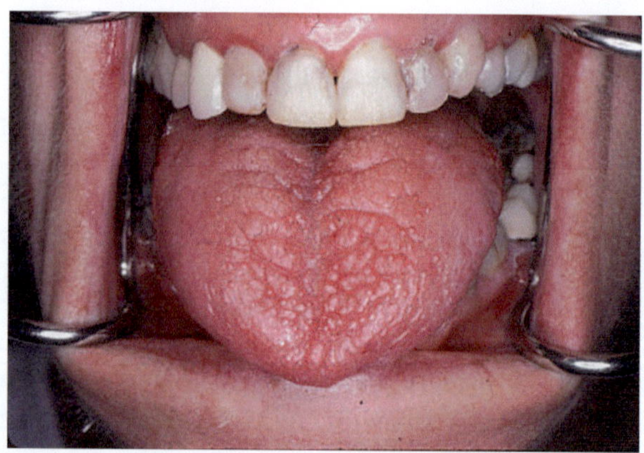

symptom while 89% will present with both dry eyes and dry mouth [13]. Histologically, a lymphocytic proliferation replaces secreting lacrimal and salivary acini (Fig. 7.6). Hyposecretion of the lacrimal and salivary glands then becomes a clinical issue. Hypolacrimation, with its failure to adequately lubricate the eye, leads to ocular surface chronic inflammation. Dry eye syndrome, also known as keratoconjunctivitis sicca, is characterized by erythema, photosensitivity, and an itching or foreign body sensation in the eye [14]. Often patients volunteer the information that they cannot produce tears during a crying event. Corneal and conjunctival abnormalities develop from the inadequate lacrimal lubrication and can be identified by an ophthalmologist via dye staining and a slit-lamp examination.

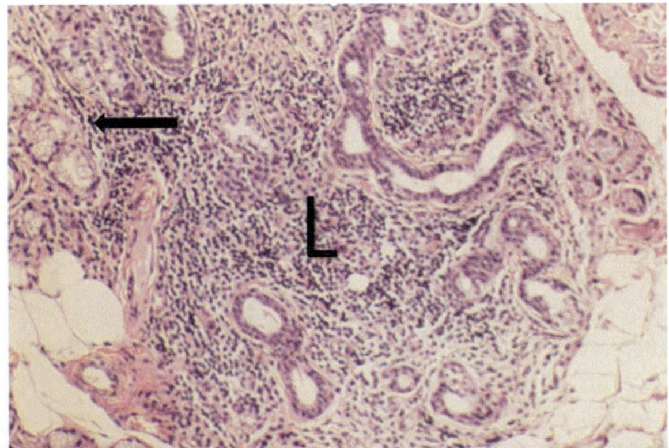

Fig. 7.6 Sjögren syndrome. Labial biopsy. Lymphocytic infiltration (L) replacing normal mucus-secreting glands (arrow)

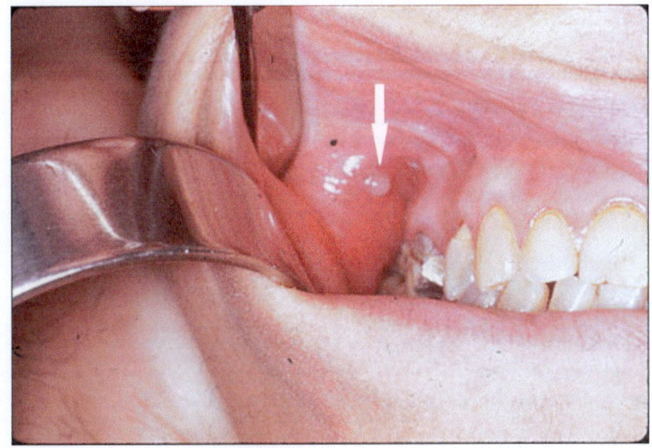

Fig. 7.7 Sjögren syndrome. Gel-like saliva adhering to buccal mucosa (arrow)

The hyposalivation associated with SS involves both whole unstimulated and whole stimulated salivary production and is a result of lymphocytic replacement of secreting acini. If any saliva can be expressed from the parotid gland orifice, it will be observed to be gel-like (Fig. 7.7) and it will adhere to the surrounding mucosa. A dry erythematous oral mucosa evolves. Salivary pooling, normally seen in the anterior mouth floor, will not be present. Difficulty with swallowing and dysgeusia develop. With the loss of saliva's lubricating ability, oral burning becomes a frequent complaint. Oral candidiasis and an increase in dental caries can be anticipated. A cobblestone (Fig. 7.5) or an atrophic tongue may also be observed in the absence of sufficient saliva.

Clinically, the major salivary glands, mostly the parotid gland (PG) and less frequently the submandibular and sublingual glands, may become swollen. The PG unilaterally and at times bilaterally is affected. The PG swellings and the associated discomfort may mimic the symptomatology that is seen in chronic parotitis (CP). As in CP, the decreased salivation and flow in SS patients result in a failure of ductal lavage, setting the stage for an ascending ductal infection by oral bacteria. The consequent duct wall inflammatory scarring and stricture formation narrow the duct lumen, impede the flow of the already SS decreased saliva, and encourage stagnation and additional cycles of ascending infection. These SS swellings of the PG caused by infection will also be recognized by the presence of a suppurative exudate exiting from the intraoral PG duct ostium and by periods of pain and more swelling when the patient stimulates the gland by eating. What has occurred in these SS patients is that a CP has developed secondarily and is now superimposed upon the original SS damaged PG (Fig. 7.8). During periods of remission, some PG fullness is usually present reflecting the residual inflammatory changes initiated by both the CP and SS.

Occasionally, in addition to PG symptomatology in SS imitating the clinical picture observed in CP, some SS patients will be seen with a persistent and painless PG swelling that mimics a neoplasm (Figs. 7.9 and 7.10). Such patients should be viewed with a high degree of suspicion regarding the possible onset of a non-Hodgkin lymphoma, usually a B cell mucosa-associated lymphoid tissue (MALT) lymphoma (Fig. 7.10c). These lymphomas tend to develop in organs where the

Fig. 7.8 (**a**) Sjögren syndrome. Patient A. Painful right parotid swelling. (**b**) Sjögren syndrome. Patient A. Multiple cervical carious lesions. (**c**) Sjögren syndrome. Patient A. Pus exiting right parotid duct orifice (arrow). (**d**) Sjögren syndrome. Patient A. Sialogram demonstrates duct inflammation with segmentation ("sausaging") combined with sialectic sialographic pattern characteristically seen in Sjögren syndrome

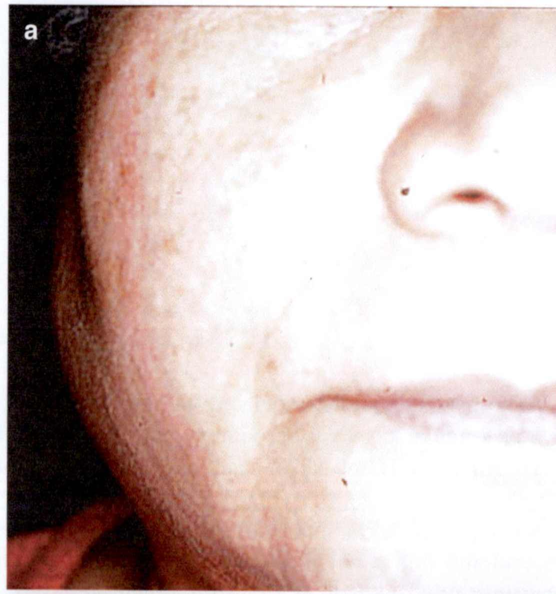

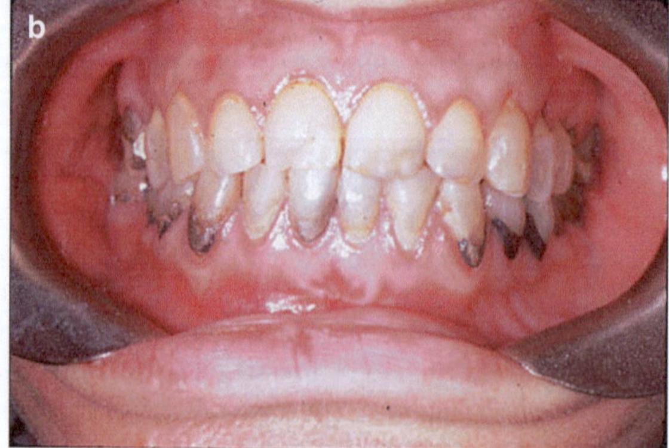

Fig. 7.8 (continued)

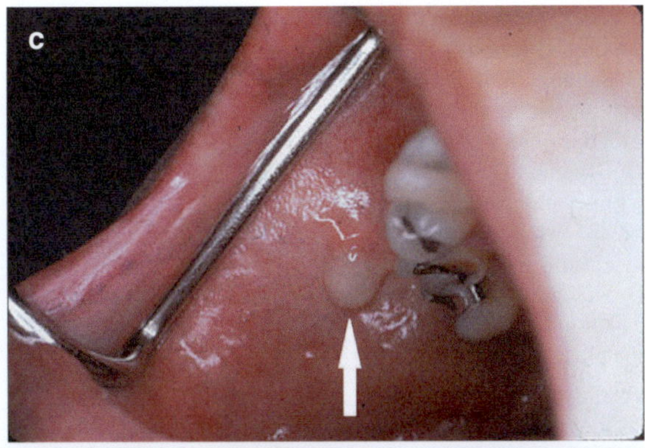

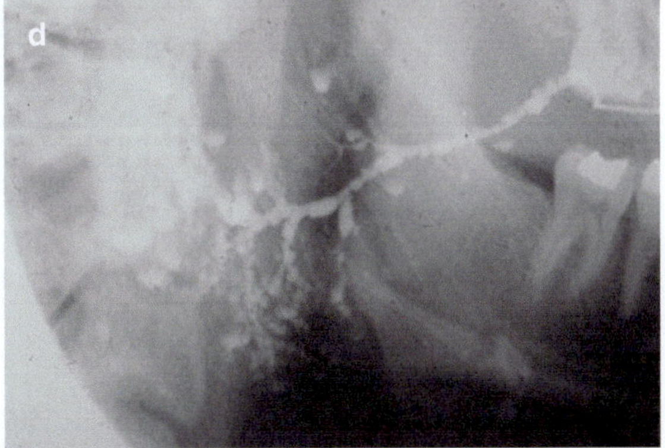

disease is active and salivary glands serve as a frequent site [10]. Therefore, SS patients with persistent PG swellings should be routinely evaluated for the existence of a MALT lymphoma. The PG is almost exclusively involved, maybe because of a B cell proliferation that originates from the PG's intraglandular lymph nodes. Lymph nodes are not normally found in other salivary glands. SS patients have a 14- to 20-fold increased risk of developing lymphoma compared with the general population [5, 7]. About 5–10% of SS patients eventually develop a lymphoma, with persistent painless salivary gland swellings and lymphadenopathies being the main clinical predictors [7, 10, 13]. Biologic risk factors for the development of an SS initiated lymphoma include the presence of a cryoglobulinemia, purpura, rheumatoid factor, hypocomplementemia, CD4 T-cell lymphocytopenia, and hepatosplenomegaly [7, 10]. Patients with these features require close follow-up because of their increased susceptibility to lymphoma.

Fatigue is a common problem seen in 70–80% of SS patients [10]. A dry respiratory tract seen in SS patients results in vocal hoarseness, while a coughing problem results from tracheal dryness. Loss of the secretory ability of the lubricating mucous glands lining the respiratory tree can cause rhinitis, pharyngitis, or laryngitis. Arthralgias in up to 75% of SS patients and myalgias are also commonly seen in association with SS. Loss of vaginal secretions causes dyspareunia. Raynaud's phenomenon has been reported in 10–20% of SS patients and usually precedes sicca symptomatology [10]. Liver, renal, nervous system, and some gastrointestinal

Fig. 7.9 (**a**) Sjögren syndrome. Patient B. Painless right and left parotid swellings. (**b**) Sjögren syndrome. Patient B. Dry mouth, cobblestone tongue, and dental breakdown. (**c**) Sjögren syndrome. Patient B. Sialogram demonstrates a classic sialectic pattern in the presence of a normal parotid duct

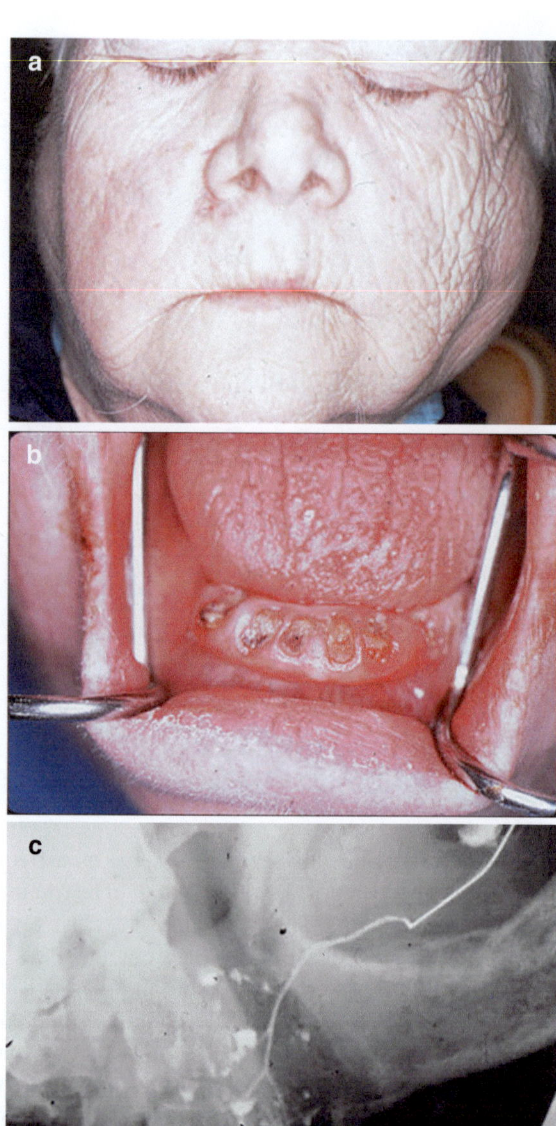

involvement have also been reported in association with SS [5, 10]. Diminished secretions of the digestive tract's exocrine glands may cause hypochlorhydria and pancreatic problems [10].

Serologically, antinuclear antibody (ANA), rheumatoid factor (RF), anti-SSA/Ro, and anti-SSB/La are frequent findings in SS. However, both elevated ANA titers and RF are non-specific for SS. Anti-SSA/Ro is positive in 74% of SS patients, while anti-SSB/La is positive in 52% of SS patients [15]. A decision has been made by a combined European and American rheumatologic consensus group to utilize anti-SSA/Ro as the sole serologic linchpin in SS diagnosis [10, 16].

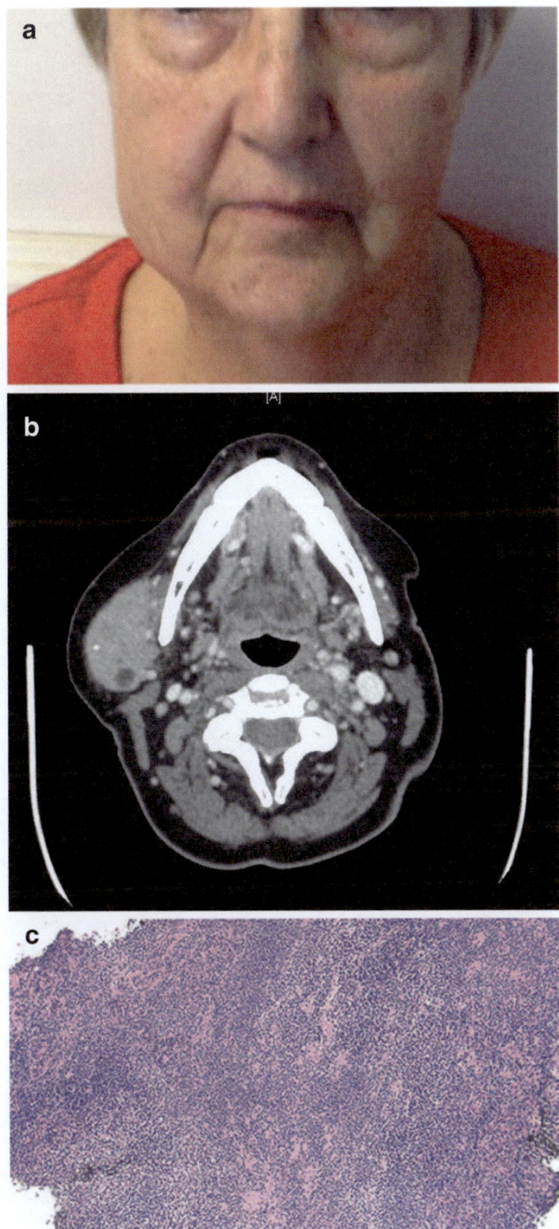

Fig. 7.10 (**a**) Patient C. Right parotid swelling. MALT lymphoma in patient with Sjögren syndrome. (**b**) Patient C. CT scan. Right parotid swelling (P). MALT lymphoma. (**c**) Patient C. Histology. MALT lymphoma. Parotid gland

Imaging can be of value in the diagnosis of SS. The oldest procedure, sialography, has drawbacks in that it is invasive and involves technical skill, patient cooperation, and the patient's exposure to radiation. However, the procedure has value because it will clearly delineate duct distribution and outline. A sialectic pattern, which varies from fine stippling to a more gross globular pattern, will be observed (Fig. 7.11). Cyst-like dilations of the ducts from the effects of salivary retention cause these stippled/globular spherical pools of contrast imaged by the sialogram. This

Fig. 7.11 (**a**) Sialogram depicting normal parotid duct arborization. (**b**) Sjögren syndrome. Sialogram. Punctate sialectasis. (**c**) Sjögren syndrome. Sialogram. Globular sialectasis. (**d**) Sjögren syndrome. Sialogram. Bilateral globular sialectasis

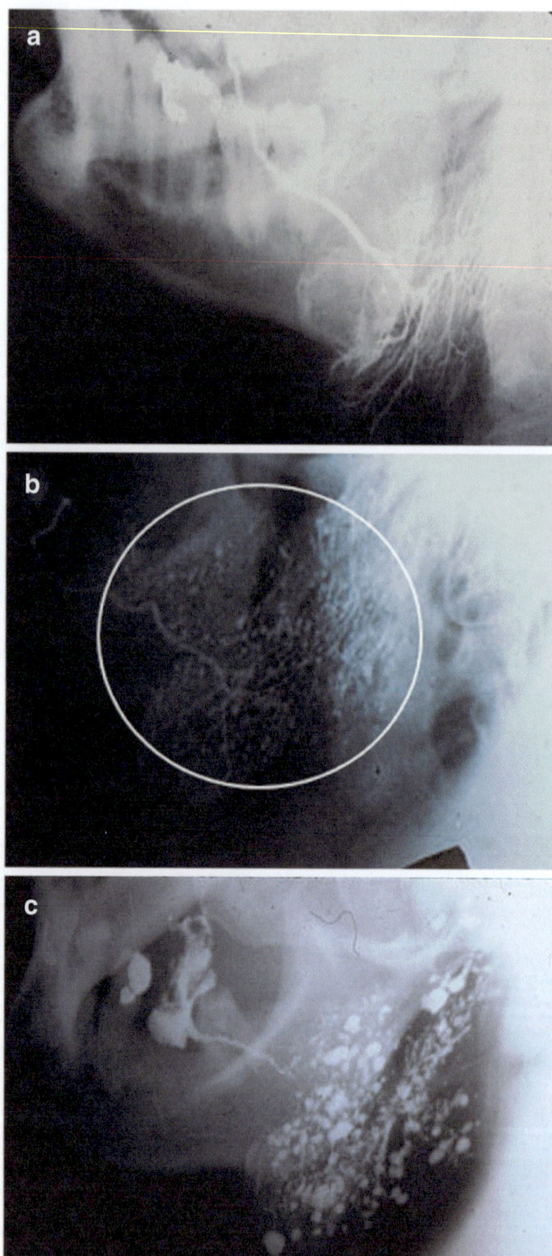

Fig. 7.11 (continued)

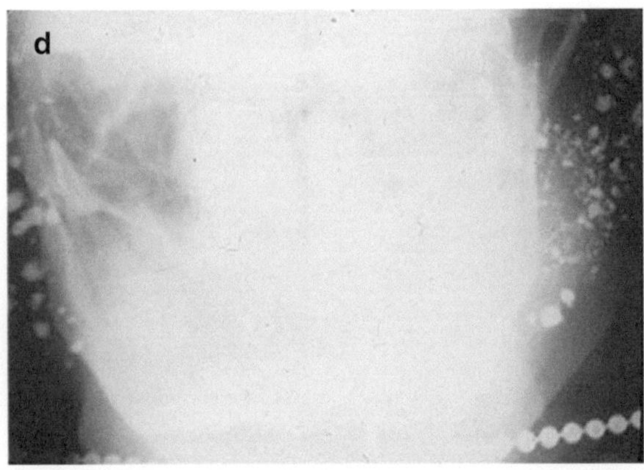

sialographic pattern probably originates from a duct metaplasia that is induced by the infiltrating lymphoproliferation associated with SS. The metaplasia is manifested by a thickening of the duct epithelium which in turn causes luminal narrowing. Salivary retention develops and results in cyst-like duct dilations. If a history of a secondary ascending infection is present, multiple stricturing of the Stensen duct, mimicking a string of sausages, from inflammatory scarring will also be observed (Fig. 7.8d).

Close scrutiny of a parotid CT scan in SS will show multiple small lucencies that represent the duct dilations seen in sialectasis. The MRI of an SS compromised PG will reveal a heterogeneous signal-intensity distribution on T1- and T2-weighted images. The multiple hypointense and hyperintense areas present a salt-and-pepper appearance [17]. Ultrasound has proven to be the most frequent imaging technique used as an aid in attaining an SS diagnosis (Fig. 7.12). Multiple hypoechoic areas, from lymphocytic foci and/or duct dilations with parenchymal inhomogeneity, will be noted involving the four main salivary glands [7, 17–19]. Sialendoscopy represents a new means of viewing the duct system of an SS involved PG and aids in the diagnosis of patients with sicca symptomatology. A pale poorly vascularized duct wall and a narrowed lumen obstructed by mucus plugs and debris will be visualized by the endoscope [17].

There are several characteristic histologic features associated with SS involvement of the salivary glands. PG biopsies reveal the presence of B and T cell lymphocytes clustering around the striated ducts (Fig. 7.6). In milder lesions, T cells predominate, whereas B cells become the dominant lymphocyte in the more advanced SS cases [19, 20]. Lymphoepithelial lesions, defined as hyperplastic ductal epithelium with infiltrating lymphocytes, develop. Progression to complete ductal obstruction with the formation of a solid mass [9, 17], referred to as an epimyoepithelial island [19] (Fig. 7.13), can be anticipated. These islands of obliterated ducts are seen in a sea of lymphocytes. Acinar atrophy, duct dilations, and

Fig. 7.12 Sjögren
syndrome. Ultrasound
demonstrates hypoechoic
areas in a background of
parenchymal
inhomogeneity

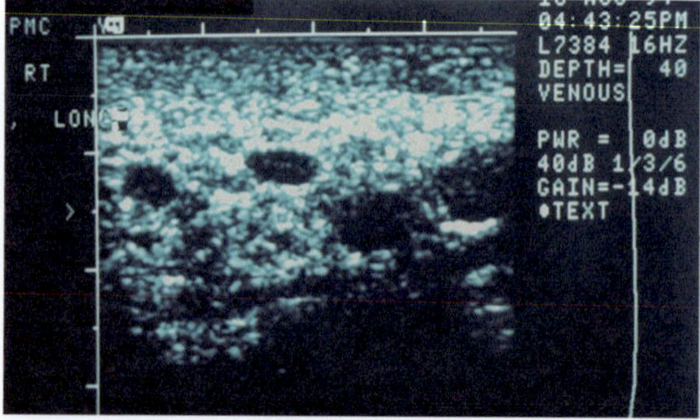

Fig. 7.13 Sjögren
syndrome. Microscopic
view of epimyoepithelial
island

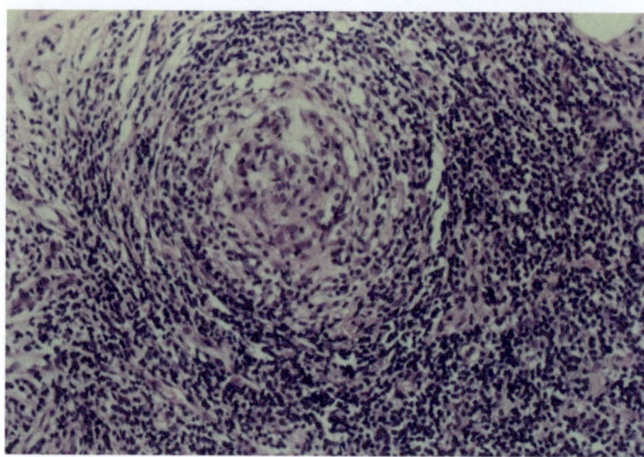

fibrosis accompany lymphoproliferation. Germinal centers, ectopically located in a
salivary gland, represent a higher degree of disease activity and serve as harbingers
of lymphoma. The lymphoma results from aggressive B cell proliferation and is
most frequently a MALT lymphoma but can be a nodal marginal zone lymphoma or
a diffuse large B-cell lymphoma [10].

Numerous classification criteria for the signs/symptoms required for a diagnosis
of primary SS have been proposed. Previously, the diagnostic requirements included
both objective and subjective symptoms. Problems developed because many of the
subjective symptoms often proved to be anecdotal. They were difficult to objectively verify for substantiation of an SS diagnosis because they were only subjective
in nature. Therefore an international consensus group, representing a range of clinical specialties, was convened to establish objective standards for an SS diagnosis.
This group of rheumatologic/SS clinicians formulated a set of classification criteria
for SS that used guidelines established by the American College of Rheumatology
(ACR) and the European League Against Rheumatism (EULAR) [16]. The group
assigned weighted scores of 1–3 points to five objective signs/symptoms associated
with SS. Emphasis was placed on the histologic presence of a focal lymphocytic

sialadenitis (Fig. 7.6) and the presence of serologic anti-SSA/Ro. A total point score of 4 or more was established as a prerequisite for the diagnosis of primary SS [16]. The five test criteria with their scores can be listed as follows:

1. The serologic presence of anti-SSA/Ro **(3 points)**. The presence of anti-SSB/La is not included because it mostly occurs in the presence of anti-SSA while it rarely occurs alone.
2. A positive labial salivary gland histologic finding **(3 points)**. Foci of lymphocytic infiltration into the salivary gland must be present. A focus is defined as a grouping of 50 or more lymphocytes in a 4 mm^2 of tissue (Fig. 7.6) [21]. At least one focus must be present to signal participation in a diagnosis of primary SS. A 6–9% false positive rate will be found in normal controls [19]. Major salivary gland biopsies are avoided because of the possible associated surgical complications (facial nerve palsy, fistula, and cosmetic issues). Besides, the simplicity of performing a labial salivary gland biopsy makes it a procedure of choice (Fig. 7.14).
3. A positive ocular staining score **(1 point)**. This score is determined by the ophthalmologist. Any existing corneal ulcerations or conjunctival damage is examined with a slit lamp, and the intensity of each is scored after staining with fluorescein and lissamine green, respectively. A combined score of 5 or more in at least one eye is required for positive inclusion in SS diagnosis.
4. A Schirmer test is positive **(1 point)** if 5 mm or less of a standardized filter paper strip, held in place beneath the lower eyelid, is moistened in 5 min in at least one eye [22].
5. An unstimulated whole saliva flow rate of only 0.1 mL/min or less is collected over a 15-min span [10, 23] **(1 point)**.

Because there is no specific cure for SS, treatment is usually directed at ameliorating symptoms of the exocrinopathy and controlling the systemic manifestations of the disease. Hydroxychloroquine (HCQ), an anti-inflammatory and anti-malarial

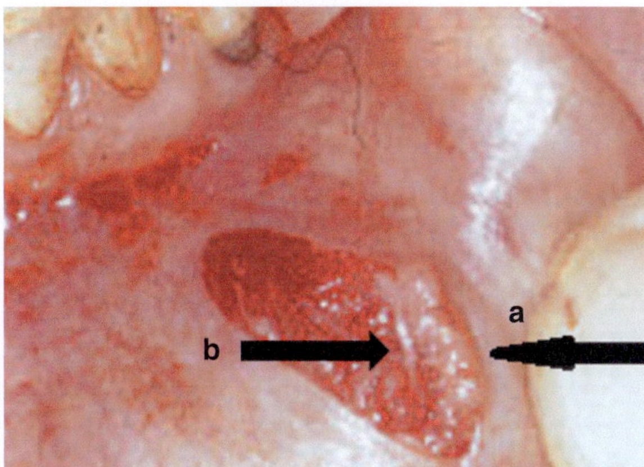

Fig. 7.14 Labial gland (arrow A) biopsy. Linear glistening structure (arrow B) is a mental nerve filament

drug, has been advocated as an agent that can improve SS symptoms. However, clinical trials have failed to confirm its therapeutic value [7]. Regardless, HCQ can be helpful in the management of the arthralgias that develop in SS [5–7, 10]. Provided that some residual functioning salivary gland tissue is present, the cholinergic agonists pilocarpine or cevimeline will kick start surviving secreting acini into overdrive and result in some alleviation of the dry mouth. Glucocorticoids or immunosuppressants can be prescribed when the viscera are damaged [6].

Besides its diagnostic value, sialendoscopy can be therapeutically utilized to treat SS. The instrument can function to irrigate salivary ducts, wash out contained ductal debris, dilate the duct, break up strictures, and infuse steroids to combat inflammation. Therefore, sialendoscopy will serve, at least to a limited extent, to improve SS symptomatology. The procedure facilitates ductal drainage and discourages the effects of a continued invasion of the PG by ascending infections. Immunosuppressants and rituximab have some limited success in controlling the systemic organ manifestations seen in patients with SS [7, 10]. Rituximab can cause B cell depletion and may have value in the treatment of B cell lymphomas associated with SS [6, 19]. B cell activating factor (BAFF), produced by immune and epithelial cells [10], is concerned with B cell maturation and it enhances the immune response. Consequently, BAFF blocking agents such as belimumab may be effective in SS treatment [7, 24]. These blocking agents can be used in conjunction with the standard chemotherapeutic medications (cyclophosphamide, doxorubicin, vincristine, and prednisolone) for treating the salivary gland B cell lymphomas that may develop in SS [5].

Adjunctive aids for the care of the significant oral dryness include mouthwashes, artificial salivas, and oral lubricants. Patients should be encouraged to frequently sip water and use sugarless sour candy and/or sugarless chewing gum, both of which act as salivary stimulants. Fluorides should be used to control the increased caries that results from hyposalivation (Fig. 7.15). Abstinence from smoking and alcohol is to be encouraged. If possible, anticholinergic medications prescribed for unrelated systemic problems are to be avoided.

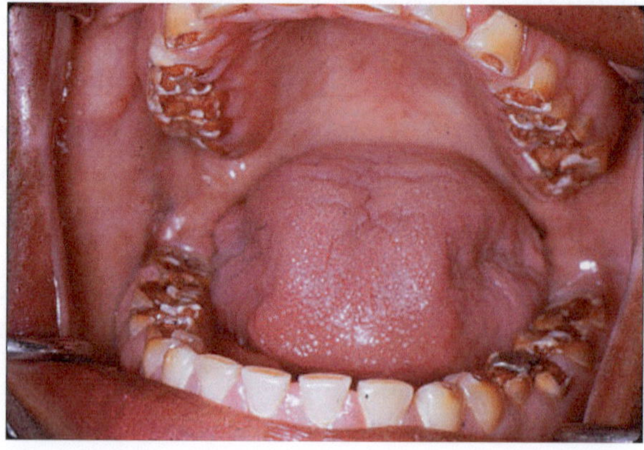

Fig. 7.15 Sjögren syndrome. Rampant caries

Immunoglobulin G4-Related Disease (IgG4-RD)

Immunoglobulin G4-related disease (IgG4-RD) represents a constellation of immune-mediated diseases that affect multiple organs. Although any organ can be involved, the pancreas, salivary glands, lacrimal glands, lung, lymph nodes, retroperitoneum, and kidney are most vulnerable. IgG4-RD is a fibroinflammatory condition of unknown etiology. It has been suggested that an unknown immune trigger incites a soft tissue B cell infiltration into multiple organ structures with the B cells subsequently differentiating into plasma cells [25]. This histopathologic picture and the presence of tumor-like sclerosing masses in the involved organs are characteristic of this disease entity. The organ involvement can develop synchronously or metachronously.

The concept of IgG4-RD was originally formulated by Hamano et al. in 2001 [26], when they noted a rise in serum IgG4 levels in patients with autoimmune pancreatitis (AIP). Subsequently, several other conditions, previously thought to be unrelated, were found to occur concurrently with AIP while simultaneously possessing similar clinical and pathological signs and symptoms. After the pancreas, the second most common site of an IgG4-RD presentation is the head and neck area [27] with the salivary glands being frequently involved. The wide variety of IgG4-RDs includes Riedel thyroiditis, interstitial pneumonitis, interstitial nephritis, lymphadenopathies, and retroperitoneal fibrosis. Küttner tumor (KT) and Mikulicz disease (MD), entities that involve the salivary glands, have also been recognized as part of the IgG4-RD spectrum [27–29].

Because IgG4-RD represents a newly recognized disease, its statistical incidence awaits future investigation. Males in a ratio of 3:1 [30] are more often seen with the disease than women. However, when the condition is limited to the head and neck area (24% of the time), females are more commonly involved [25, 28, 31]. Although IgG4-RD can develop in children, adults over 50 years of age are the typical group seen with the disease [32, 33].

Because no specific serologic markers for IgG4-RD have been found, diagnosis is challenging. Symptomatology is varied and is dependent on the extent of the disease and the organ that is involved. Clinical, radiologic, and serologic findings offer diagnostic clues that are helpful, but not sufficiently substantive to verify a diagnosis of IgG4-RD without histologic evidence. Therefore, an international consensus group was convened to create a diagnostic protocol. The group established the following five pathologic conditions whose presence in a surgical specimen provided guidelines for an accurate and meaningful diagnosis [29, 30]:

1. A dense lymphoplasmacytic infiltrate into the involved organ
2. Tissue fibrosis with a storiform pattern
3. Obliterative phlebitis
4. Abundant infiltrating IgG4-positive plasma cells
5. IgG4 to IgG plasma cell ratio exceeding 40% on immunohistochemistry

Items 1–3 represent the classic pathologic features of IgG4-RD, while items 4 and 5 are not specific for IgG4-RD but do serve as contributory diagnostic evidence. Besides these microscopic findings, diffuse tumor-like firm masses are present clinically in the involved organs. The serology will reveal elevated levels of IgG4 (>135 mg/dL) in 60–70% of the IgG4-RD patients [27]. This serologic finding is supportive, but nonspecific for IgG4-RD because similar elevated levels can be found in a variety of infectious, inflammatory, and neoplastic conditions. By itself, an elevated serum IgG4 has only a positive predictive value of 34% [25] for IgG4-RD. An eosinophilia may also be present and serves as adjunctive diagnostic evidence [29, 33]. Serologic elevated levels of the erythrocyte sedimentation rate and C-reactive protein also occur but again are non-specific markers of IgG4-RD [29]. A confident diagnosis of IgG4-RD awaits the histopathologic substantiation from a surgical specimen.

Salivary gland (SG) involvement in IgG4-RD is frequently present. In a retrospective review of 493 IgG4-RD patients, Wallace et al. [34] found that 38% had SG symptomatology. Isolated firm painless bilateral submandibular salivary gland (SMSG) swellings were the most common presenting sign (Fig. 7.16). The stimulus for a patient visit emanates from a concern regarding the SMSG's persistent swelling. The SMSG swellings are often accompanied by bilateral lacrimal gland swellings. Liu et al. [35] reviewed 428 positive IgG4-RD patients and reported that those patients who had SG disease (IgG4-SG) had their disease symptoms confined to the head and neck regions with frequent involvement of the lacrimal glands. The lacrimal gland, parotid gland (PG), and SMSG are usually involved together, but in different combinations [33]. Systemic disease manifestations tend to be present in the absence of SG disease [35].

Although the SMSG is the salivary gland that is usually affected by IgG4-RD, the parotid and sublingual glands, as well as the minor salivary glands, have occasionally been compromised by the disease. The SMSG swelling usually has a

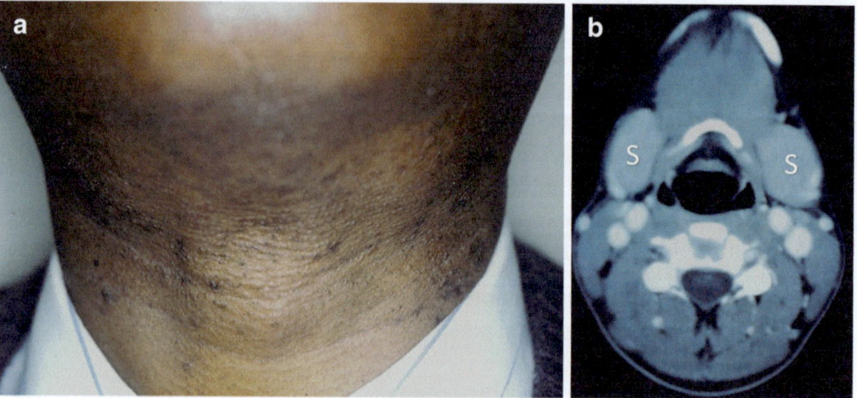

Fig. 7.16 (**a**) Immunoglobulin G4-related salivary gland disease (IgG4-SD). Patient D. Bilateral submandibular gland swelling. (**b**) IgG4-SD. Patient D. CT scan demonstrates bilateral enlarged submandibular glands (S)

long-standing unrelenting history. There is no history of fluctuation in gland size in association with meals and pain is not an issue. Palpation indicates each SMSG is well-circumscribed, firm, and painless, such that it closely resembles a neoplasm. A moderate hyposalivation is present [29, 33] because of the acinar replacement by the pathology associated with IgG4-RD.

As stated, KT and MD have been accepted into the spectrum of IgG4-RD. According to the new diagnostic classification, KT and MD are thought to be expressions of IgG4-RD in the SG and are considered variations of IgG4-related sialadenitis [27]. The chronic sclerosing sialadenitis seen in KT is similar to the pathologic fibrotic pattern associated with IgG4-RD of the SMSG, and the presence of many IgG4-positive plasma cells in KT adds to the similarity. Patients with KT do not show involvement of other organs. It is possible that KT represents an early or immature form of IgG4-RD. KT usually involves the SMSG unilaterally, but bilateral cases do exist. Clinically, KT is a painless circumscribed SG mass that is considered a pseudotumor because of its clinical similarity to a true tumor. MD differs clinically from KT in that it involves the SMSG bilaterally, while it also causes bilateral symmetrical swellings of the parotid and lacrimal glands. It may be accompanied by oral and ocular dryness [27]. Histologically, MD reveals a benign and significant tumor-like invasion by IgG4-bearing plasma cells with hyperplastic germinal center formation within the glands [27, 29].

Diagnosis of IgG4-SG disease is clinched with the microscopic findings (Fig. 7.17). Total examination of a surgical biopsy of an involved SMSG will reveal an abundant lymphoplasmacytic and IgG4 positive plasma cell infiltration, a preserved glandular lobular architecture, large lymphoid follicles with hypercellular germinal centers, some sparing of the salivary ducts, and a mild acinar destruction [29]. Storiform fibrosis and obliterative phlebitis are inconsistently seen in the SGs [29]. Occasionally, because of concerns with cosmetics or with danger to the mandibular marginal branch of the facial nerve, a labial salivary gland biopsy has been

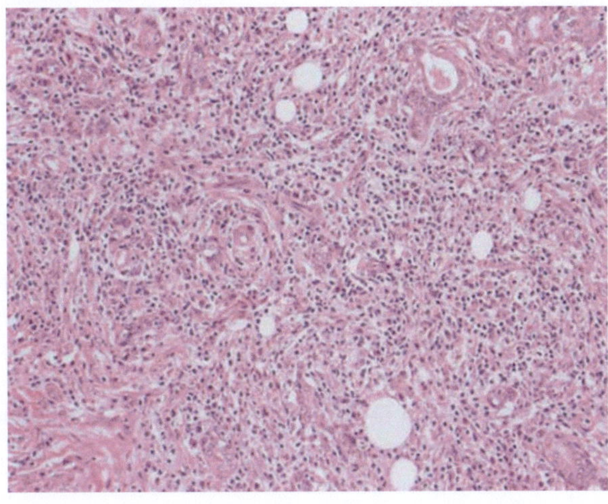

Fig. 7.17
IgG4-SD. Extensive infiltration of lymphocytes and plasma cells into a fibrous stroma. (Deshpande V, et al. Modern Pathol 2012;25:1181)

performed as an alternative to an SMSG diagnostic surgical biopsy [36]. Positive results have been obtained, but the sensitivity of the labial salivary biopsy is low [27].

Imaging of the SMSG depicts an enlarged gland with a non-specific pattern that is consistent with a non-specific fibro-inflammatory process [25]. Definitive IgG4-RD imaging diagnostic characteristics are not available. However, imaging derives its usefulness by differentiating IgG4-SG disease from a possible malignancy or infectious disease [27]. Imaging must be integrated into the clinical, serologic, and pathologic findings in order to aid in diagnosis.

The disease should be treated early in its development prior to the onset of an organ dysfunction caused by any accompanying extensive fibrosis. However, in IgG4-RD patients with asymptomatic lymphadenopathy, slight SG enlargement, and even with incidentally detected lung nodules, watchful waiting with re-evaluation every 6 months is a therapeutic option [28, 33]. Glucocorticoids have proven to be an effective therapy for a symptomatically active IgG4-RD. Quick resolutions usually result, but remissions do occur [29]. Immunosuppressants (methotrexate, azathioprine, cyclosporin, and tacrolimus) can be used with the glucocorticoid for better results [37]. Rituximab can be prescribed therapeutically in combination with a corticosteroid and it also has been advocated for maintenance therapy [29, 33]. After treatment, a long-term survival period of 20 years can be expected [25].

Primary Biliary Cholangitis

Primary biliary cholangitis (PBC), formerly known as primary biliary cirrhosis, is an autoimmune liver disease characterized by the presence of antimitochondrial antibodies (AMA) and a progressive intrahepatic bile duct destruction leading to cirrhosis and eventual liver failure. The exact etiology of this autoimmune disease remains an enigma. However, the presence of a PBC familial history, urinary tract infection, or smoking along with environmental factors is reported to be associated with PBC pathogenesis [38–40]. The disease predominantly involves women in the sixth decade of their life [38, 39], who are often found to be subjectively asymptomatic but have unsuspected elevations of liver enzymes. This relatively benign state may last for many years, but progression in 2–4 years is recognized in most patients when fatigue, itching, and jaundice develop. A female-to-male ratio of 10:1 and a prevalence of 33.8 per 100,000 in the Japanese population have been reported [39, 41].

The most common early PBC symptom is fatigue, which is present in 80% of the patients [38]. Jaundice and pruritus from cholestasis are also present in a high percentage of PBS patients [42]. A decreased bone density, with features of osteopenia and osteoporosis, has been reported and results from cholestatic-induced malabsorption of vitamin D [38, 39]. Additionally, investigation will usually uncover the co-existence of other autoimmune diseases in the majority of PBC patients. Most commonly, Sjögren syndrome (SS) and autoimmune thyroiditis are present, but systemic lupus erythematosus, systemic sclerosis, and rheumatoid arthritis have also been recognized [43]. Occasionally, hepatocellular carcinomas are encountered in PBC patients [39]. A confident PBC diagnosis is based on the presence of two of three of the following objective criteria: high AMA titers, elevated liver enzymes, and positive histology.

The presence of AMA in 90–100% of the PBC patients is a key component in PBC diagnosis. Diagnosis is based on the existence of AMA in titers of 1:40 or higher [39, 40, 44]. The consistent presence of elevated cholestatic enzymes (alkaline phosphatase, glutamyl transferase, and bilirubin) also serves as PBC markers [38, 39]. Serologically, hyperlipidemia is present in 80% of PBC patients [40]. Biopsy specimens will demonstrate a non-suppurative cholangitis and a bile duct destruction that progresses to cirrhosis within 4 years [42, 45]. Histologically, a florid lymphocytic infiltration will also be noted in the liver.

Abdominal imaging does not contribute to the diagnosis of PBC, but ultrasound studies can serve to rule out other causes of cholestatic disease. Ultrasound can also help in monitoring and assessing the severity of liver damage [42].

Fortunately, drug therapy is available for managing PBC. The treatment does not offer a cure, but disease progression will be slowed significantly. Ursodeoxycholic acid (UDCA) therapy has proven to be an effective therapeutic agent. Obeticholic acid and fenofibrate have been used in conjunction with UDCA [42]. The drugs function to lower serum levels of bilirubin and alkaline phosphatase. Nevertheless, PBC advances in most patients to liver cirrhosis and liver failure, but the rate of its advance varies. End-stage liver disease mandates a need for a liver transplant [38, 42].

A close relationship between PBC and SS exists. These two autoimmune diseases can demonstrate similar immunological destruction of the epithelium of the salivary and lacrimal glands, the bile ducts, and even urinary tract epithelium, a phenomenon referred to as epithelitis [46]. Liver disease has proven to be a common non-exocrine feature of primary SS [47, 48] with 6.6% of 410 SS patients reported to have PBC [44]. Conversely, the prevalence of SS in PBC patients has been reported to be in the range of 34–81% [39, 43, 44, 48]. The sicca signs, hyposalivation (Fig. 7.18), and hypolacrimation, which are present in this PBC group, tend to be milder than what is seen in classic primary SS patients [48]. Regardless, the hyposalivation is sufficient to cause extensive caries, oral burning, dysphagia, and a cobblestone or an atrophic tongue, while the hypolacrimation will cause subjective burning and itching sensations in the eyes. PBC patients who had biopsies of their labial salivary glands, a significant procedure in SS diagnosis, were reported to demonstrate the typical microscopic focal mononuclear cell infiltrations associated with SS in 14 of 15 specimens [49]. A detailed review of SS will be found in the beginning of this chapter.

Parotid sialography has also been used as a tool to investigate PBC patients. Sialectasis, a droplet pattern characteristically seen in SS, was observed in 9 of 14 PBC patients [50], while another report indicated 18 of 22 PBC patients demonstrated sialectasis sialographically (Fig. 7.19) [51].

A curative regimen for any co-existing SS is not available. Therefore, the sicca and its sequelae that develop in PBC patients are treated palliatively as outlined in the previous section on SS. Because of the very high correlation between PBC and

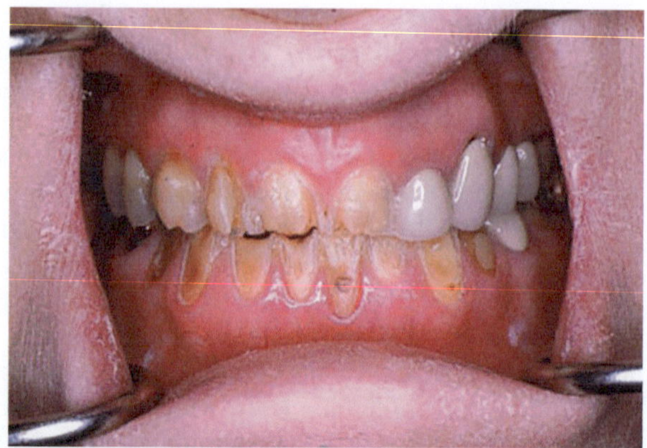

Fig. 7.18 Primary biliary cholangitis. Dry mouth and lips with enamel loss

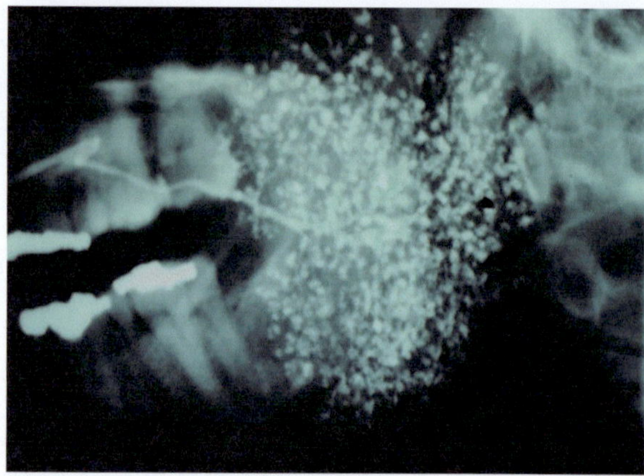

Fig. 7.19 Primary biliary cholangitis. Parotid sialogram reveals sialectic pattern

SS, an evaluation of tear and salivary production should be performed once PBC has been diagnosed. The progress to corneal ulceration from the frequent presence of hypolacrimation or oral problems from decreased salivation can be discouraged with an early diagnosis and the use of cholinergic drugs. Artificial salivas, lubricants, and mouthwashes are available as adjunctive aids in combating oral dryness. Fluorides can be prescribed to control the increased incidence of caries caused by hyposalivation.

Graft-Versus-Host Disease

Graft-versus-host disease (GvHD) (GvHD) is an autoimmune complication commonly encountered after an allogeneic hematopoietic stem cell transplantation (HSCT). The transplantation procedure is usually performed therapeutically for patients with acute lymphatic or acute myeloid leukemias or high-risk myelodysplastic syndrome [52, 53]. In GvHD, the donated cells view the recipient's body as foreign when the transplant is received from an HLA-mismatched related donor or from an HLA-matched unrelated donor. GvHD occurs in 40–70% of the transplant patients if the donor is unrelated and 25–45% of the recipients if the HLA-matched donor is related [53, 54]. The pathogenesis of GvHD is based on donor graft T lymphocytes that recognize antigenic disparities between the donor and recipient and cause damage via cytotoxicity to a variety of the recipient's tissues and organs [54]. Therefore, the severity of GvHD damage correlates with the number of T cells transfused [55].

Acute and chronic forms of GvHD exist, each with its own clinical features. Acute GvHD usually develops as an acute inflammatory syndrome within 100 days of the transplant procedure [56]. Although chronologically acute GvHD occurs earlier than the chronic form, diagnosis is more accurately based on their clinical presentation. The symptomatology of acute GvHD classically includes skin changes resembling widespread lichen planus and liver and gastrointestinal involvement [55]. Rarely are the oral tissues involved in acute GvHD, whereas oral problems are quite common in chronic GvHD with oral lesions reported in 45–83% of chronic GvHD patients [53, 57].

Numerous organ and tissue involvements, a persistence of years, and a variable severity are characteristics of chronic GvHD. Chronic GvHD is characterized by chronic inflammation and fibrosis and is considered an autoimmune-like multisystemic disease [53, 54, 57]. It is a significant complication encountered by long-term survivors of HSCT, and it occurs in approximately half of the HSCT recipients [53, 58]. Chronic GvHD may develop as a progression from an existing acute form, after resolution of acute GvHD or de novo [54]. Symptoms of chronic GvHD, initiated by infiltrating T cells, can become manifest in the oral cavity, gastrointestinal tract, liver, skin, respiratory tract, eyes, genitals, and musculoskeletal and nervous systems [55]. Salivary gland (SG) involvement, lichen planus-like oral mucosal lesions, and a reduction in the extent of mouth opening due to cutaneous sclerosis are hallmarks of chronic GvHD oral expression [58, 59]. Clinically, the oral mucosa will demonstrate white striae, ulcers, or erythema [57]. Desquamative gingivitis, characterized by erythema, erosion, and friable loss of superficial epithelium, can develop [53].

Because major and minor SGs are implicated in the symptomatology of chronic GvHD, a review of salivary flow rates was performed for chronic GvHD patients [60]. A mean reduction of 55–90% in whole unstimulated salivary flow was found and was responsible for complaints of a dry mouth [54, 61]. Another study of 101 chronic GvHD patients revealed that 77% had hyposalivation, and significantly, it was almost always associated with hypolacrimation [61]. These sicca symptoms clinically mirror Sjögren syndrome (SS). Differentiation can be achieved by determining the absence of the diagnostic SS autoantibodies in chronic GvHD patients. Histopathologically, both major and minor salivary glands in patients with chronic

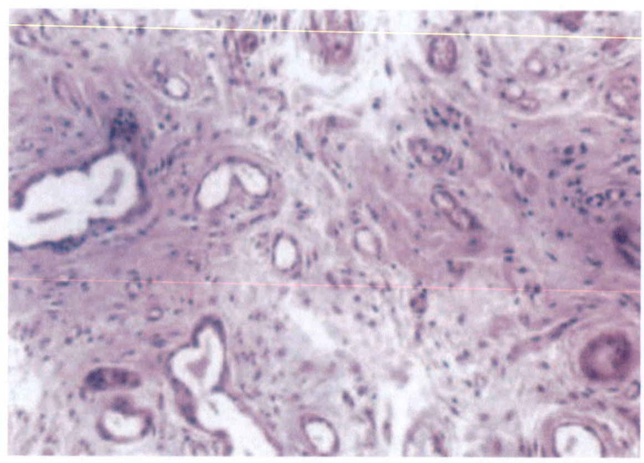

Fig. 7.20 Chronic graft-versus-host disease. Salivary gland biopsy. Loss of acini, fibrosis, and duct dilation. (Alborghetti MP, et al. J Oral Pathol Med 2005;34:486)

GvHD will demonstrate an infiltration of lymphocytes that is accompanied by duct dilation, parenchymal loss, and fibrosis (Fig. 7.20) [54, 60]. The lymphocytic infiltration is less intense than that seen in SS [60]. The level of pathologic change correlates directly with the level of hyposalivation. In addition to the decreased salivary quantity, sialochemical changes can occur in chronic GvHD and are reported to include higher concentrations of sodium, magnesium, albumin, immunoglobulin G, and total protein [61].

As stated, minor SG pathology, as well as major SG disease, can be associated with chronic GvHD. In addition to a lymphocytic infiltration in minor SGs, superficial oral mucoceles can occasionally occur at the oral mucosa's epithelial-connective tissue interface. These mucoceles tend to be asymptomatic, small, tense, translucent vesicles; occur in clusters mainly on the soft palate and buccal mucosa; and burst spontaneously [57] (Fig. 7.21). They are not preceded by local trauma. The oral lichenoid mucosal changes seen in chronic GvHD probably play a significant role in the development of these superficial mucoceles [62]. A full discussion of these superficial mucoceles can be found in Chap. 18.

The treatment regimen for chronic GvHD usually involves the prolonged use of immunosuppressives. Complete responses have been obtained in approximately 50% of the patients [54]. For oral dryness, the sialogogic agents, pilocarpine or cevimeline, can be prescribed because of their cholinergic ability. Sugarless chewing gum or sour candy will also serve to stimulate residual parenchyma. Artificial salivas, oral lubricants, and mouthwashes are available for adjunctive palliative therapy. Because candidiasis is encouraged by dry mouth and immunosuppression, antifungals should be available as part of the therapeutic regimen. Fluoride therapy is recommended to discourage increases in caries that may be the by-product of hyposalivation. Because the lesions associated with chronic GvHD can undergo malignant transformation, long-term follow-up is indicated.

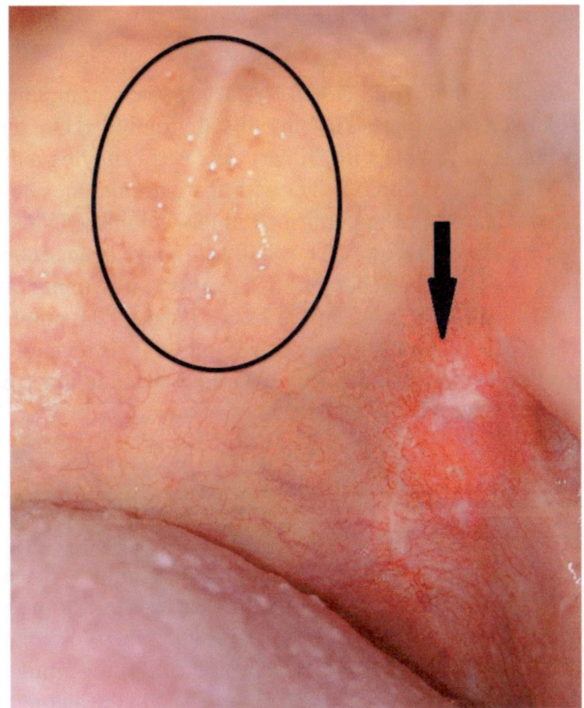

Fig. 7.21 Chronic graft-versus-host disease. Palate. Superficial mucoceles (circled) and lichenoid lesion (arrow)

Diabetes (Type I)

Blood sugar levels are regulated by the hormone insulin, produced by the pancreas. Autoimmune disease (AID) of the pancreas causes the immune system's destruction of the insulin-producing pancreatic cells and results in type I diabetes, whose peak age incidence is around 13 or 14 years. The cause of the immune system's misdirection is unknown. Women, as well as certain ethnic groups, seem to be more susceptible. A familial association may play a role in the onset of AID of the pancreas, and environmental factors may contribute. Type 2 diabetes does not have an autoimmune background. It usually develops in adults when normally produced insulin is not used properly by the body. These patients are considered to have a metabolic disease that causes insulin resistance.

Diabetic patients with persistent and painless bilateral parotid gland swellings have frequently been seen in the Salivary Gland Center. Their history and clinical examination facilitate a diagnosis of sialadenosis, initiated by diabetes. A review of sialadenosis and its relation to diabetes can be found in Chap. 9.

Autoimmune Thyroid Disease

Autoimmune thyroid disease (ATD) is a very common autoimmune condition confronted by humans. Hashimoto's thyroiditis (HT) represents the most frequent expression of ATD with Graves' disease occupying a distant second place.

The relationship of ATD with the autoimmune Sjögren syndrome (SS) is well known and has been confirmed in the Columbia University Salivary Gland Center (SGC). Patients with ATD, usually HT, have been seen in the SGC. They were seen because of the presence of SS. Therefore, it is important to be aware that ATD can occasionally be found in the background of the autoimmune SS patient and vice versa. The relationship between SS and ATD is reviewed in Chap. 10. SS also merits its own section and has been separately listed in this Chap. 7.

Myasthenia Gravis

Myasthenia gravis (MG) is a chronic autoimmune disease characterized by a disorder of neuromuscular function that causes skeletal muscle weakness. Disruption in neuromuscular transmission develops when circulating autoantibodies block/destroy acetylcholine (ACH) receptors, thus preventing the release of ACH. Because ACH is the key neurotransmitter involved in the autonomic nervous system innervation of the salivary glands, a decrease in secretory stimulation and volume might be anticipated in undiagnosed MG patients. However, no information regarding the possible presence of hyposalivation in MG was obtained from a literature review.

The Columbia University Salivary Gland Center (SGC) has had the opportunity to examine several MG patients whose complaint concerned hypersalivation. These patients were being treated with various inappropriate dosages of acetylcholinesterase (ACHE) inhibitors. Consequently, increased secretory activity from overdosage developed because of the prolonged presence of the ACH nerve transmitter. Treatment required adjustment in the prescribed dosage of the ACHE inhibitor.

Surprisingly, because the MG patients seen in the SGC only had concerns centering around hypersalivation, a further discussion of MG and the reason for the increased salivation can be found in the section on hypersalivation in Chap. 2.

References

1. Angum F, Khan T, Kaler J, Siddiqui L, Hussain A. The prevalence of autoimmune disorders in women: a narrative review. Cureus. 2020;12(5):e8094. Published 2020 May 13. https://doi.org/10.7759/cureus.8094.
2. Hayter SM, Cook MC. Updated assessment of the prevalence, spectrum and case definition of autoimmune disease. Autoimmun Rev. 2012;11(10):754–65. https://doi.org/10.1016/j.autrev.2012.02.001.

3. Sjögren H. Zur Kenntnis der keratoconjunctivitis sicca. Keratitis filiformis bei Hypofunktion der Tränendrüsen. Acta Ophthalmol. 1933;2:1–15.

4. Sebastian A, Szachowicz A, Wiland P. Classification criteria for secondary Sjögren's syndrome. Current state of knowledge. Reumatologia. 2019;57(5):277–80. https://doi.org/10.5114/reum.2019.89520.

5. Bowman SJ. Primary Sjögren's syndrome. Lupus. 2018;27(1_suppl):32–5. https://doi.org/10.1177/0961203318801673.

6. Chen X, Wu H, Wei W. Advances in the diagnosis and treatment of Sjogren's syndrome. Clin Rheumatol. 2018;37(7):1743–9. https://doi.org/10.1007/s10067-018-4153-8.

7. Mariette X, Criswell LA. Primary Sjögren's syndrome. N Engl J Med. 2018;378(10):931–9. https://doi.org/10.1056/NEJMcp1702514.

8. Brito-Zerón P, Acar-Denizli N, Zeher M, et al. Influence of geolocation and ethnicity on the phenotypic expression of primary Sjögren's syndrome at diagnosis in 8310 patients: a cross-sectional study from the Big Data Sjögren Project Consortium. Ann Rheum Dis. 2017;76(6):1042–50. https://doi.org/10.1136/annrheumdis-2016-209952.

9. Qin B, Wang J, Yang Z, et al. Epidemiology of primary Sjögren's syndrome: a systematic review and meta-analysis. Ann Rheum Dis. 2015;74(11):1983–9. https://doi.org/10.1136/annrheumdis-2014-205375.

10. Negrini S, Emmi G, Greco M, et al. Sjögren's syndrome: a systemic autoimmune disease. Clin Exp Med. 2022;22(1):9–25. https://doi.org/10.1007/s10238-021-00728-6.

11. Reveille JD, Wilson RW, Provost TT, Bias WB, Arnett FC. Primary Sjögren's syndrome and other autoimmune diseases in families. Prevalence and immunogenetic studies in six kindreds. Ann Intern Med. 1984;101(6):748–56. https://doi.org/10.7326/0003-4819-101-6-748.

12. Selmi C, Gershwin ME. Chronic autoimmune epithelitis in Sjögren's syndrome and primary biliary cholangitis: a comprehensive review. Rheumatol Ther. 2017;4(2):263–79. https://doi.org/10.1007/s40744-017-0074-2.

13. Baldini C, Pepe P, Quartuccio L, et al. Primary Sjogren's syndrome as a multi-organ disease: impact of the serological profile on the clinical presentation of the disease in a large cohort of Italian patients. Rheumatology (Oxford). 2014;53(5):839–44. https://doi.org/10.1093/rheumatology/ket427.

14. Kuklinski E, Asbell PA. Sjogren's syndrome from the perspective of ophthalmology. Clin Immunol. 2017;182:55–61. https://doi.org/10.1016/j.clim.2017.04.017.

15. Patel R, Shahane A. The epidemiology of Sjögren's syndrome. Clin Epidemiol. 2014;6:247–55. Published 2014 Jul 30. https://doi.org/10.2147/CLEP.S47399.

16. Shiboski CH, Shiboski SC, Seror R, et al. 2016 American College of Rheumatology/European League Against Rheumatism classification criteria for primary Sjögren's syndrome: a consensus and data-driven methodology involving three international patient cohorts. Ann Rheum Dis. 2017;76(1):9–16. https://doi.org/10.1136/annrheumdis-2016-210571.

17. van Ginkel MS, Glaudemans AWJM, van der Vegt B, et al. Imaging in primary Sjögren's syndrome. J Clin Med. 2020;9(8):2492. Published 2020 Aug 3. https://doi.org/10.3390/jcm9082492.

18. Huang PH, Chen DY. Diagnostic value of the salivary gland ultrasonography scoring system in patients with primary Sjogren's syndrome. J Med Ultrasound. 2021;29(4):235–6. Published 2021 Dec 15. https://doi.org/10.4103/jmu.jmu_144_21.

19. Liao R, Yang HT, Li H, et al. Recent advances of salivary gland biopsy in Sjögren's syndrome. Front Med (Lausanne). 2022;8:792593. Published 2022 Jan 10. https://doi.org/10.3389/fmed.2021.792593.

20. Mielle J, Tison A, Cornec D, Le Pottier L, Daien C, Pers JO. B cells in Sjögren's syndrome: from pathophysiology to therapeutic target [published online ahead of print, 2019 Feb 15]. Rheumatology (Oxford) 2019;key332. https://doi.org/10.1093/rheumatology/key332.

21. Daniels TE, Cox D, Shiboski CH, et al. Associations between salivary gland histopathologic diagnoses and phenotypic features of Sjögren's syndrome among 1,726 registry participants. Arthritis Rheum. 2011;63(7):2021–30. https://doi.org/10.1002/art.30381.

22. Whitcher JP, Shiboski CH, Shiboski SC, et al. A simplified quantitative method for assessing keratoconjunctivitis sicca from the Sjögren's syndrome international registry. Am J Ophthalmol. 2010;149(3):405–15. https://doi.org/10.1016/j.ajo.2009.09.013.

23. Navazesh M, Kumar SK, University of Southern California School of Dentistry. Measuring salivary flow: challenges and opportunities. J Am Dent Assoc. 2008;139 Suppl:35S–40S. https://doi.org/10.14219/jada.archive.2008.0353.

24. De Vita S, Quartuccio L, Seror R, et al. Efficacy and safety of belimumab given for 12 months in primary Sjögren's syndrome: the BELISS open-label phase II study. Rheumatology (Oxford). 2015;54(12):2249–56. https://doi.org/10.1093/rheumatology/kev257.

25. Behzadi F, Suh CH, Jo VY, Shanmugam V, Morgan EA, Guenette JP. Imaging of IgG4-related disease in the head and neck: a systematic review, case series, and pathophysiology update. J Neuroradiol. 2021;48(5):369–78. https://doi.org/10.1016/j.neurad.2021.01.006.

26. Hamano H, Kawa S, Horiuchi A, et al. High serum IgG4 concentrations in patients with sclerosing pancreatitis. N Engl J Med. 2001;344(10):732–8. https://doi.org/10.1056/NEJM200103083441005.

27. Kamiński B, Błochowiak K. Mikulicz's disease and Küttner's tumor as manifestations of IgG4-related diseases: a review of the literature. Reumatologia. 2020;58(4):243–50. https://doi.org/10.5114/reum.2020.98437.

28. Olmos RD, Rodrigues MAVM, Ferreira CR, Etrusco RCF, Romagnolli C. IgG4-related disease: a diagnostic challenge. Autops Case Rep. 2021;11:e2021312. Published 2021 Aug 20. https://doi.org/10.4322/acr.2021.312.

29. Skillington SA, Ogden MA. IgG4-related disease and the salivary glands: a review of pathophysiology, diagnosis, and management. Otolaryngol Clin North Am. 2021;54(3):497–508. https://doi.org/10.1016/j.otc.2021.02.002.

30. Deshpande V, Zen Y, Chan JK, et al. Consensus statement on the pathology of IgG4-related disease. Mod Pathol. 2012;25(9):1181–92. https://doi.org/10.1038/modpathol.2012.72.

31. Wang L, Zhang P, Zhang X, et al. Sex disparities in clinical characteristics and prognosis of immunoglobulin G4-related disease: a prospective study of 403 patients. Rheumatology (Oxford). 2019;58(5):820–30. https://doi.org/10.1093/rheumatology/key397.

32. Ruberto E, Gangemi E, Covello R, Pellini R, Vidiri A. MRI features in submandibular gland chronic sclerosing sialadenitis: a report of three cases and imaging findings. Iran J Otorhinolaryngol. 2020;32(113):397–401. https://doi.org/10.22038/ijorl.2020.47418.2583.

33. Karadeniz H, Vaglio A. IgG4-related disease: a contemporary review. Turk J Med Sci. 2020;50(SI-2):1616–31. Published 2020 Nov 3. https://doi.org/10.3906/sag-2006-375.

34. Wallace ZS, Zhang Y, Perugino CA, et al. Clinical phenotypes of IgG4-related disease: an analysis of two international cross-sectional cohorts. Ann Rheum Dis. 2019;78(3):406–12. https://doi.org/10.1136/annrheumdis-2018-214603.

35. Liu Y, Xue M, Wang Z, et al. Salivary gland involvement disparities in clinical characteristics of IgG4-related disease: a retrospective study of 428 patients. Rheumatology (Oxford). 2020;59(3):634–40. https://doi.org/10.1093/rheumatology/kez280.

36. Tachibana T, Orita Y, Wani Y, et al. Application of lip biopsy for the histological diagnosis of immunoglobulin G4-related disease [published online ahead of print, 2020 Nov 4]. Ear Nose Throat J. 2020;101(8):547–51. https://doi.org/10.1177/0145561320971932.

37. Omar D, Chen Y, Cong Y, Dong L. Glucocorticoids and steroid sparing medications monotherapies or in combination for IgG4-RD: a systematic review and network meta-analysis. Rheumatology (Oxford). 2020;59(4):718–26. https://doi.org/10.1093/rheumatology/kez380.

38. Selmi C, Bowlus CL, Gershwin ME, Coppel RL. Primary biliary cirrhosis. Lancet. 2011;377(9777):1600–9. https://doi.org/10.1016/S0140-6736(10)61965-4.

39. Tanaka A. Current understanding of primary biliary cholangitis. Clin Mol Hepatol. 2021;27(1):1–21. https://doi.org/10.3350/cmh.2020.0028.

40. Pandit S, Samant H. Primary biliary cholangitis. In: StatPearls. Treasure Island: StatPearls Publishing; 2022.

41. Sood S, Gow PJ, Christie JM, Angus PW. Epidemiology of primary biliary cirrhosis in Victoria, Australia: high prevalence in migrant populations. Gastroenterology. 2004;127(2):470–5. https://doi.org/10.1053/j.gastro.2004.04.064.

42. Laschtowitz A, de Veer RC, Van der Meer AJ, Schramm C. Diagnosis and treatment of primary biliary cholangitis. United European Gastroenterol J. 2020;8(6):667–74. https://doi.org/10.1177/2050640620919585.

43. Floreani A, Franceschet I, Cazzagon N, et al. Extrahepatic autoimmune conditions associated with primary biliary cirrhosis. Clin Rev Allergy Immunol. 2015;48(2–3):192–7. https://doi.org/10.1007/s12016-014-8427-x.

44. Hatzis GS, Fragoulis GE, Karatzaferis A, Delladetsima I, Barbatis C, Moutsopoulos HM. Prevalence and longterm course of primary biliary cirrhosis in primary Sjögren's syndrome. J Rheumatol. 2008;35(10):2012–6.

45. Locke GR 3rd, Therneau TM, Ludwig J, Dickson ER, Lindor KD. Time course of histological progression in primary biliary cirrhosis. Hepatology. 1996;23(1):52–6. https://doi.org/10.1002/hep.510230108.

46. Selmi C, Meroni PL, Gershwin ME. Primary biliary cirrhosis and Sjögren's syndrome: autoimmune epithelitis. J Autoimmun. 2012;39(1–2):34–42. https://doi.org/10.1016/j.jaut.2011.11.005.

47. Matsumoto T, Morizane T, Aoki Y, et al. Autoimmune hepatitis in primary Sjogren's syndrome: pathological study of the livers and labial salivary glands in 17 patients with primary Sjogren's syndrome. Pathol Int. 2005;55(2):70–6. https://doi.org/10.1111/j.1440-1827.2005.01790.x.

48. Zhu Y, Ma X, Tang X, Hua B. Liver damage in primary biliary cirrhosis and accompanied by primary Sjögren's syndrome: a retrospective pilot study. Cent Eur J Immunol. 2016;41(2):182–7. https://doi.org/10.5114/ceji.2016.60993.

49. Hansen BU, Lindgren S, Eriksson S, et al. Clinical and immunological features of Sjögren's syndrome in patients with primary biliary cirrhosis with emphasis on focal sialadenitis. Acta Med Scand. 1988;224(6):611–9. https://doi.org/10.1111/j.0954-6820.1988.tb19634.x.

50. Alarcón-Segovia D, Díaz-Jouanen E, Fishbein E. Features of Sjögren's syndrome in primary biliary cirrhosis. Ann Intern Med. 1973;79(1):31–6. https://doi.org/10.7326/0003-4819-79-1-31.

51. Golding PL, Smith M, Williams R. Multisystem involvement in chronic liver disease. Studies on the incidence and pathogenesis. Am J Med. 1973;55(6):772–82. https://doi.org/10.1016/0002-9343(73)90258-1.

52. Passweg JR, Baldomero H, Basak GW, et al. The EBMT activity survey report 2017: a focus on allogeneic HCT for nonmalignant indications and on the use of non-HCT cell therapies. Bone Marrow Transplant. 2019;54(10):1575–85. https://doi.org/10.1038/s41409-019-0465-9.

53. Haverman TM, Raber-Durlacher JE, Raghoebar II, et al. Oral chronic graft-versus-host disease: what the general dental practitioner needs to know. J Am Dent Assoc. 2020;151(11):846–56. https://doi.org/10.1016/j.adaj.2020.08.001.

54. Nagler RM, Nagler A. Salivary gland involvement in graft-versus-host disease: the underlying mechanism and implicated treatment. Isr Med Assoc J. 2004;6(3):167–72.

55. Ferrara JL, Deeg HJ. Graft-versus-host disease. N Engl J Med. 1991;324(10):667–74. https://doi.org/10.1056/NEJM199103073241005.

56. Nassereddine S, Rafei H, Elbahesh E, Tabbara I. Acute graft *versus* host disease: a comprehensive review. Anticancer Res. 2017;37(4):1547–55. https://doi.org/10.21873/anticanres.11483.

57. Elad S, Aljitawi O, Zadik Y. Oral graft-versus-host disease: a pictorial review and a guide for dental practitioners. Int Dent J. 2021;71(1):9–20. https://doi.org/10.1111/idj.12584.

58. van Leeuwen SJM, Potting CMJ, Huysmans MDNJM, Blijlevens NMA. Salivary changes before and after hematopoietic stem cell transplantation: a systematic review. Biol Blood Marrow Transplant. 2019;25(6):1055–61. https://doi.org/10.1016/j.bbmt.2019.01.026.

59. Noce CW, Gomes A, Copello A, et al. Oral involvement of chronic graft-versus-host disease in hematopoietic stem cell transplant recipients. Gen Dent. 2011;59(6):458–64.

60. Imanguli MM, Atkinson JC, Mitchell SA, et al. Salivary gland involvement in chronic graft-versus-host disease: prevalence, clinical significance, and recommendations for evaluation [published correction appears in Biol Blood Marrow Transplant. 2016 Jun;22(6):1147]. Biol Blood Marrow Transplant. 2010;16(10):1362–9. https://doi.org/10.1016/j.bbmt.2010.03.023.
61. Norhagen G, Engström PE, Björkstrand B, Hammarström L, Smith CI, Ringdén O. Salivary and serum immunoglobulins in recipients of transplanted allogeneic and autologous bone marrow. Bone Marrow Transplant. 1994;14(2):229–34.
62. García-F-Villalta MJ, Pascual-López M, Elices M, Daudén E, García-Diez A, Fraga J. Superficial mucoceles and lichenoid graft versus host disease: report of three cases. Acta Derm Venereol. 2002;82(6):453–5. https://doi.org/10.1080/000155502762064610.

Chapter 8
Granulomatous Inflammation

Louis Mandel

Abstract Granulomatous inflammation is a distinctive form of chronic inflammation characterized by the presence of tumor-like masses of granulomas. Sarcoidosis represents a non-caseating granulomatous disease that primarily involves the lungs. However, it is not unusual for sarcoidosis to also involve the salivary glands, with the parotid gland being the gland most often compromised. Tuberculosis, another granulomatous disease, differs from sarcoidosis in that it is a caseating granulomatous disease. Tuberculous intraglandular and paraglandular lymphadenopathies can involve the parotid gland area while swelling in the submandibular gland area is caused by paraglandular lymphadenopathies. Granulomatosis with polyangiitis (Wegener's), a potentially lethal granulomatous disease, is characterized by caseating granulomas of the upper and lower respiratory tracts, vasculitis of the small blood vessels and the presence of glomerulonephritis.

Introduction

Inflammation is a complex tissue, vascular, and lymphatic response to an irritant whose purpose is to localize and destroy the irritant and set the stage for repair. An irritant can be defined as an agent that interferes with normal cellular metabolism. Acute inflammation represents an immediate response to the irritant and is characterized by an increased movement from the blood of plasma and leukocytes to the area of injury (Fig. 8.1). Chronic inflammation is a prolonged response to an irritant whose histologic features include a variety of mononuclear cells (lymphocytes, plasma cells, and macrophages), fibroblasts, and blood vessels that replace the initial acute influx of leukocytes.

Granulomatous inflammation (GI) represents a distinctive form of chronic inflammation that is characterized by the presence of tumor-like masses of granulomas. Histologically, these granulomas consist of macrophages, giant cells, and

143

L. Mandel, *Clinical Management of Salivary Gland Disorders*,
https://doi.org/10.1007/978-3-031-50012-1_8

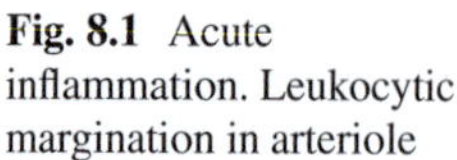

Fig. 8.1 Acute inflammation. Leukocytic margination in arteriole

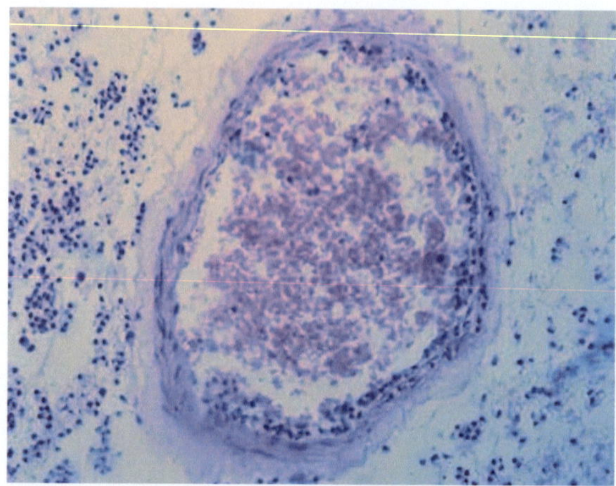

lymphocytes. Activated macrophages within the granuloma are referred to as epithelioid cells because of their resemblance to epithelial cells. The granulomas act to form a barrier around the offending irritant. The resulting granulomatous wall is persistent and forms when the irritant resists routine physiologic destruction via the body's normal inflammatory mechanisms.

The broad and most common causes of GI include infection, foreign bodies, and autoimmune diseases [1]. Tuberculosis, leprosy, and histoplasmosis represent granulomatous diseases that are incited by infectious agents. Foreign body granulomas represent reactions to inert materials (sutures, splinters, etc.) without an adaptive immune response. Immune responses are the result of a variety of conditions, most commonly an autoimmune disease such as sarcoidosis. The respiratory tract serves as a common site for the onset of GI. Tuberculosis and granulomatosis with polyangiitis (GPA) (Wegener's granulomatosis) represent necrotizing forms of GI that affect the respiratory tract, while sarcoidosis is a non-necrotizing variety that also mainly involves the respiratory system [2].

Sarcoidosis

Sarcoidosis is a multisystem non-caseating granulomatous disease that primarily manifests itself via pulmonary infiltrations and bilateral hilar lymphadenopathy. The lung is the most common organ affected by sarcoidosis and its presence, albeit often silent, can be radiographically demonstrated in 90% of the patients [3]. The exact etiology of sarcoidosis has not been determined. However, the prevailing theory is that various unidentified antigens, either infectious or environmental, can cause an exaggerated immune reaction in a genetically susceptible host [4]. In the United States, sarcoidosis has a prevalence of 10–40 cases/100,000 with females, particularly Blacks, being most susceptible [5] (Fig. 8.2). Young adults in the 20- to 40-year age category represent the largest group of sarcoidosis patients [6, 7].

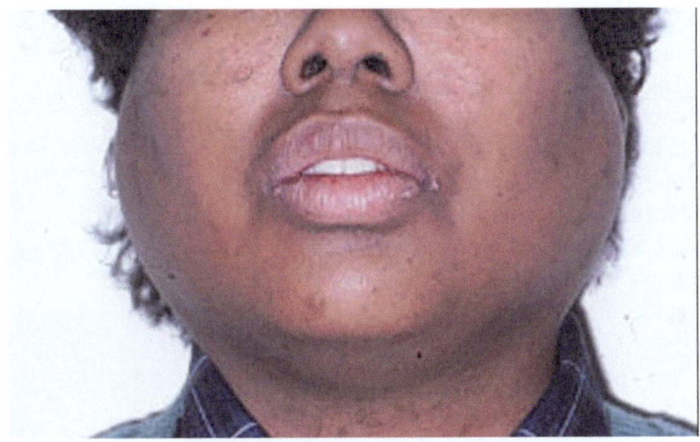

Fig. 8.2 Sarcoidosis with bilateral parotid gland involvement

Coughing, dyspnea, and chest pain are subjective complaints that accompany the disease and signal pulmonary involvement. Although chest films will substantiate lung involvement in the vast majority of sarcoidosis patients, normal chest films have been seen in 8–10% of the patients during their first examination [8]. Extrapulmonary disease is commonly present in lung-positive and lung-negative patients and most often can involve organs such as the skin, eyes, liver, spleen, and salivary glands. Although any organ can be involved, the lung represents the dominant injured structure. Spontaneous recovery has been reported in 50–66% of the patients [4, 9], but advanced pulmonary disease with pulmonary fibrosis has been observed in 1–5% of the patients [10]. In addition, malignant lymphoproliferations (lymphoma) occur 5.5 times more frequently in sarcoidosis patients than in the normal population [8]. The most common associated malignancy is Hodgkin's lymphoma occurring in an older patient with chronic sarcoidosis.

It is not unusual for sarcoidosis to involve a major salivary gland. Salivary gland swellings develop and are usually bilateral (Figs. 8.3 and 8.4) but can be unilateral (Fig. 8.5) in presentation. Palpation reveals the gland to be firm and painless. Fluctuation in size with meals does not occur. Hyposalivation may be a feature [8, 9, 11, 12]. The parotid gland (PG) has been estimated to be involved in 6% of sarcoidosis patients [7, 12]. The submandibular salivary gland (SMSG) is involved to a lesser extent and its involvement can occur with or without PG enlargement. The minor salivary glands are also affected by the disease process. Biopsies of the labial salivary glands demonstrate diagnostic granulomas in 50–58% of sarcoidosis patients [4, 11, 13].

Sarcoidal disease of the salivary glands manifests itself in a variety of patterns. The most common pattern is represented by systemic symptomatology and a major salivary gland swelling with histologic involvement of the minor salivary glands. Such patients generally have previously been diagnosed with sarcoidosis because of their respiratory signs and symptoms and varied organ involvement. A second pattern of salivary gland involvement is characterized by the absence of clinical PG/SMSG problems. These patients with known sarcoidosis may not show major salivary gland swellings, but microscopic sections of biopsied minor salivary glands will often demonstrate the hallmark granulomas. When examining this patient

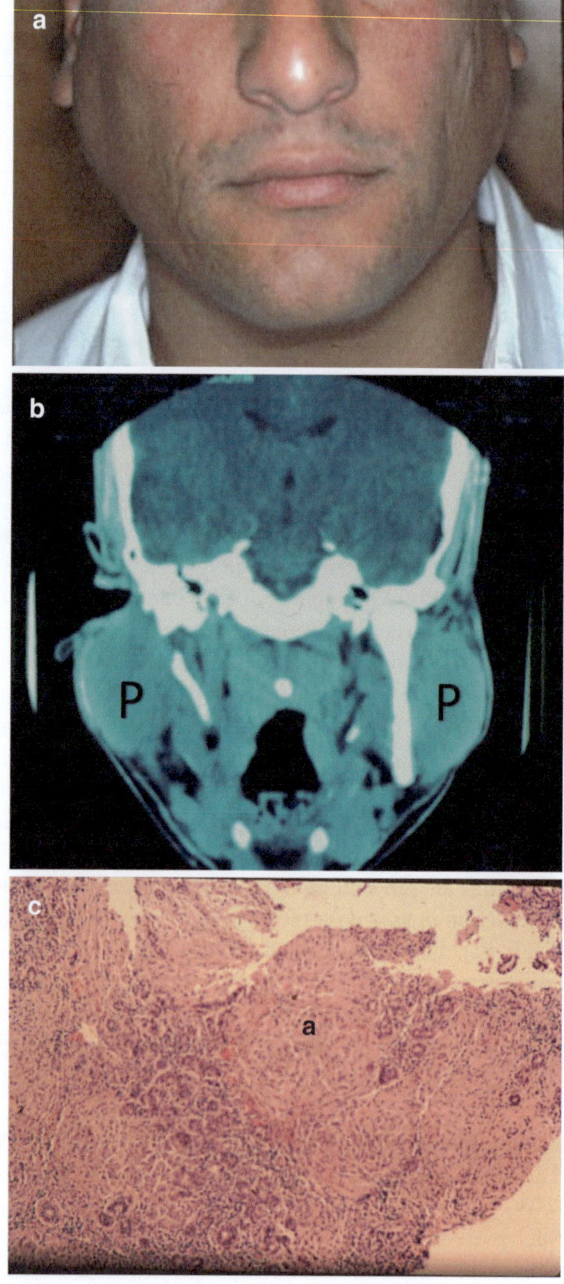

Fig. 8.3 (**a**) Sarcoidosis. Patient A. Bilateral parotid gland hypertrophy. (**b**) Sarcoidosis. Patient A. CT scan reveals bilaterally enlarged parotid glands (P). (**c**) Sarcoidosis. Patient A. Labial salivary gland biopsy. Granuloma (**a**) replacing normal glandular tissue

group, Cahn et al. [14] demonstrated granulomas in 38% of the palatal gland specimens, while Nessan and Jacoway [13] found sarcoidal granulomas in 58% of the examined labial salivary glands.

Patients with uveoparotid fever, also known as Heerfordt's syndrome, represent a third clinical category that is observed in recognized cases of systemic

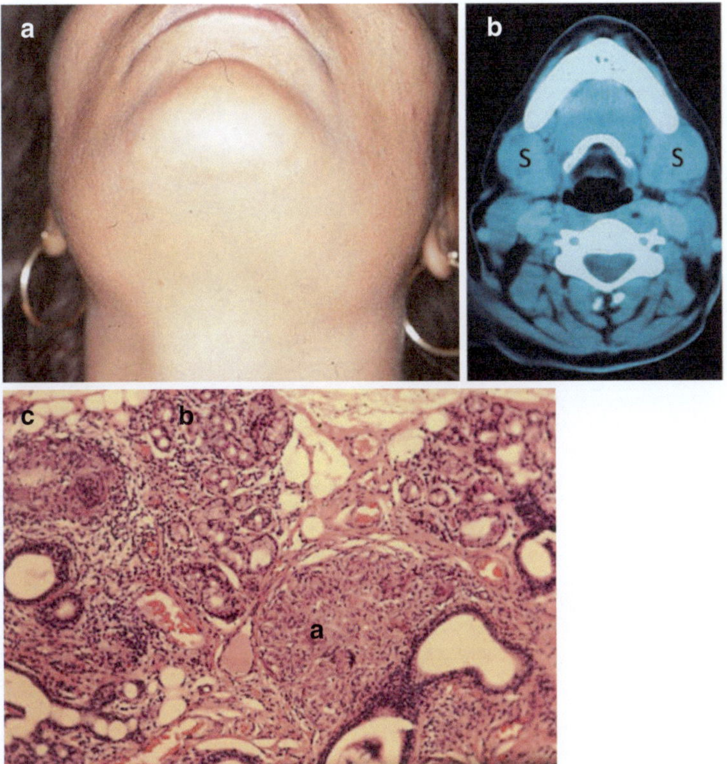

Fig. 8.4 (a) Sarcoidosis. Patient B. Bilateral submandibular gland swelling. (b) Sarcoidosis. Patient B. CT scan. Bilaterally enlarged submandibular glands (S). (c) Sarcoidosis. Patient B. Labial salivary gland biopsy. Granuloma (a) and glandular tissue (b) are present

sarcoidosis. Uveoparotid fever is identified by a triad of symptoms [10]: inflammation of the eye's uveal tract, bilateral PG swelling, and cranial nerve involvement, usually a facial palsy from a direct granulomatous infiltration into cranial nerve VII. Fever is an adjunctive symptom that may accompany the triad.

The fourth clinical salivary gland picture seen in sarcoidosis patients is those who demonstrate granulomatous infiltration into major and minor salivary glands with major salivary gland swellings in the absence of systemic symptoms of sarcoidosis. The major salivary gland swellings (PG and/or SMSG) may thus act as a clinical herald for the existence of a silent systemic sarcoidosis. These patients seek care because of the cosmetic distress caused by the persistently enlarged salivary gland.

No serologic finding is available to make a confident diagnosis for the existence of sarcoidosis. Angiotensin-converting enzyme (ACE) levels can be of some help. ACE is secreted by the lung's endothelial cells and alveolar macrophages as well as the granuloma's epithelioid cells [7, 15]. Levels of ACE are markedly elevated in 60% of sarcoidosis patients [3, 7] and the levels parallel the total body mass of granulomas. Unfortunately, the test is nonspecific because it is positive in other granulomatous entities such as miliary tuberculosis and leprosy. Some diagnostic

Fig. 8.5 (**a**) Sarcoidosis. Patient C. Unilateral involvement. Left submandibular salivary gland. (**b**) Sarcoidosis. Patient C. Sialogram. Duct arborization absent because of replacement by granulomatous infiltration

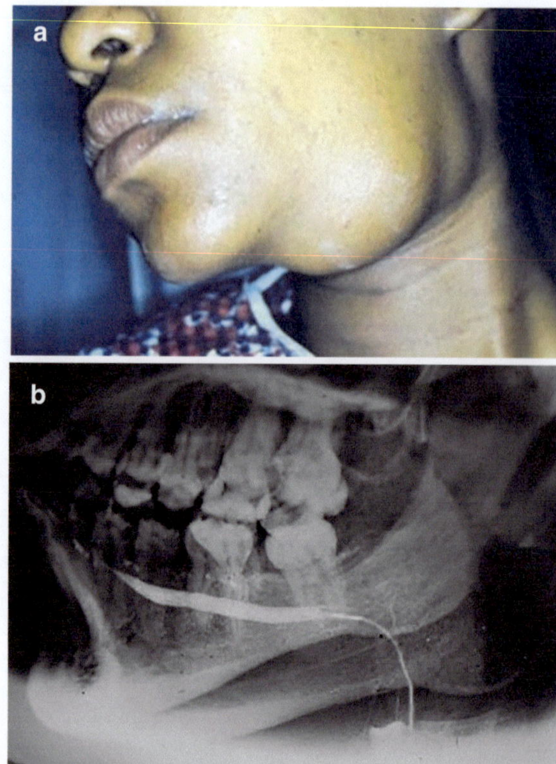

aids may be obtained from hypercalcemia that has been reported to be present in sarcoidosis [4, 9].

The diagnosis of sarcoidosis is based on the described clinical signs and symptoms. CT or MRI offers limited diagnostic help because imaging usually only reveals a solitary mass in the PG or SMSG which cannot be distinguished from a true neoplasm. Alternatively, the granulomas in the major salivary glands may appear as multiple nodular masses. Diagnostic imaging information is best obtained with a radioisotope scan using gallium 67 citrate. The gallium is picked up by the acute and chronic areas of inflammation. Patients with sarcoidosis will demonstrate the panda sign because, when the radioisotope scan is viewed, deposits of gallium will be seen in the nasopharynx (nose), bilaterally in the lacrimal glands (eyes), and bilaterally in the PGs (cheeks). This distribution of gallium isotope will now mimic the facial appearance of a panda. The panda sign is positive in 79% [5] of sarcoidosis patients, but it can also be seen in lymphomas, Sjogren's syndrome, and even HIV.

After the clinical and radiologic findings, the third leg for sarcoidosis diagnosis is the histologic demonstration of the classic granuloma. Essentially, a non-caseating granuloma consisting of masses of epithelioid cells and a scattering of giant cells will be observed. Lymphocytes act as the peripheral border for the granuloma. A fourth diagnostic leg includes the need to eliminate from consideration other granulomatous diseases such as histoplasmosis, blastomycosis, berylliosis, tuberculosis, and foreign bodies. Special staining can be utilized as aids to rule out these non-sarcoidal granulomatous diseases.

The Kveim-Siltzbach reaction is an old and interesting diagnostic sarcoidosis test that is not frequently utilized [4]. Homogenates of allogenic sarcoidal lymph node tissue are injected intradermally into the patient. In sarcoidosis, nodular eruptions will develop at the injection site within a few weeks. Biopsies of the nodules will demonstrate granulomas that are identical to sarcoidosis granulomas. The test has proven to be positive in 80% of sarcoidosis patients [11].

Prompt therapeutic intervention is required to avoid granuloma multiplication and progression. Organ dysfunction and ultimately organ failure from hyaline fibrosis [7] result if the disease is not treated and allowed to advance. If the eye is involved, blindness may result. Therefore, the presence of uveitis demands aggressive therapeutic intervention. A 1% mortality rate has also been reported [10] and results from pulmonary fibrosis accompanied by pulmonary hypertension [4]. Spontaneous remission can occur in many patients (reported to vary from 10–30% [16] to 50–66% [4, 9]) over a 12- to 36-month time span [4]. Remission of major salivary gland swellings can also occur [17]. Once medical treatment has been decided upon, immunosuppressive medications are administered. Minimal steroid doses are prescribed in order to avoid steroid toxicity. The immunosuppressive methotrexate and cyclophosphamide have been used as supplements to avoid steroid toxicity [4] or when steroids have proven to be ineffective. Recently, monoclonal antibodies such as infliximab (Fig. 8.6), adalimumab, or etanercept [4, 9] have been introduced into the therapeutic regimen [16]. These monoclonal antibodies act against tumor necrosing factor alpha (TNFα). Circulating levels of this factor increase in sarcoidosis and may be responsible for the intensity of the granulomatous inflammation. Infliximab acts by binding to TNFα and thereby blocks its interaction with TNFα receptor sites [15]. Care must be taken when prescribing these monoclonal medications because they may activate latent tuberculosis and encourage secondary infection [11].

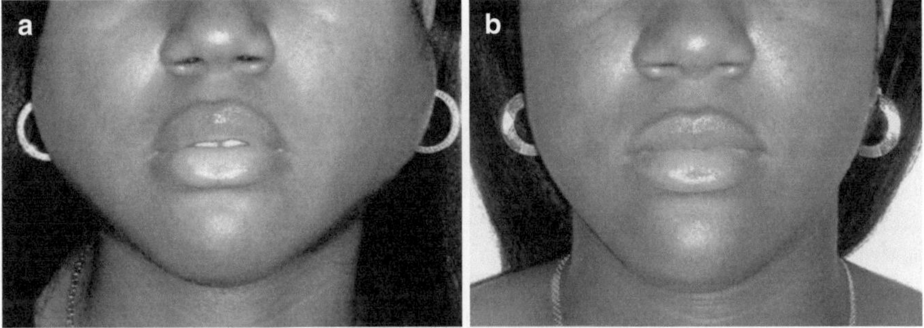

Fig. 8.6 (a) Sarcoidosis. Patient D. Bilateral parotid gland swelling. (Mandel L, et al. JADA 2005;136:1282). (b) Sarcoidosis. Patient D. Resolution of bilateral parotid swelling after treatment with infliximab. (Mandel L, et al. JADA 2005;136:1282)

Granulomatosis with Polyangiitis (Wegener's Granulomatosis)

Granulomatosis with polyangiitis (GPA), previously known as Wegener's granulomatosis, is a potentially lethal systemic disease characterized by necrotizing granulomatosis that involves the upper and lower respiratory tracts, vasculitis of the small blood vessels, and the presence of co-existing glomerulonephritis [18]. GPA has a reported incidence of 5–10 cases per 1,000,000 people [18] with the upper respiratory tract involved in 72% of the cases and the lower respiratory tract and kidney involved in 61% and 47% of the cases, respectively [19]. Males, whose mean age is 52 years, represent the predominant group of GPA patients [20]. Multiple other organs (skin, breast, nervous system, and gastrointestinal tract) can play into the GPA symptom complex. However, the first symptom is usually associated with otorhinolaryngological structures with head and neck involvement (nose, ear, eye, mouth, and salivary glands) occurring in 90% of the patients [21].

Most patients seek care because of their developing respiratory complaints. Maxillary sinusitis is the major feature of GPA's upper respiratory tract involvement. In addition, nasal obstruction, nasal bone destruction, epistaxis, rhinorrhea, and a saddle nose may be present. The lower respiratory tract pathology manifests itself as pathologic lesions of the lung which can be visualized with routine pulmonary radiographs. Coughing and hemoptysis can be anticipated. Kidney disease (glomerulonephritis) can lead to kidney failure if prompt treatment is not instituted. Constitutional symptoms such as fever, fatigue, myalgias, and arthralgias are to be expected. Serologically, antineutrophil cytoplasm antibodies (ANCA) are usually present [18]. However, an initial absence of ANCA has been recorded in 15–33% of the patients [22].

The criteria for GPA diagnosis has been established by the American College of Rheumatology [23]. At least two of the following four criteria must be present:

1. Maxillary sinus involvement
2. A lung X-ray that shows nodules, cavities, or infiltrate
3. Urinary sediment with hematuria
4. Histologic granulomas within an artery or in the perivascular area of an artery or arteriole

However, clinical practice usually bases the diagnosis on both the presence of ANCA and the biopsy findings of an affected organ. ANCA activates circulating neutrophils to adhere to a vessel's endothelial cells and induces endothelial degranulation which serves to bring about significant granulomatous changes in the vessel wall [24]. The developing vasculitis also narrows the vascular lumen and decreases blood flow. The decreased vascular supply leads to organ failure and bone destruction.

The salivary glands can be implicated in GPA disease. The parotid gland (PG) is involved 78% of the time (Fig. 8.7), and the submandibular (SMSG) and sublingual glands are involved 36% and 2.5% of the time, respectively [19, 20]. It is not unusual for the PG to be the only salivary gland to show signs of GPA, while it may also prove to be the forerunner of the disease process [19, 20]. Unilateral and bilateral painful persistently swollen PGs may develop. Simultaneous swellings of the PG

Fig. 8.7 Granulomatosis with polyangiitis. Left parotid swelling

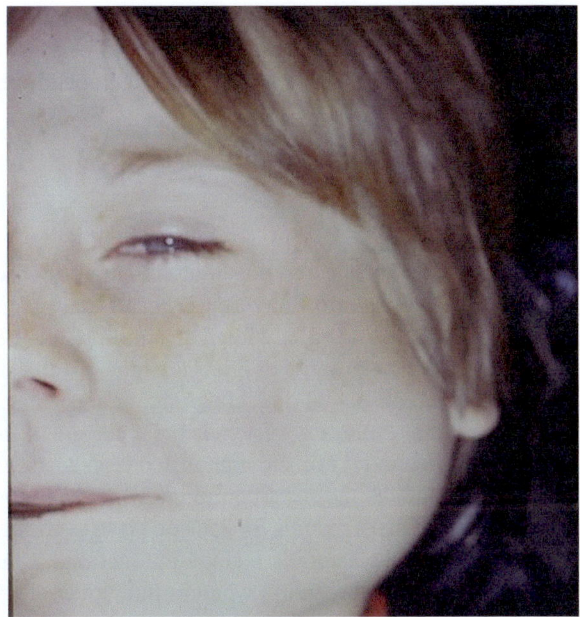

Fig. 8.8 Granulomatosis with polyangiitis. Parotid biopsy demonstrates necrosis with granulomatous inflammation. (Kenis I, et al. IMAJ 2013;15:186)

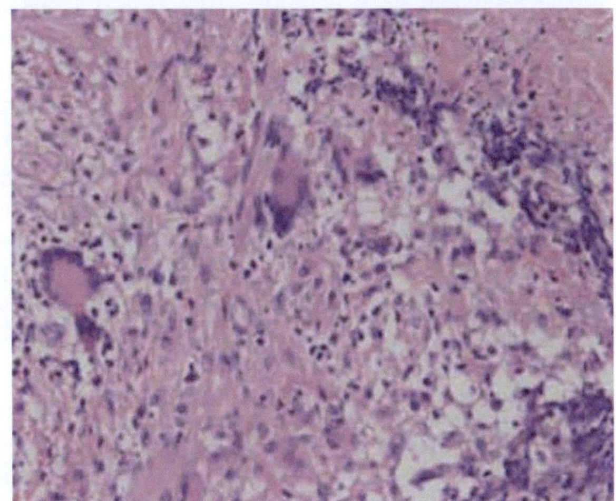

and SMSG may also be present [21]. Facial palsy has been reported to be a complication in 41% of the patients with PG disease [20].

Unfortunately, there are no distinguishing features of GPA that can be ascertained from imaging. Imaging (CT/MRI) of a PG with GPA will demonstrate an enlarged salivary gland whose swelling can originate from a diffuse or localized GPA [8]. Because of the decreased vascularity, contrast enhancement will be minimal and serves to indicate intraglandular ischemia [20]. Any existing adjacent areas of bone destruction will also be visualized. Imaging functions to eliminate the common PG misdiagnoses of infection or neoplasm. Histologically, necrosis and granulomatous inflammation will be observed involving the salivary glands (Fig. 8.8).

Although GPA can be fatal, prompt treatment with prednisone and cyclophosphamide has resulted in a remission rate of 90% with a 10-year survival [25]. Rituximab has recently been added to the therapeutic regimen [18].

Tuberculosis

Tuberculosis (TB) is a necrotizing granulomatous disease, caused by *Mycobacterium tuberculosis* that can affect any organ, but its main focus is the pulmonary system. Globally, it is a leading killer with over a million fatalities every year [26]. Infection is transmitted when airborne droplets are inhaled after being released by a contaminated individual during talking, coughing, or sneezing.

Although the respiratory system is the main site of infection (Fig. 8.9), extrapulmonary TB infection is not uncommon and represents 20–25% of TB cases [26, 27]. TB lymphadenitis is the most common form of extrapulmonary TB, and in countries such as India, it accounts for 35% of TB cases [28]. The unusual epidemiologic features of TB lymphadenitis include the fact that it manifests more frequently in females in a young age group, whereas pulmonary TB is more often seen in older males [28].

The head and neck comprise 10% of TB's extrapulmonary sites [29] with involvement of the cervical lymph nodes, referred to as scrofula, being its most frequent expression (Fig. 8.10). The majority of these nodes are located in the submandibular region, a posterior triangle of the neck, and the supraclavicular area. Positive lymph nodes are also present in the PG, mostly in its superficial lobe. Healing of the tuberculous nodes often results in dystrophic calcification.

M. tuberculosis can survive in the body without causing overt signs and symptoms. However, activation with symptomatology can develop. Tuberculous involvement of an intraglandular or paraglandular PG lymph node may originate from hematogenous or lymphatic spread from a lung focus or even from closely positioned adjacent contaminated nodes. Additionally, sputum contaminated by pulmonary foci or by oral TB lesions can enter the PG via the duct orifice [30, 31]. Once

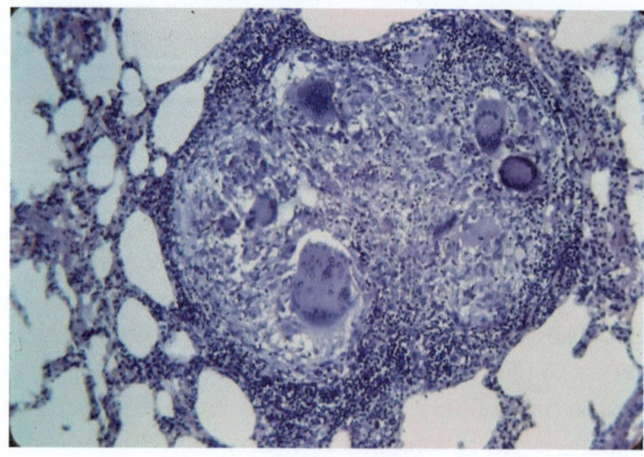

Fig. 8.9 Tuberculosis. Tuberculous granuloma with giant cells in the lung

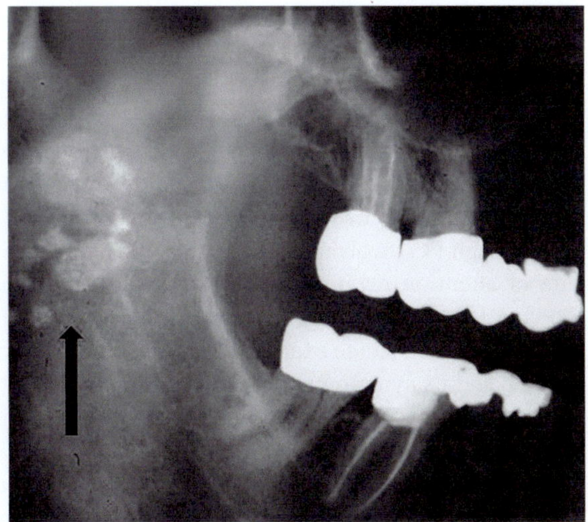

Fig. 8.10 Tuberculosis. Calcified cervical lymph nodes superimposed on ramus (arrow)

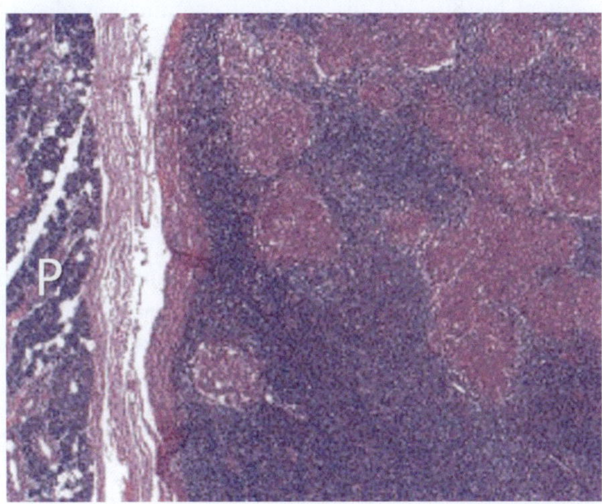

Fig. 8.11 Tuberculosis. Granulomatous inflammation in lymph node abutting parotid gland (P). (Birkent H, et al. J Med Case Rep 2008;2:62)

the PG is involved, it clinically manifests its symptomatology either as the more common localized nodular form of PG swelling or as the rare diffuse form of PG swelling [30–32]. The PG swelling in the localized form is due to intraparotid lymph node involvement (Fig. 8.11). Diffuse PG involvement reflects an infectious secondary spread to the gland's parenchyma from infected lymph nodes [29, 33] or contaminated sputum. The localized form originating from PG nodal disease simulates a neoplasm, while the uncommon diffuse parenchymal variety resembles acute or chronic sialadenitis.

If TB of the salivary glands becomes a problem, the PG is usually involved. When the PG is affected, the swellings will be evident in the pre-tragal area or just below the ear. The overlying skin is not erythematous and its temperature is normal. Submandibular salivary glands have on occasion been infected [34]. The 30- to

50-year age category [35], with a somewhat greater incidence in females [36], seems to be the group most frequently seen with PG TB. The PG is unilaterally involved, but bilateral PG disease is always a possibility. The PG is the only salivary gland that contains lymph nodes within its parenchyma. The PG lymphadenopathy caused by TB is painless, but, with time, an abscess with associated pain and sinus formation can develop. It is not unusual for patients with TB of the PG to have no signs of pulmonary or systemic disease [33, 37].

Although PG involvement in TB is a relatively rare condition, it demands a measure of attention regarding its presence. A long-standing history of a firm slow-growing PG swelling may mimic a neoplasm and can lead to a misdiagnosis with needless surgery. Acute exacerbations of the PG tuberculous lymphadenitis can also develop and its symptomatology will simulate an acute parotitis. An accurate clinical diagnosis involves a variety of investigative techniques. The results of fine needle aspiration biopsy (FNAB) are often non-specific when examining the limited acquired tissue histologically or microbiologically for the guilty acid-fast bacillus. A PCR study [36, 38, 39] can be performed on the acquired FNAB tissue. PCR has proven to be a very effective tool in the diagnostic armamentarium. The patient's medical history and the physical examination also play key roles in diagnosis. Naturally, the gold standard for diagnosis is a microscopic study that demonstrates a caseous granuloma with epithelioid cells, Langerhans giant cells, and lymphocytes that involve the lymph nodes of the PG's superficial lobe. Parenchymal involvement with a decrease in ductal and acinar clusters is rare [38] and if present probably results from infected sputum or intraglandular nodal spread.

Imaging (CT/MRI) can serve as a useful adjunctive tool for differential diagnosis, but a consistent and clear pathognomonic picture has not been observed [31]. Tuberculous lymphadenitis, as observed in imaging studies, has been described as a multilocular nodal mass with central lucency and a thick smooth-walled corrugated enhancing rim [38]. Unfortunately, TB of the PG lymph nodes is usually misdiagnosed initially as a tumor.

Recognition of tuberculous PG disease is imperative because it will serve to avoid a misdiagnosis and it will negate a surgical therapeutic approach that would sacrifice the superficial lobe of the PG. Early diagnosis is facilitated by always maintaining a suspicion of the presence of TB parotitis. Once a tuberculous diagnosis is made, therapy can be initiated. A regimen of isoniazid, rifampicin, pyrazinamide, and ethambutol has met with success [32].

References

1. Mukhopadhyay S, Farver CF, Vaszar LT, et al. Causes of pulmonary granulomas: a retrospective study of 500 cases from seven countries. J Clin Pathol. 2012;65(1):51–7. https://doi.org/10.1136/jclinpath-2011-200336.
2. Shah KK, Pritt BS, Alexander MP. Histopathologic review of granulomatous inflammation. J Clin Tuberc Other Mycobact Dis. 2017;7:1–12. Published 2017 Feb 10. https://doi.org/10.1016/j.jctube.2017.02.001.

3. Blaise P, Fardeau C, Chapelon C, Bodaghi B, Le Hoang P. Minor salivary gland biopsy in diagnosing ocular sarcoidosis. Br J Ophthalmol. 2011;95(12):1731–4. https://doi.org/10.1136/bjophthalmol-2011-300129. Epub 2011 Sep 6. PMID: 21900225.
4. Mrówka-Kata K, Kata D, Lange D, Namysłowski G, Czecior E, Banert K. Sarcoidosis and its otolaryngological implications. Eur Arch Otorrinolaringol. 2010;267(10):1507–14. https://doi.org/10.1007/s00405-010-1331-y. Epub 2010 Jul 9. PMID: 20617327.
5. Kurdziel KA. The panda sign. Radiology. 2000;215(3):884–5. https://doi.org/10.1148/radiology.215.3.r00jn31884. PMID: 10831715.
6. Izumi T. Symposium: population differences in clinical features and prognosis of sarcoidosis throughout the world. Sarcoidosis. 1992;9:S105–18.
7. Surattanont F, Mandel L, Wolinsky B. Bilateral parotid swelling caused by sarcoidosis. J Am Dent Assoc. 2002;133(6):738–41. https://doi.org/10.14219/jada.archive.2002.0270. PMID: 12083650.
8. Vairaktaris E, Vassiliou S, Yapijakis C, Papakosta V, Kavantzas N, Martis C, Patsouris E. Salivary gland manifestations of sarcoidosis: report of three cases. J Oral Maxillofac Surg. 2005;63(7):1016–21. https://doi.org/10.1016/j.joms.2005.03.017. PMID: 16003631.
9. Banks GC, Kirse DJ, Anthony E, Bergman S, Shetty AK. Bilateral parotitis as the initial presentation of childhood sarcoidosis. Am J Otolaryngol. 2013;34(2):142–4. https://doi.org/10.1016/j.amjoto.2012.08.007. Epub 2012 Oct 23. PMID: 23102965.
10. Fraga RC, Kakizaki P, Valente NYS, Portocarrero LKL, Teixeira MFS, Senise PF. Do you know this syndrome? Heerfordt-Waldenström syndrome. An Bras Dermatol. 2017;92(4):571–2. https://doi.org/10.1590/abd1806-4841.20175211. PMID: 28954117; PMCID: PMC5595615.
11. Vourexakis Z, Dulguerov P, Bouayed S, Burkhardt K, Landis BN. Sarcoidosis of the submandibular gland: a systematic review. Am J Otolaryngol. 2010;31(6):424–8. https://doi.org/10.1016/j.amjoto.2009.08.001. Epub 2009 Oct 12. PMID: 20015798.
12. Radochová V, Radocha J, Laco J, Slezák R. Oral manifestation of sarcoidosis: a case report and review of the literature. J Indian Soc Periodontol. 2016;20(6):627–9. https://doi.org/10.4103/jisp.jisp_378_16. PMID: 29238144; PMCID: PMC5713087.
13. Nessan VJ, Jacoway JR. Biopsy of minor salivary glands in the diagnosis of sarcoidosis. N Engl J Med. 1979;301(17):922–4. https://doi.org/10.1056/NEJM197910253011705. PMID: 481539.
14. Cahn LR, Eisenbud L, Blake MN, Stern D. Biopsies of normal-appearing palates of patients with known sarcoidosis; a preliminary report. Oral Surg Oral Med Oral Pathol. 1964;18:342–5. https://doi.org/10.1016/0030-4220(64)90086-6. PMID: 14178910.
15. Mandel L, Wolinsky B, Chalom EC. Treatment of refractory sarcoidal parotid gland swelling in a previously reported unresponsive case. J Am Dent Assoc. 2005;136(9):1282–5. https://doi.org/10.14219/jada.archive.2005.0345. PMID: 16196234.
16. Wu JJ, Schiff KR. Sarcoidosis. Am Fam Physician. 2004;70(2):312–22. PMID: 15291090.
17. Fatahzadeh M, Rinaggio J. Diagnosis of systemic sarcoidosis prompted by orofacial manifestations: a review of the literature. J Am Dent Assoc. 2006;137(1):54–60. https://doi.org/10.14219/jada.archive.2006.0021. PMID: 16456999.
18. Wojciechowska J, Krajewski W, Krajewski P, Kręcicki T. Granulomatosis with polyangiitis in otolaryngologist practice: a review of current knowledge. Clin Exp Otorhinolaryngol. 2016;9(1):8–13. https://doi.org/10.21053/ceo.2016.9.1.8. Epub 2016 Mar 7. PMID: 26976020; PMCID: PMC4792240.
19. Kikuchi R, Aoshiba K, Nakamura H. Salivary gland enlargement as an unusual imaging manifestation of granulomatosis with polyangiitis involving the head and neck region. AJR Am J Roentgenol. 2016;206(6):W94. https://doi.org/10.2214/AJR.16.16042. Epub 2016 Mar 21. PMID: 26998726.
20. Green I, Szyper-Kravitz M, Shoenfeld Y. Parotitis as the presenting symptom of Wegener's granulomatosis: case report and meta-analysis. Isr Med Assoc J. 2013;15(3):188–92. PMID: 23662387.
21. Barrett AW. Wegener's granulomatosis of the major salivary glands. J Oral Pathol Med. 2012;41(10):721–7. https://doi.org/10.1111/j.1600-0714.2012.01141.x.

22. Ceylan A, Asal K, Çelenk F, Köybaşioğlu A. Parotid gland involvement as a presenting feature of Wegener's granulomatosis. Singapore Med J. 2013;54(9):e196–8. https://doi.org/10.11622/smedj.2013183.

23. Leavitt RY, Fauci AS, Bloch DA, Michel BA, Hunder GG, Arend WP, Calabrese LH, Fries JF, Lie JT, Lightfoot RW Jr, et al. The American College of Rheumatology 1990 criteria for the classification of Wegener's granulomatosis. Arthritis Rheum. 1990;33(8):1101–7. https://doi.org/10.1002/art.1780330807. PMID: 2202308.

24. Nahlieli O. Wegener's granulomatosis and the salivary glands. Isr Med Assoc J. 2013;15(3):178–9. PMID: 23662384.

25. Bülbül Y, Ozlü T, Oztuna F. Wegener's granulomatosis with parotid gland involvement and pneumothorax. Med Princ Pract. 2003;12(2):133–7. https://doi.org/10.1159/000069111. PMID: 12634471.

26. Landegger LD. Tuberculous abscesses in the head and neck region. Diagnostics (Basel). 2022;12(3):686. Published 2022 Mar 11. https://doi.org/10.3390/diagnostics12030686.

27. Garg R, Verma SK, Mehra S, Srivastawa AN. Parotid tuberculosis. Lung India. 2010;27(4):253–5. https://doi.org/10.4103/0970-2113.71969. PMID: 21139728; PMCID: PMC2988182.

28. Handa U, Mundi I, Mohan S. Nodal tuberculosis revisited: a review. J Infect Dev Ctries. 2012;6(1):6–12. Published 2012 Jan 12. https://doi.org/10.3855/jidc.2090.

29. Thakur J, Thakur A, Mohindroo N, Mohindroo S, Sharma D. Bilateral parotid tuberculosis. J Glob Infect Dis. 2011;3(3):296–9. https://doi.org/10.4103/0974-777X.83543. PMID: 21887065; PMCID: PMC3162820.

30. Papadogeorgakis N, Mylonas AI, Kolomvos N, Angelopoulos AP. Tuberculosis in or near the major salivary glands: report of 3 cases. J Oral Maxillofac Surg. 2006;64(4):696–700. https://doi.org/10.1016/j.joms.2005.11.035. Erratum in: J Oral Maxillofac Surg 2006 May;64(5):873. PMID: 16546652.

31. Maurya MK, Kumar S, Singh HP, Verma A. Tuberculous parotitis: a series of eight cases and review of literature. Natl J Maxillofac Surg. 2019;10(1):118–22. https://doi.org/10.4103/njms.NJMS_34_18. PMID: 31205402; PMCID: PMC6563638.

32. Kim YH, Jeong WJ, Jung KY, Sung MW, Kim KH, Kim CS. Diagnosis of major salivary gland tuberculosis: experience of eight cases and review of the literature. Acta Otolaryngol. 2005;125(12):1318–22. https://doi.org/10.1080/00016480510012246. PMID: 16303681.

33. Mert A, Ozaras R, Bilir M, Cicek Y, Tabak F, Tahan V, Ozturk R. Primary tuberculosis of the parotid gland. Int J Infect Dis. 2000;4(4):229–30. https://doi.org/10.1016/s1201-9712(00)90115-2. PMID: 11231188.

34. Hashemi P, Rashidi A, Razmpa E. Tuberculosis of major salivary glands: report of a 7-year experience in Tehran, Iran. Int J Infect Dis. 2007;11(4):368–9. https://doi.org/10.1016/j.ijid.2006.09.006. Epub 2007 Feb 28. PMID: 17331779.

35. Babazade F, Mortazavi H, Jalalian H. Parotid tuberculosis: a forgotten suspicion (a case report and literature review). Int J Dermatol. 2012;51(5):588–91. https://doi.org/10.1111/j.1365-4632.2011.05014.x. PMID: 22515584.

36. Cataño JC, Robledo J. Tuberculous lymphadenitis and parotitis. Microbiol Spectr. 2016;4(6). https://doi.org/10.1128/microbiolspec.TNMI7-0008-2016. PMID: 28084205.

37. Vyas S, Kaur N, Yadav TD, Gupta N, Khandelwal N. Tuberculosis of parotid gland masquerading parotid neoplasm. Natl J Maxillofac Surg. 2012;3(2):199–201. https://doi.org/10.4103/0975-5950.111381. PMID: 23833498; PMCID: PMC3700157.

38. Zhang D, Li X, Xiong H, Yang C, Lv F, Huang X, Li Q, Tang Z, Luo T. Tuberculosis of the parotid lymph nodes: clinical and imaging features. Infect Drug Resist. 2018;11:1795–805. https://doi.org/10.2147/IDR.S164993. PMID: 30349336; PMCID: PMC6188200.

39. Dhingra S, Juneja R. Diverse clinical presentations of tubercular parotitis in children: case series with review of literature. Sudan J Paediatr. 2021;21(1):67–75. https://doi.org/10.24911/SJP.106-1588918898. PMID: 33879946; PMCID: PMC8025998.

Chapter 9
Sialadenosis

Louis Mandel

Abstract Sialadenosis is usually seen as a chronic persistent asymptomatic bilateral hypertrophy of the parotid glands (PG). The condition occurs in patients with diabetes, alcoholism or malnutritional syndromes. It is believed that the common denominator that unites these systemic problems under one umbrella is that they all present with a peripheral neuropathy of the autonomic nerve supply to the salivary glands. A demyelinating neuropathy involving the sympathetic system develops. Excessive intracellular protein production and/or a failure to signal its secretion results. Individual acinar cells become engorged with intracellular protein. Cellular enlargement occurs and leads to the clinically visible PG hypertrophy.

Introduction

Sialadenosis or sialosis is a chronic diffuse non-inflammatory non-neoplastic salivary gland condition characterized by persistent bilateral parotid gland (PG) enlargements that are usually painless. The submandibular and minor salivary glands are infrequently involved [1]. Sialadenosis can develop in association with a variety of systemic conditions that include diabetes mellitus, alcoholism, and malnutrition and can even occur idiopathically [2–6]. The leading hypothesis that unites these disparate systemic entities, under the umbrella of sialadenosis, is that they all have a peripheral neuropathy of the autonomic nerve supply to the salivary glands [7, 8].

The autonomic nerve supply to the PG involves both parasympathetic and sympathetic innervations. Parasympathetic activity is related to fluid and electrolyte secretion, whereas sympathetic innervation is concerned with intracellular protein synthesis and secretion. It is believed that patients with sialadenosis develop a demyelinating neuropathy involving sympathetic innervation [7, 9]. The neuropathy results in excessive intracellular protein production and/or a failure to signal its

L. Mandel, *Clinical Management of Salivary Gland Disorders*, https://doi.org/10.1007/978-3-031-50012-1_9

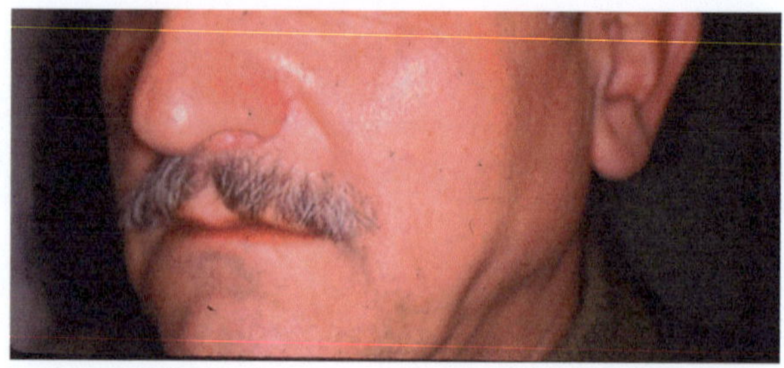

Fig. 9.1 Sialadenosis in diabetic. Left parotid gland swelling

secretion. Consequently, individual acinar cells become engorged with intracytoplasmic protein granules. The granule accumulation (zymogen) results in the enlargement of individual acinar cells, and in turn the acini increase in size [7] which leads to clinically visible PG hypertrophy (Fig. 9.1).

Parenchymal acini are formed by groups of 7–10 secreting pyramidal cells grouped around the lumen of an intercalated duct. An individual acinus normally measures approximately 40 μm in diameter [7], but, in sialadenosis, the acinus can expand up to 100 μm [5, 6]. It has also been suggested that the development of hypertrophy of individual acini may be facilitated by defective myoepithelial cells that fail to mechanically support the acinus and allow acinar cell expansion [9, 10]. Furthermore, it is possible that cellular aquaporin water channels play a role in the pathophysiologic events that lead to sialadenosis by creating a disturbance in cell volume regulation [1, 11].

Patients with sialadenosis usually present themselves with prolonged histories of painless bilateral, occasionally unilateral, symmetrical PG swellings. The most common clinical manifestation of sialadenosis is the bilateral swelling of the PGs [12]. Most patients are between 40 and 70 years of age, with no sex predilection evident [12, 13]. The swellings do not fluctuate in size in tandem with eating, and there are no subjective complaints regarding salivary volume. Questioning reveals that patients usually but not always have a history of diabetes (Figs. 9.2 and 9.3), an alcohol-incited liver disease (Figs. 9.4, 9.5, 9.6, 9.7, and 9.8), or a malnutritional syndrome (Figs. 9.9 and 9.10). Their decision to seek medical care is most often prompted by their cosmetic concerns or anxiety regarding the origin of the facial swelling.

Extraorally when palpated, the swellings are noted to follow the anatomic outline of the PG. No pain is elicited, and the tissue tone is normal. Cervical lymphadenopathy is not present. Intraorally, the mucosa is normally moist. When massaged extraorally, each PG will produce an aqueous clear salivary return that is visible intraorally at the respective parotid duct orifice. The Columbia University Salivary Gland Center has observed increased PG secretory volumes in patients with sialadenosis. Substantiation for this observational clinical finding can be obtained from the fact that, in humans, a positive correlation has been found to exist between increased flow rate and increased PG size [14, 15]. Therefore, it should not be surprising that enlarged secretory acinar cells produce larger secretory volumes that may be further augmented by pathologically increased parasympathetic stimulation.

Fig. 9.2 (**a**) Sialadenosis. Patient A. Diabetes. Bilateral asymptomatic parotid swelling. (**b**) Sialadenosis. Patient A. Diabetes. CT scan. Bilateral parotid (P) hypertrophy. (**c**) Sialadenosis. Patient A. Diabetes. Fine-needle-aspiration biopsy demonstrates enlarged acinus

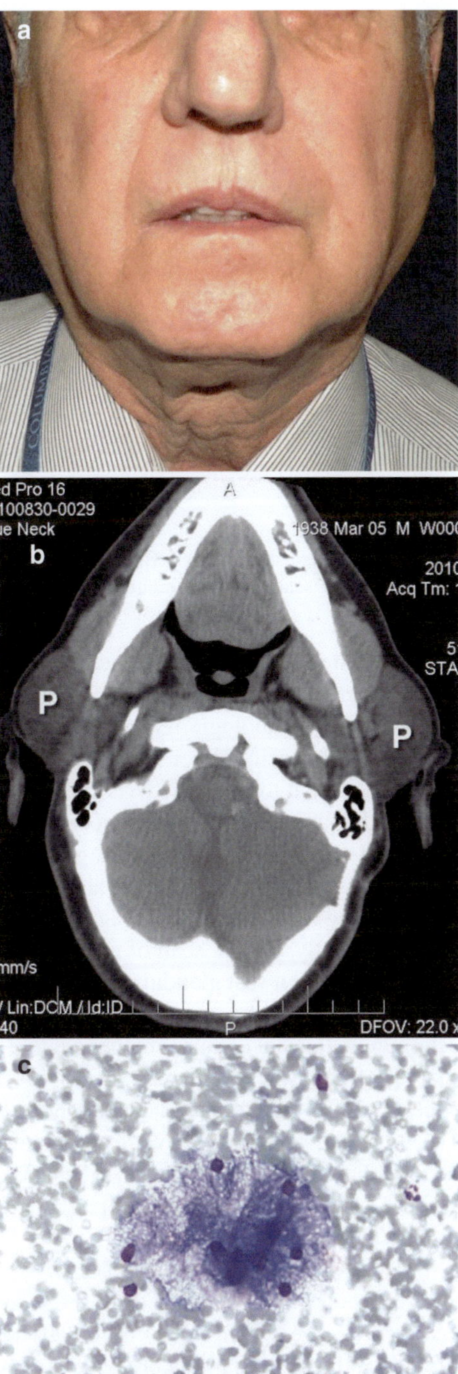

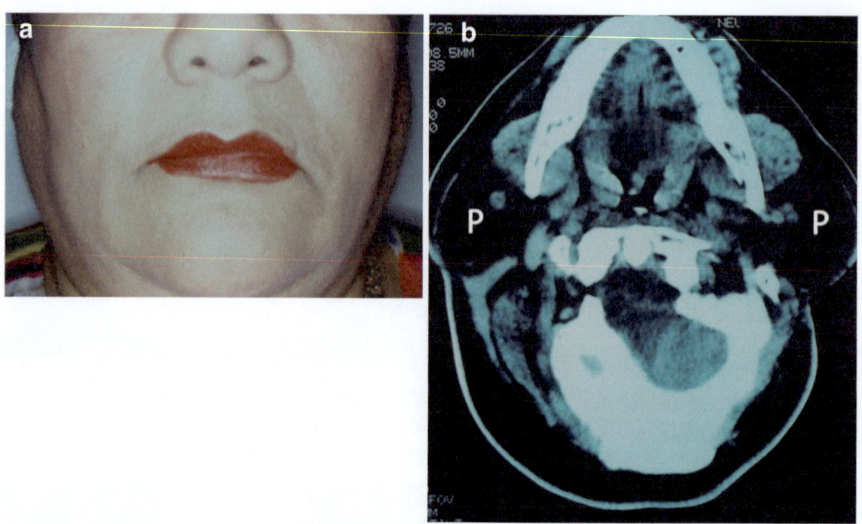

Fig. 9.3 (**a**) Sialadenosis. Patient B. Diabetes. Bilateral parotid swelling. (**b**) Sialadenosis. Patient B. Diabetes. CT scan images of bilateral lucent parotid glands (P)

The existence of sialadenosis can receive adjunctive diagnostic aid from a CT scan performed without contrast. Bilateral PG enlargement will readily be observed, but no specific pathologic features will be present. In addition, there usually is an increased PG density. When a normal PG is viewed on a CT scan, it has a lucency that may cause it to have a "Swiss cheese-like" appearance. The lucency represents the fact that approximately 25% of the PG bulk is occupied by adipose tissue [16, 17]. With the hypertrophy of the glandular acini, lucent fat is replaced by the expanding enlarged parenchymal acini causing the PG to approach the density of the adjoining masseter muscle (Figs. 9.2b, 9.4b, and 9.7b).

Occasionally, the CT scan of a patient with sialadenosis will reveal a lucent PG that results from a vast glandular infiltration of adipose tissue (Figs. 9.3b and 9.8b). The causation for the parenchymal replacement by fat has not been definitively determined. It is not certain whether a fatty PG represents an end stage of sialadenosis [12, 18] caused by a disturbance in fat metabolism following the initial acinar hypertrophy or an alternate independent pathway in the evolution of sialadenosis.

Ultrasound imaging of sialadenosis shows glandular hyperechogenicity with no focal lesions. Sialography will reveal normal duct caliber and distribution. However, because of the glandular hypertrophy, the ducts will be widely dispersed over the enlarged PG (Fig. 9.4c).

Fine needle aspiration biopsy (FNAB) specimens can harvest cells that testify to the increased acinar size (Figs. 9.2c and 9.4d) [7, 19]. A densely granular cytoplasm that involves the acinar cells with basally positioned nuclei will also be observed. Atypical cells and inflammatory cells are characteristically absent [13]. If the sialadenosis is a result of fat infiltration, the FNAB will reveal an elevated presence of adipose cells that can readily be imaged and confirmed by a CT scan.

Information derived from available investigative procedures is crucial in reaching a diagnosis of sialadenosis. A search for co-existing related systemic diseases is

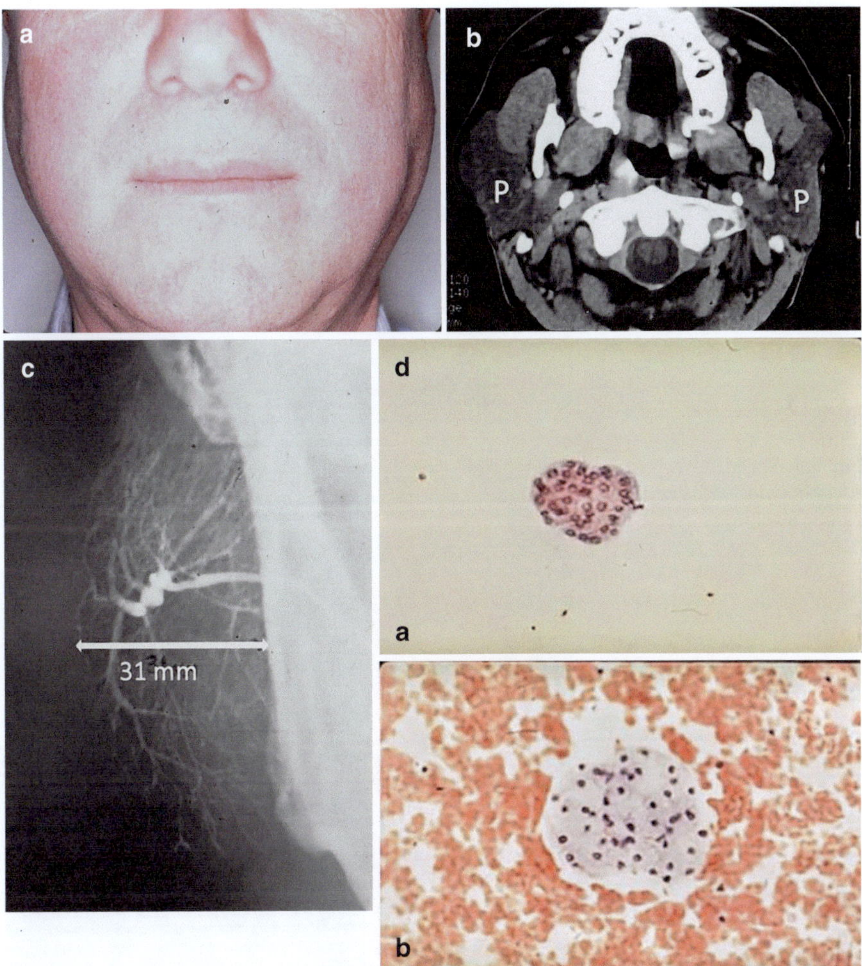

Fig. 9.4 (**a**) Sialadenosis. Patient C. Alcohol (whiskey). Bilateral parotid swelling. (**b**) Sialadenosis. Patient C. Alcohol. CT scan. Bilateral parotid (P) hypertrophy. (**c**) Sialadenosis. Patient C. Alcohol. Sialogram, anterior–posterior view. Distance from ramus is 31 mm (normal 25 mm), indicating parotid enlargement. (**d**) Sialadenosis. Patient C. Fine-needle-aspiration biopsy. Normal-sized acinus (**a**). Enlarged acinus (**b**)

an imperative facet in the diagnosis of sialadenosis. Integrating the patient's medical history with the clinical signs and symptoms of the glandular swelling is a mandatory procedure. The enlarged PG and its homogeneously increased CT imaged density will support a diagnosis of sialadenosis. Further evidence substantiating the presence of sialadenosis can be derived from the FNAB cytologic findings of enlarged acini.

Effective therapeutic management of the PG hypertrophy associated with sialadenosis is not available. Because sialadenosis is usually partnered with a systemic disorder, treatment must incorporate care of the underlying medical condition. Some diminution in gland size may be achieved with treatment of the co-existing

Fig. 9.5 Sialadenosis. Alcohol (vodka). Bilateral parotid swelling

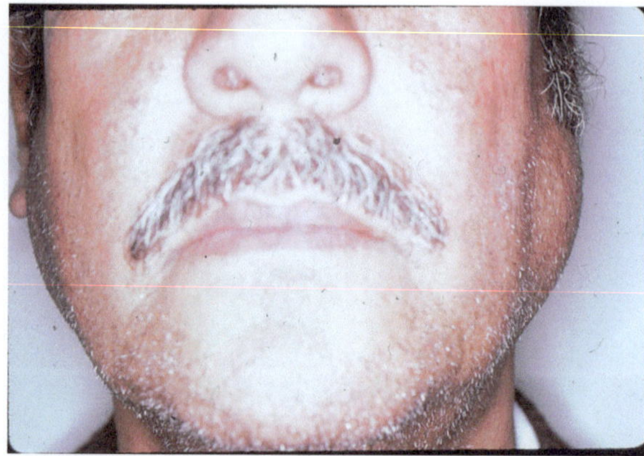

Fig. 9.6 Sialadenosis. Alcohol (wine). Bilateral parotid swelling

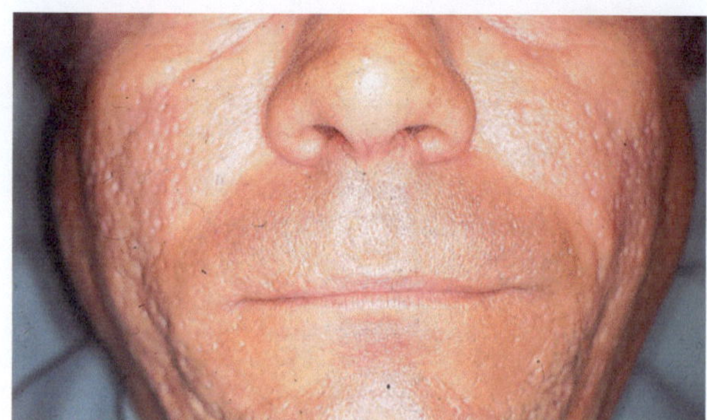

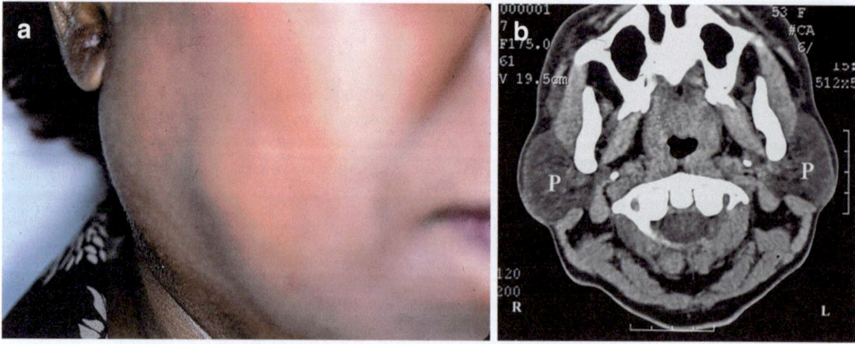

Fig. 9.7 (**a**) Sialadenosis. Patient D. Alcohol (beer). Right parotid swelling (left was also enlarged) in a prodigious beer drinker. (**b**) Sialadenosis. Patient D. Alcohol. The patient drank considerable amounts of beer. CT scan reveals bilaterally enlarged parotid glands (P)

Fig. 9.8 (**a**) Sialadenosis. Patient E. Alcohol (whiskey). Bilateral parotid swelling. (**b**) Sialadenosis. Patient E. Alcohol. CT scan. Bilateral large lucent parotid glands (P)

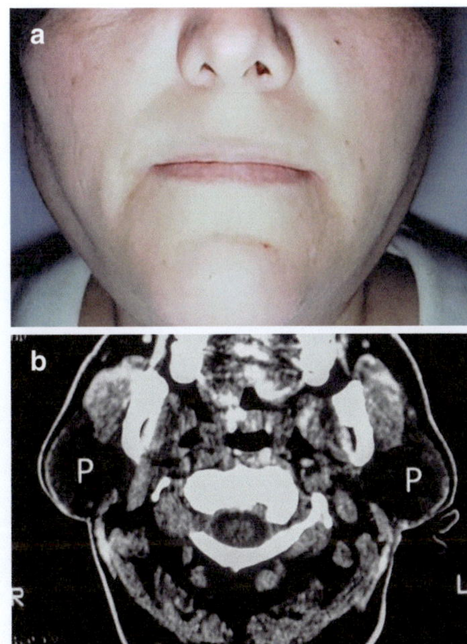

Fig. 9.9 (**a**) Anorexia nervosa. Patient F. Right parotid swelling. (**b**) Anorexia nervosa. Patient F. Left parotid swelling

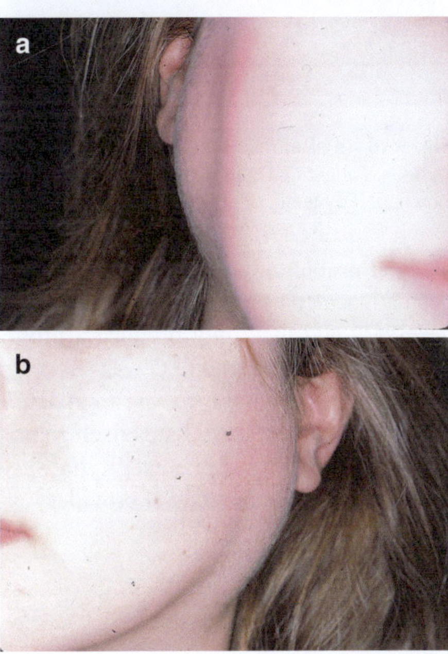

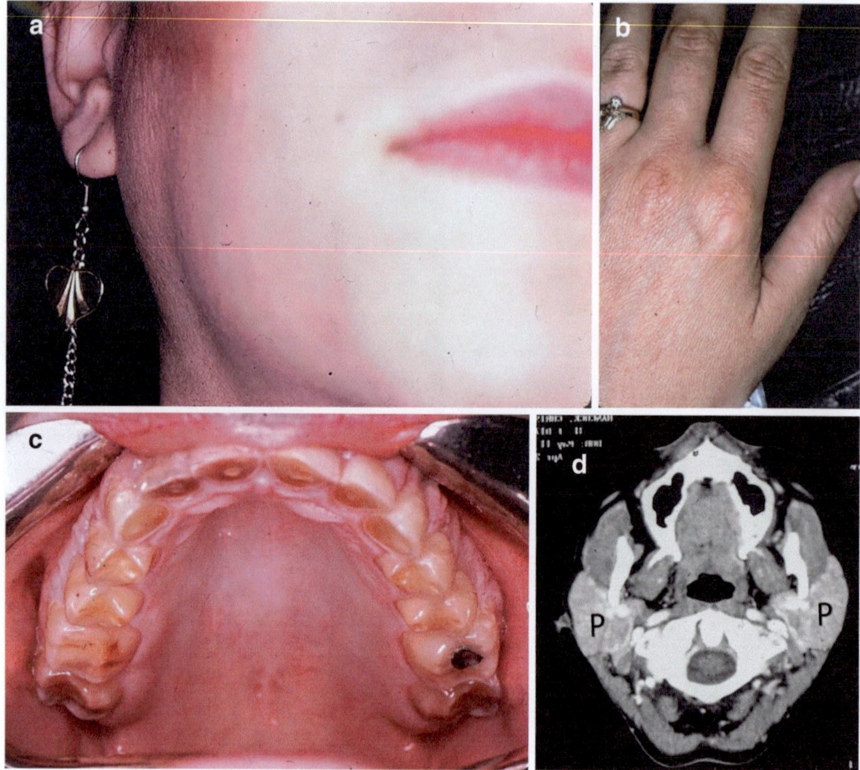

Fig. 9.10 (**a**) Bulimia. Patient G. Right parotid swelling (left parotid was also swollen). (**b**) Bulimia. Patient G. Calluses in knuckle area (Russel's sign). (**c**) Bulimia. Patient G. Dental corrosion maxillary teeth. (**d**) Bulimia. CT scan. Enhanced enlarged parotids (P) in active bulimia

medical problem, but total resolution is not usually attained. Botulinum toxin has been advocated as a means of causing glandular atrophy, but repeated injections are necessary and they only produce a limited successful outcome [10, 18]. Surgical reduction of the enlarged PG was advocated for cosmetic reasons in the past, but its morbidity has discouraged this approach. Fortunately, the benign nature of PG sialadenosis therapeutically lends itself to no treatment tinctured with observation and reassurance. However, the underlying systemic condition always requires attention from the appropriate medical provider.

Diabetic Sialadenosis

In 2018, diabetes was estimated to involve 34 million people in the United States with about one-quarter of those over 65 years of age suffering from the abnormality [20]. Diabetes is a defect in carbohydrate metabolism caused in one of two ways. Type 1 diabetes is a deficiency in pancreatic insulin production that results from an autoimmune involvement of the pancreas and is usually seen in childhood or the teenage years. Type 2 diabetes, often associated with obesity, develops in adults as a result of the body's ineffective use of normally produced pancreatic insulin. This insulin resistance in type 2 is responsible for 90% of the diabetic cases. Both type 1 and 2 diabetes are characterized by hyperglycemia which is associated with a greater risk of heart disease, peripheral neuropathy, stroke, blindness, kidney disease, and amputations.

A relationship between diabetes and sialadenosis has been noted, but infrequently reported. Sialadenosis occurs in approximately 25–49% of diabetic patients [1, 21], while 49% of patients with sialadenosis have diabetes (Figs. 9.1, 9.2, and 9.3) [21]. As in all cases of sialadenosis, the bilateral parotid gland (PG) swellings that are present are persistent, subjectively painless, do not fluctuate in size, and when palpated are normal in tone. Submandibular gland involvement is rarely observed. Intraorally, the salivary return from each PG can be seen to be increased, but normal in quality when each gland is massaged extraorally.

As per the studies of Donath and Seifert [7], the pathophysiology of PG hypertrophy is thought to be caused by peripheral autonomic demyelinating neuropathy. The glandular effects of this neuropathy have been explained in the introduction to this chapter (Fig. 9.2). The CT scan of a PG with sialadenosis has also been summarized.

Because autonomic nerve fibers are small, defects in these nerves tend to appear early in the evolution of diabetic neuropathy [22]. This fact may be the explanation for the occasional occurrence of PG sialadenosis prior to the onset of the more overt signs of diabetes. Fatty replacement of PG parenchyma has also been noted in diabetic patients. The fat infiltration may result from a diabetic disturbance in lipid metabolism, the mechanism of which is not fully understood [12, 23, 24], or an alternate route to the development of sialadenosis (Fig. 9.3).

Other than botulinum toxin injections that are marginally helpful, there is no specific treatment available for PG hypertrophy [14]. Care should be directed toward diabetic control with the knowledge that only some minimal improvement in PG size can be obtained. The known benign course of PG diabetic sialadenosis mandates a "hands-off" treatment supplemented with patient reassurance.

Alcoholic Sialadenosis

Chronic alcoholism is one of the main causes of bilateral parotid gland (PG) sialadenosis (Figs. 9.4, 9.5, 9.6, 9.7, and 9.8). Alcohol-induced PG sialadenosis occurs in 30–80% of patients who have cirrhosis [18], while its reported incidence drops to 10% in patients who have non-cirrhotic alcohol-damaged livers [25]. The toxic liver effect of ethanol is what initiates liver cirrhosis.

The PG and occasionally the submandibular gland are affected in most cases of chronic alcohol abuse. Characteristically, it is when the liver pathology progresses to hepatic cirrhosis that the histologic features of sialadenosis materialize in the PG. It has also been suggested that nutritional deficiencies, brought about by a disturbance in metabolism incited by a diseased liver and exacerbated by alcoholism, are underlying factors in the pathophysiology of alcoholic sialadenosis [26]. Acinar hypertrophy, with a resulting increase in PG size, develops from an autonomic demyelinating polyneuropathy that causes cytoplasmic protein granule accumulation within individual secreting parenchymal cells (Figs. 9.2c and 9.4d). This pathophysiologic pathway [7] for all causes of sialadenosis has been generally accepted and has been described in the beginning of this chapter. The clinical signs and symptoms of alcohol-provoked PG sialadenosis, as well as the histology, can also be found at the beginning of this chapter.

Occasionally, as in diabetic sialadenosis, imaging of alcoholic sialadenosis will depict a hypertrophied PG that is totally lucent, reflecting the replacement of secreting acini by adipocytes (Fig. 9.8b). As previously stated in the beginning of this chapter, it is believed that acinar cell hypertrophy and fat infiltration may represent different pathways to sialadenosis [7]. It has also been reported that, in the acute stage of alcoholic sialadenosis, cellular enlargement develops, while the chronic stage is represented by progression to a marked fatty infiltration of the PG [27]. The mechanism of this progression is not fully understood, but poor liver function in alcoholism is known to cause a disturbance in fat metabolism that may manifest itself as an increased PG fat content.

With the recognition of an alcohol-induced sialadenosis and because of an assumed associated liver pathology, a medical referral becomes mandatory. Medical therapy results in some decrease in liver disease and PG size, but the long-term PG prognosis varies.

Nutritional Disorders and Sialadenosis

Sialadenosis has been observed and reported in patients afflicted by malnutritional conditions (Figs. 9.9 and 9.10) [1, 4, 12, 18, 28]. Any disorder that affects the digestion of food or its absorption over a prolonged period may result in sialadenosis [3]. Nutritional disorders such as starvation, anorexia nervosa (AN) (Fig. 9.9), pellagra, and kwashiorkor are some of the conditions that can lead to sialadenosis [28]. Bulimia may represent yet another causative factor in nutritional sialadenosis (Fig. 9.10).

The pathophysiology, signs, and symptoms of the sialadenosis seen in anorexia/malnutrition are those that have been outlined earlier in this chapter. Because bulimic PG sialadenosis may originate from a different pathophysiologic pathway, it has been listed and reviewed independently.

Successful treatment is aimed at rectifying the underlying nutritional deficit. Resolution of the PG hypertrophy has not been reported, but some resolution probably occurs following diet normalization.

Anorexia Nervosa

Eating disorders have become a relatively common problem in our society, particularly among young women, less often in males, seeking to have the ideal figure. These disorders include anorexia nervosa (AN) (Fig. 9.9), bulimia nervosa (BN)

(Fig. 9.10), and a high incidence of crossover between AN and BN. AN is considered a form of self-starvation that can be life-threatening without intervention. People with AN have an abnormally low body weight, a disproportionate fear of gaining weight, and a distorted body image of themselves. Superimposed upon these issues, significant mental distress develops as the individual tries to cope with everyday common emotional problems. Patients with AN have been referred to the Salivary Gland Center, because of the presence of a bilateral PG hypertrophy, whose diagnosis has eluded the primary practitioner. Occasionally, the submandibular salivary gland is involved. The patient usually expresses an overwhelming concern regarding the cosmetic issue and becomes disproportionately focused on the altered facial appearance caused by the PG swellings.

The etiology, symptomatology, and imaging of the PG enlargements in AN are those seen in sialadenosis and have been reviewed in the beginning of this chapter. Hyposalivation may be present but probably represents the effect of the patient's dehydration from a self-perpetuated starvation diet combined with the use of prescribed anti-depressant medications.

Therapy for AN involves a team approach. Hospitalization may be necessary if cardiac arrhythmias, electrolyte imbalances, or dehydration have developed. Psychologic care is imperative and requires input from the family. With a return to a normal diet, the resolution of the PG sialadenosis can occur with the passage of time.

Bulimia

Bulimia or "ox hunger" is characterized by episodes of binge eating, during which there is a large intake of food over a short time span, followed by induced vomiting and occasional periods of fasting. It is characteristically seen in young women who have a false body image of themselves as being obese. Feelings of low self-esteem and guilt develop and the bulimic resorts to dieting. Attempts at dieting to lose weight often are not very successful and lead to hunger, which in the susceptible individual causes an eating binge. Self-induced vomiting is initiated to counter any weight gain initiated by binge eating. Once the individual realizes that any binge-created weight gain can be nullified by vomiting, there is less tendency to limit the binge/emetic cycles. A natural progression is to binge and vomit not only when hungry but also when tense, stressed, or anxious [29]. Emetics, laxatives, and diuretics are frequently used as adjuncts to further aid weight loss. The criteria for a diagnosis of bulimia require three major components. Primarily, it includes recurrent episodes of binge eating with the patient's awareness that there has been a loss of control. Second, signs of depression are present, and finally, there is no known associated physical disorder.

The average intake of food during a binge is 3400 calories with some patients ingesting as much as 50,000 calories in a day [30]. The mean age of a bulimic is 22.6 years with the problem having been present for approximately 6 years [30].

The occurrence of bulimia, highest in young females, has an incidence that varies from 2 to 12% [31, 32], while among college women, it is as high as 19% [33]. Males are reported to represent 5–10% of the bulimics [29, 34]. The binge/vomiting cycles, usually carried out in secret, may be practiced as few as twice a day and as frequently as 20 times each day [29, 35].

The Columbia University Salivary Gland Center has had frequent referrals of bulimic patients who were seen because of the presence of parotid gland (PG) swellings (Fig. 9.10a). It has been reported [36] that 18–68% of bulimic patients have bilateral PG, occasionally unilateral, enlargement that can be accompanied by some submandibular gland involvement. The frequency of occurrence and severity of the PG swellings are directly proportional to the frequency of vomiting. Initially, the PG swellings are intermittent, but persistent swellings tend to develop in chronic bulimics after an early period of waxing and waning [37]. Because vomiting is precipitated over prolonged time periods by insertion of fingers into the mouth, calluses on the dorsum of the hand in the knuckle region may occasionally be seen (Russell's sign) (Fig. 9.10b).

The patient's request for medical attention emanates from a concern regarding the origin of the facial swelling as well as the cosmetic issue. The persistent PG swelling is usually painless, and there is no fluctuation in size from the salivary stimulus of eating. Palpation of the enlarged PG causes no pain and reveals that the tissue tone is normal. No cervical lymphadenopathy is present. Intraorally, the mucosa is normally moist. Extraoral massage of the PG produces salivary returns that clinically seem to be elevated from normal-appearing parotid duct orifices.

A clinical clue pointing to bulimia is the dental corrosion that is most visible on the palatal aspect of the maxillary anterior teeth (Fig. 9.10c). The repeated exposure of these tooth surfaces to the emetically regurgitated acidic vomitus causes chemical corrosion with enamel and dentin destruction (perimylolysis). The palatal mucosa should also be examined. On occasion, the pathologic entity sialometaplasia necrotica (SN) will be present involving the palatal soft tissues. This somewhat rare finding in bulimic patients was first reported by Schoning et al. [38]. Subsequently, sporadic reports of SN in bulimics have been made [39]. However, the etiologic relationship of SN to bulimia has not been defined.

A serum electrolyte study can be helpful in diagnosing a secretive bulimic patient [40–42]. In bulimics, serum electrolyte loss, brought about by the frequent and persistent emetic episodes and the adjunctive use of laxatives and diuretics, may become clinically evident. Hypokalemia and hypochloremia can develop. Their levels of loss are in direct proportion to the frequency of the vomiting/purging episodes [40, 41] and may even require hospitalization.

CT scan imaging will reveal the presence of an enlarged PG with the absence of inflammation and neoplasms. As in sialadenosis, the PG approaches the density of the masseter muscle. The image reflects the increase in PG parenchymal density and results from individual acini enlargement and replacement of normally present lucent adipose tissue. Another reason for augmented PG visibility is related to the gland's vascularity which is increased in the active bulimic. The increased number of vessels with their contained contrast serves to enhance the PG (Fig. 9.10d).

Histologically, as observed in sialadenosis, the acini of the PG of a bulimic are significantly enlarged and engorged with protein granules. The acini nuclei are depressed basally, and only a mild scattered lymphocytic infiltration is present [43]. A decreased fat cell content is also present resulting from its replacement by the acinar hypertrophy.

The exact etiological cause of the parotidomegaly seen in bulimia is thought to be a result of the same autonomic neuropathy seen in the varied systemic causes of sialadenosis. However, it is also possible that the PG hypertrophy may represent a work hypertrophy resulting from the multiple vomiting episodes that induce increased PG cholinergic activity leading to cellular enlargement [36, 44].

Treatment of the PG swelling in bulimics is aimed at eliminating the emetic episodes. Psychiatric care may be necessary, and it should entail individual, group, family, and behavioral therapies. The PG swellings will usually subside once emesis stops, but the process can be slow and at times the PG hypertrophy will not resolve [45]. Only 50% of patients with bulimia show resolution of the PG swellings after 10 years [18]. Botulinum toxin to interrupt PG innervation and decrease gland size has had only limited success [10, 18].

Idiopathic Sialadenosis

Although it has been generally accepted that sialadenosis can be precipitated by the development of an autonomic demyelinating neuropathy initiated by diabetes, chronic alcoholism, or malnutrition, there are some patients with sialadenosis that do not have a background of any of these disorders [1, 6, 28, 46–49]. Despite having the classic signs and symptoms of sialadenosis, no underlying allied medical condition can be found. Only after a detailed examination, which includes a thorough medical history, social history, physical and clinical examinations, serology, imaging, and cytology, can the known and established clinical causes of sialadenosis be eliminated. Thereupon these patients can be classified into the idiopathic category. Continued observation is warranted because of the possible eventual development of symptomatology associated with the late onset of a sialadenosis-inciting systemic disease.

Imaging findings and the treatment for the issues related to PG hypertrophy that are idiopathic in origin have been addressed in the previous discussion on sialadenosis and can be found at the beginning of this chapter.

Medications

Sialadenosis resulting from adverse drug reactions is rare. Medications that have been listed as causative agents of sialadenosis frequently include valproic acid, an anticonvulsant used in the treatment of epilepsy [50, 51]. Antihypertensives (guanethidine, reserpine, and nifedipine), psychotropic agents, and bronchodilators have also been implicated in the development of sialadenosis [1, 12, 50, 52]. However, the exact mechanism by which these drugs induce sialadenosis remains an enigma.

References

1. Scully C, Bagán JV, Eveson JW, Barnard N, Turner FM. Sialosis: 35 cases of persistent parotid swelling from two countries. Br J Oral Maxillofac Surg. 2008;46(6):468–72. https://doi.org/10.1016/j.bjoms.2008.01.014.
2. Borsanyi SJ. Chronic asymptomatic enlargement of the parotid glands. Ann Otol Rhinol Laryngol. 1962;71:857–67. https://doi.org/10.1177/000348946207100401.
3. Som PM, Shugar JM, Train JS, Biller HF. Manifestations of parotid gland enlargement: radiographic, pathologic, and clinical correlations. Part I: the autoimmune pseudosialectasias. Radiology. 1981;141(2):415–9. https://doi.org/10.1148/radiology.141.2.7291566.
4. Chilla R. Sialadenosis of the salivary glands of the head. Adv Otorhinolaryngol. 1981;26:1.
5. Ascoli V, Albedi FM, De Blasiis R, Nardi F. Sialadenosis of the parotid gland: report of four cases diagnosed by fine-needle aspiration cytology. Diagn Cytopathol. 1993;9(2):151–5. https://doi.org/10.1002/dc.2840090208.
6. Henry-Stanley MJ, Beneke J, Bardales RH, Stanley MW. Fine-needle aspiration of normal tissue from enlarged salivary glands: sialosis or missed target? Diagn Cytopathol. 1995;13(4):300–3. https://doi.org/10.1002/dc.2840130405.
7. Donath K, Seifert G. Ultrastructural studies of the parotid glands in sialadenosis. Virchows Arch A Pathol Anat Histol. 1975;365(2):119–35. https://doi.org/10.1007/BF00432384.
8. Chilla R. Sialadenosis of the salivary glands of the head. Studies on the physiology and pathophysiology of parotid secretion. Adv Otorhinolaryngol. 1981;26:1.
9. Ihrler S, Rath C, Zengel P, Kirchner T, Harrison JD, Weiler C. Pathogenesis of sialadenosis: possible role of functionally deficient myoepithelial cells. Oral Surg Oral Med Oral Pathol Oral Radiol Endod. 2010;110(2):218–23. https://doi.org/10.1016/j.tripleo.2010.03.014.
10. Jeon YT, Hong MP, Lee SJ, Shin GC, Choi J, Lim JY. Efficacy and safety of intraglandular botulinum toxin injections for treatment of sialadenosis. Clin Otolaryngol. 2021;46(5):1131–5. https://doi.org/10.1111/coa.13788.
11. Mandic R, Teymoortash A, Kann PH, Werner JA. Sialadenosis of the major salivary glands in a patient with central diabetes insipidus—implications of aquaporin water channels in the pathomechanism of sialadenosis. Exp Clin Endocrinol Diabetes. 2005;113(4):205–7. https://doi.org/10.1055/s-2005-837555.
12. Guan G, Won J, Mei L, Polonowita A. Extensive adipose replacement of the parotid glands: a case report and literature review. Oral Surg. 2020;13:41–7.
13. Jagtap SV, Aramani SS, Mane A, Bonde V. Sialosis: cytomorphological significance in the diagnosis of an uncommon entity. J Cytol. 2017;34(1):51–2. https://doi.org/10.4103/0970-9371.197620.
14. Ono K, Morimoto Y, Inoue H, Masuda W, Tanaka T, Inenaga K. Relationship of the unstimulated whole saliva flow rate and salivary gland size estimated by magnetic resonance image in healthy young humans. Arch Oral Biol. 2006;51(4):345–9. https://doi.org/10.1016/j.archoralbio.2005.09.001.
15. Ono K, Inoue H, Masuda W, et al. Relationship of chewing-stimulated whole saliva flow rate and salivary gland size. Arch Oral Biol. 2007;52(5):427–31. https://doi.org/10.1016/j.archoralbio.2006.10.021.
16. Scott J, Flower EA, Burns J. A quantitative study of histological changes in the human parotid gland occurring with adult age. J Oral Pathol. 1987;16(10):505–10. https://doi.org/10.1111/j.1600-0714.1987.tb00681.x.

17. Kelly SA, Black MJ, Soames JV. Unilateral enlargement of the parotid gland in a patient with sialosis and contralateral parotid aplasia. Br J Oral Maxillofac Surg. 1990;28(6):409–12. https://doi.org/10.1016/0266-4356(90)90041-i.
18. Davis AB, Hoffman HT. Management options for sialadenosis. Otolaryngol Clin North Am. 2021;54(3):605–11. https://doi.org/10.1016/j.otc.2021.02.005.
19. Donath K. Wangenschwellung bei Sialadenose. HNO. 1979;27:113.
20. United States Department of Health and Human Services. National Diabetes Statistic Report 2020. Estimates of diabetes and its burden in the United States.
21. Russotto SB. Asymptomatic parotid gland enlargement in diabetes mellitus. Oral Surg Oral Med Oral Pathol. 1981;52(6):594–8. https://doi.org/10.1016/0030-4220(81)90075-x.
22. Dejgaard A. Pathophysiology and treatment of diabetic neuropathy. Diabet Med. 1998;15(2):97–112. https://doi.org/10.1002/(SICI)1096-9136(199802)15:2<97::AID-DIA523>3.0.CO;2-5.
23. Rao SK, Rao YK. Parotid biopsies in young diabetics. J Indian Med Assoc. 1979;72(4):77–9.
24. Tüzün E, Hatemi AC, Memişoğlu K. Possible role of gangliosides in salivary gland complications of diabetes. Med Hypotheses. 2000;54(6):910–2. https://doi.org/10.1054/mehy.1999.0978.
25. Proctor GB, Shori DK. The effect of ethanol on salivary glands. In: Preedy VR, Watson RR, editors. Alcohol and the gastrointestinal tract. Boca Raton: CRC Press; 1996. p. 111–22.
26. Guggenheimer J, Close JM, Eghtesad B. Sialadenosis in patients with advanced liver disease. Head Neck Pathol. 2009;3(2):100–5. https://doi.org/10.1007/s12105-009-0113-6.
27. Mandel L, Vakkas J, Saqi A. Alcoholic (beer) sialosis. J Oral Maxillofac Surg. 2005;63(3):402–5. https://doi.org/10.1016/j.joms.2004.04.034.
28. Pape SA, MacLeod RI, McLean NR, Soames JV. Sialadenosis of the salivary glands. Br J Plast Surg. 1995;48(6):419–22. https://doi.org/10.1016/s0007-1226(95)90233-3.
29. Casper RC. The pathophysiology of anorexia nervosa and bulimia nervosa. Annu Rev Nutr. 1986;6:299–316. https://doi.org/10.1146/annurev.nu.06.070186.001503.
30. Mitchell JE, Pyle RL, Eckert ED. Frequency and duration of binge-eating episodes in patients with bulimia. Am J Psychiatry. 1981;138(6):835–6. https://doi.org/10.1176/ajp.138.6.835.
31. Rauch SD, Herzog DB. Parotidectomy for bulimia: a dissenting view. Am J Otolaryngol. 1987;8(6):376–80. https://doi.org/10.1016/s0196-0709(87)80023-6.
32. Rockwell WJ. Eating disorders: evaluation and treatment. N C Med J. 1988;49(10):533–5.
33. Pyle RL, Mitchell JE, Eckert E. The incidence of bulimia in freshman college students. Int J Eat Disord. 1988;2:75.
34. Mitchell JE, Seim HC, Colon P, Pomeroy C. Medical complications and medical management of bulimia. Ann Intern Med. 1987;107:71.
35. Jacobs MB, Schneider JA. Medical complications of bulimia: a prospective evaluation. Q J Med. 1985;54(214):177–82.
36. Garcia Garcia B, Dean Ferrer A, Diaz Jimenez N, Alamillos Granados FJ. Bilateral parotid sialadenosis associated with long-standing bulimia: a case report and literature review. J Maxillofac Oral Surg. 2018;17(2):117–21. https://doi.org/10.1007/s12663-016-0913-7.
37. Ahola SJ. Unexplained parotid enlargement: a clue to occult bulimia. Conn Med. 1982;46(4):185–6.
38. Schöning H, Emshoff R, Kreczy A. Necrotizing sialometaplasia in two patients with bulimia and chronic vomiting. Int J Oral Maxillofac Surg. 1998;27(6):463–5. https://doi.org/10.1016/s0901-5027(98)80039-8.
39. Aframian DJ. Anorexia/bulimia-related sialadenosis of palatal minor salivary glands. J Oral Pathol Med. 2005;34(6):383. https://doi.org/10.1111/j.1600-0714.2005.00313.x.
40. Wolfe BE, Metzger ED, Levine JM, Jimerson DC. Laboratory screening for electrolyte abnormalities and anemia in bulimia nervosa: a controlled study. Int J Eat Disord. 2001;30(3):288–93. https://doi.org/10.1002/eat.1086.
41. Setnick J. Micronutrient deficiencies and supplementation in anorexia and bulimia nervosa: a review of literature. Nutr Clin Pract. 2010;25(2):137–42. https://doi.org/10.1177/0884533610361478.

42. Barron LJ, Barron RF, Johnson JCS, et al. A retrospective analysis of biochemical and haematological parameters in patients with eating disorders. J Eat Disord. 2017;5:32. Published 2017 Oct 2. https://doi.org/10.1186/s40337-017-0158-y.
43. Coleman H, Altini M, Nayler S, Richards A. Sialadenosis: a presenting sign in bulimia. Head Neck. 1998;20(8):758–62.
44. Mehler PS, Wallace JA. Sialadenosis in bulimia. A new treatment. Arch Otolaryngol Head Neck Surg. 1993;119(7):787–8. https://doi.org/10.1001/archotol.1993.01880190083017.
45. Nitsch A, Dlugosz H, Gibson D, Mehler PS. Medical complications of bulimia nervosa. Cleve Clin J Med. 2021;88(6):333–43. Published 2021 Jun 2. https://doi.org/10.3949/ccjm.88a.20168.
46. Borsanyi SJ, Blanchard CL. Asymptomatic parotid swelling and isoproterenol. Laryngoscope. 1962;72:1777–83. https://doi.org/10.1288/00005537-196212000-00008.
47. Ino C, Matsuyama K, Ino M, Yamashita T, Kumazawa T. Approach to the diagnosis of sialadenosis using sialography. Acta Otolaryngol Suppl. 1993;500:121–5. https://doi.org/10.3109/00016489309126194.
48. Yu YH, Park YS, Kim SH, et al. Korean J Gastroenterol. 2009;54(1):50–4. https://doi.org/10.4166/kjg.2009.54.1.50.
49. Naik K, Mandel L. Sialosis, gout induced or idiopathic? Case report. J Oral Maxillofac Surg. 2017;75(2):343–7. https://doi.org/10.1016/j.joms.2016.08.028.
50. Mauz PS, Mörike K, Kaiserling E, Brosch S. Valproic acid-associated sialadenosis of the parotid and submandibular glands: diagnostic and therapeutic aspects. Acta Otolaryngol. 2005;125(4):386–91.
51. Derin H, Derin S, Oltulu P, Özbek O, Çaksen H. Pediatric sialadenosis due to valproic acid. J Craniofac Surg. 2017;28(2):e127–9.
52. Coleman H, Altini M, Nayler S, Richards A. Sialadenosis: a presenting sign in bulimia. Head Neck. 1998;20(8):758–62. https://doi.org/10.1002/(sici)1097-0347(199812)20:8<758::aid-hed16>3.0.co;2-n. PMID: 9790300.

Chapter 10
Endocrinopathies and the Salivary Glands

Louis Mandel

Abstract The function of the endocrine system is to produce the hormones that regulate the metabolism of specific cells and organs. Any disturbance in the production or activity of these hormones will produce alterations in the physiologic activity of the target cell or organ. Abnormal symptomatology will develop and can be recognized clinically. Several endocrine conditions have a known impact upon the salivary glands. Endocrine conditions such as diabetes, autoimmune thyroid disease, polycystic ovarian syndrome and acromegaly can be associated with salivary gland abnormalities.

Introduction

The endocrine system consists mostly of glands, scattered throughout the body, that secrete hormones directly into the bloodstream. The major endocrine glands include the pituitary, thyroid, pancreas, thymus, and adrenals. A hormone is considered a regulatory substance that modulates the activity of specific cells and tissues. The endocrine gland's hormone can act in two ways. The hormone can function to control the release of another glandular hormone (the pituitary's growth hormone and its effect on the liver's release of insulin-like growth factor 1) or communicate directly with the target organ (the release of pancreatic insulin to help the liver process glucose). A disturbance in hormone production or its mode of action inevitably alters the physiologic activity of the target cell and organ resulting in an abnormal systemic symptomatology that can be recognized clinically. This chapter will review those endocrinopathies that have a direct or indirect impact on the salivary gland apparatus.

© The Author(s), under exclusive license to Springer Nature Switzerland AG 2024

L. Mandel, *Clinical Management of Salivary Gland Disorders*, https://doi.org/10.1007/978-3-031-50012-1_10

Diabetes

Diabetes mellitus is a metabolic disease characterized by chronic hyperglycemia. It is the most common endocrine problem encountered in the Western world where it has become a growing health concern. This endocrinopathy develops via two different pathways. Type 1 diabetes results from an autoimmune pancreatic condition that causes an inability to produce insulin. Type 1 diabetes usually manifests itself via a rapid onset of symptoms in children and teenagers, but it can develop in adults. Type 2 diabetes represents a more common type of diabetes accounting for 90–95% of all cases [1]. It usually develops in adults over 40 years of age and has an association with obesity, a family history, hypertension, and a sedentary lifestyle. It is slow in onset. Type 2 diabetes results from the body's failure to respond to normally produced insulin. Regardless of whether the problem is Type 1 or 2 diabetes, the resulting high blood sugar levels can lead to disorders of the vascular, neurologic, and immune systems.

Although only occasionally reported, a clear linkage between diabetes and sialadenosis has been established (Fig. 10.1). A comprehensive review of the origin of this relationship and the signs and symptoms of sialadenosis have been considered previously in Chap. 9.

Besides sialadenosis, hyposalivation represents another expression of the effect diabetes has on the salivary glands. At this point, it should be restated that the Salivary Gland Center has clinically observed increased salivary flows in patients with sialadenosis. Nevertheless, some reports indicate that the salivary flow rates in both type 1 and 2 diabetes are moderately depressed [2, 3] with the magnitude of hyposalivation in type 2 diabetes being not as severe as seen in type 1 [4]. The discrepancy may arise from the fact that different methods of salivary collection were used at different times of the day in patients with a variety of medical problems that required the use of medications that had anti-sialogogic side effects [3]. The decreased salivary flow may also originate from any existing hyperglycemia which causes a polyuria [5]. The polyuria results in increased body fluid loss. Dehydration with hyposalivation can be the end product of the polyuria. Fatty infiltration of the

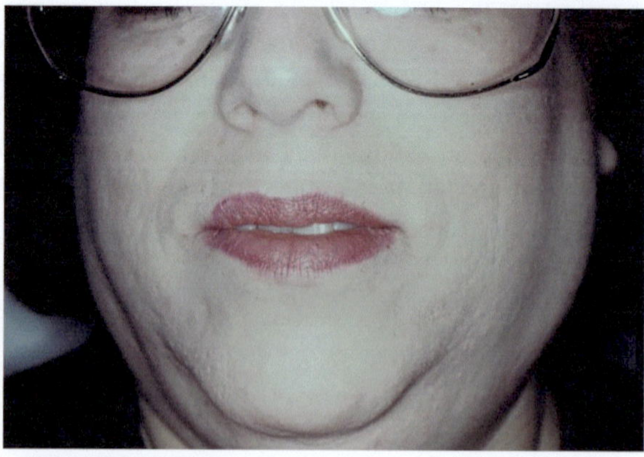

Fig. 10.1 Diabetic sialadenosis with bilateral parotid gland hypertrophy

salivary glands and even the neuropathy that accompanies diabetes may also play roles in the onset of hyposalivation [5, 6]. Nevertheless, keep in mind that the frequent older diabetic patient's subjective complaint of dry mouth (xerostomia) may have its origin from a variety of systemic conditions for which anti-sialogoguic medications have been prescribed.

Polycystic Ovarian Syndrome

Polycystic ovarian syndrome (PCOS) is a common endocrine disorder found in 4–15% of reproductive-age women [7, 8]. Family history appears to play a role in its incidence. Although there is considerable variation, the diagnosis of PCOS is based on the presence of two of the three following signs [7]:

1. Irregular menses. Infertility affects 40% of women with PCOS [8].
2. Hyperandrogenism. Androgen, a male hormone typically present in small quantities in women, is usually increased in PCOS and is the probable cause of the co-existence of hirsutism and acne. Approximately 70% of PCOS patients show signs of hirsutism [8, 9], while acne is observed in 15–30% [8].
3. Polycystic ovaries.

PCOS patients are prone to the development of the metabolic syndrome whose symptoms include obesity, dyslipidemia, hypertension, and cardiovascular disease. Insulin resistance with insulinemia and impaired glucose tolerance are also common manifestations associated with PCOS [7–9]. Diabetes has proven to be a significant risk factor in PCOS patients with 4–10% of PCOS patients reported to have type 2 diabetes [10]. Obese PCOS women are in special jeopardy because they tend to progress from normal glucose function to impaired glucose tolerance or diabetes rapidly. This fast progression to diabetes exceeds what obese women without PCOS experience [11]. The relationship of PCOS to diabetes is further highlighted by its disproportionate presence in type 1 and 2 diabetes. The prevalence of PCOS in patients with type 1 diabetes has been reported to be as high as 82%, while its incidence in type 2 diabetes is estimated at 26.7% [8].

Because PCOS patients are vulnerable to diabetes, the practitioner should be aware that sialadenosis is frequently a PCOS co-morbidity. The salivary gland manifestations associated with PCOS are those that occur in relation to sialadenosis. Sialadenosis is a painless noninflammatory persistent swelling usually involving both parotid glands (PG) (Fig. 10.2a, b) with occasional involvement of the submandibular salivary glands. The swellings do not fluctuate in size and are normal in tone when palpated. Sialadenosis may precede the diagnosis of diabetes or even develop in a controlled diabetic patient. Because the PG swellings are slow in onset and asymptomatic, other than cosmetically, their presence is not immediately noticed by the patient. A caveat exists in that, although sialadenosis is most frequently observed in diabetics and alcoholics, malnourished patients are also prone to sialadenosis. In addition, there are some sialadenosis patients who have no known underlying related systematic condition.

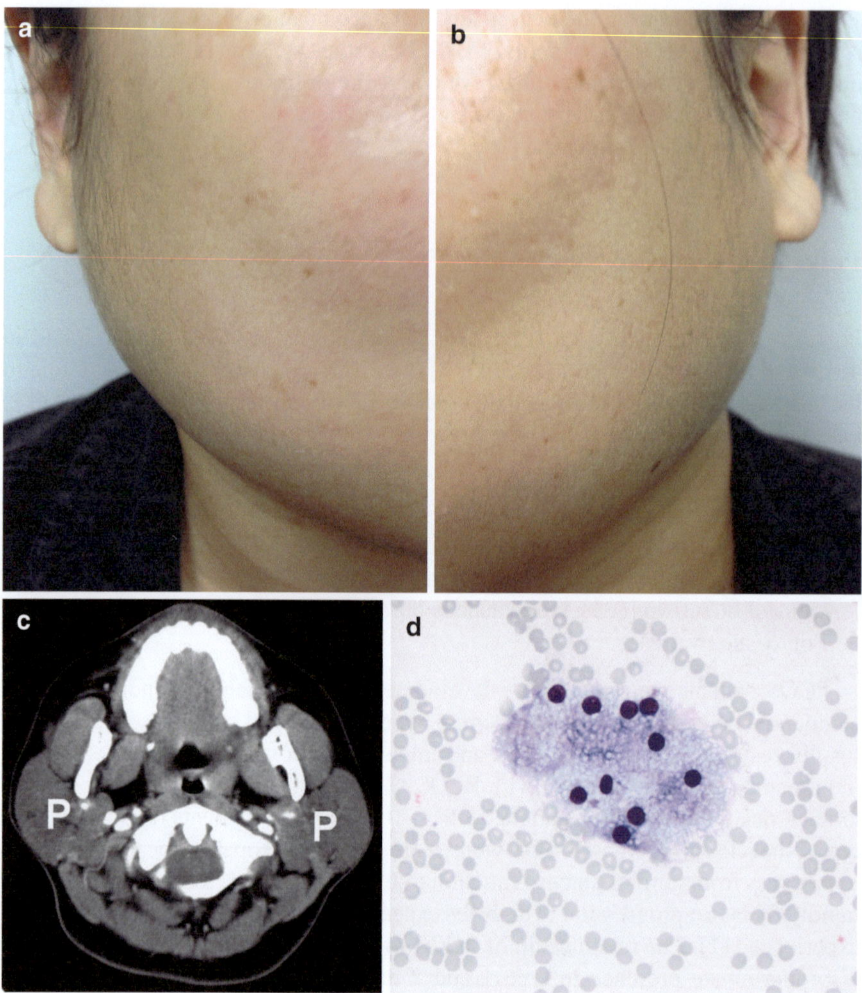

Fig. 10.2 (**a**) Polycystic ovarian syndrome (PCOS). Patient A. Right parotid hypertrophy. (**b**) PCOS. Patient A. Left parotid hypertrophy. (**c**) PCOS. Patient A. CT scan demonstrating enlarged parotids (P) with evidence of increased density. (**d**) PCOS. Patient A. Fine-needle aspiration of parotid. Acinus is enlarged measuring approximately 90 μm (normal 40 μm)

A demyelinating autonomic neuropathy affecting the sympathetic innervation to the PG has been postulated as the etiology behind the PG hypertrophy seen in sialadenosis [12]. A dysregulation of acinar cell zymogen granule synthesis leading to its increased production, with or without a failure to secrete the zymogen, causes hypertrophy of individual acinar cells (Fig. 10.2c, d). Water channel proteins, aquaporins [13], and functionally deficient myoepithelial cells [14] have also been suggested as the causes of PG acinar cell hypertrophy. An increase in acinar cell size translates into the enlarged PG that characterizes sialadenosis. Furthermore, the expanded acinar size leads to added glandular density as the enlarged acini replace normally present adipose tissue (Fig. 10.2c). A detailed discussion of the symptomatology, clinical diagnosis, imaging, histology, and pathophysiology of sialadenosis can be found in Chap. 9.

Because the pathophysiology of PCOS is not fully understood, treatment is usually centered around individual PCOS symptoms. Treatment is also focused on all metabolic consequences associated with the metabolic syndrome [15]. Oral contraceptives are administered for menstrual irregularities and hirsutism, spironolactone is prescribed for androgen excess, and a variety of medications and technical procedures are used for any existing infertility co-morbidity [8].

The chief concern of patients with PG diabetic sialadenosis centers around their facial appearance caused by the bilateral enlargement of the PG. Diabetic control with medication and diet does not effectively solve the parotidomegaly. Surgery for cosmetic reasons is rarely warranted. Because the enlargement of the PG has a known benign course, no treatment, other than reassurance and periodic observations, has become an acceptable therapeutic option.

Autoimmune Thyroid Disease

Autoimmune thyroid disease (ATD) represents the most frequent autoimmune condition that occurs in humans. It has been reported to affect 2–5% of the Western world's population [16]. The two major forms of ATD are the hypothyroidism of Hashimoto's thyroiditis (HT) and the hyperthyroidism of Graves' disease, with HT being decidedly the most common ATD [17]. The prevalence of HT increases with age, with females being the prevailing target. A genetic susceptibility and a familial association for the occurrence of HT have been accepted as causative factors. Environmental causes, such as the side effects of immunologically moderating medicaments, may also play a role in the onset of HT [18].

HT is a T-cell organ-specific ATD stemming from an impaired immune function that leads to an attack on the thyroid gland [19]. The pathophysiology of HT's thyroid gland failure involves the destruction of the follicular cells of the thyroid gland. The destructive process advances gradually, and because the thyroid gland has a synthetic reserve, euthyroidism may be maintained for years. As the thyroid destruction progresses, clinical symptoms will develop in patients. The symptomatology includes fatigue, bradycardia, weight gain, poor adaptation to cold, and a puffy face. Serologically, the thyroid-stimulating hormone level slowly rises. Often thyroid peroxidase antibodies, markers of the autoimmune process, are also present in the serum.

Ultrasound imaging usually shows an enlarged thyroid gland with a heterogeneous echotexture and multiple hypoechoic areas rather than a normal homogeneous pattern (Fig. 10.3a). Histologically, a florid lymphoplasmacytic cell infiltration is present and actively causes a replacement of the follicular cells (Fig. 10.3b). Germinal center formation and varying degrees of fibrosis will be observed. Hypervascularity may also be present.

Hashimoto's thyroiditis is more common in populations of patients who have other autoimmune disorders. Its incidence increases in patients with type 1 diabetes,

Fig. 10.3 (**a**) Hashimoto's thyroiditis. Ultrasound. Heterogeneous thyroid parenchyma with hypoechoic areas caused by lymphocytic infiltration. (**b**) Hashimoto's thyroiditis. Lymphocytic infiltration replacing thyroid follicles. (Nam YJ, et al. Endocrinol Metab 2013;28:341). (**c**) Ultrasound parotid gland. Heterogeneous and hypoechoic areas. Patient positive for Hashimoto's thyroiditis and Sjögren syndrome

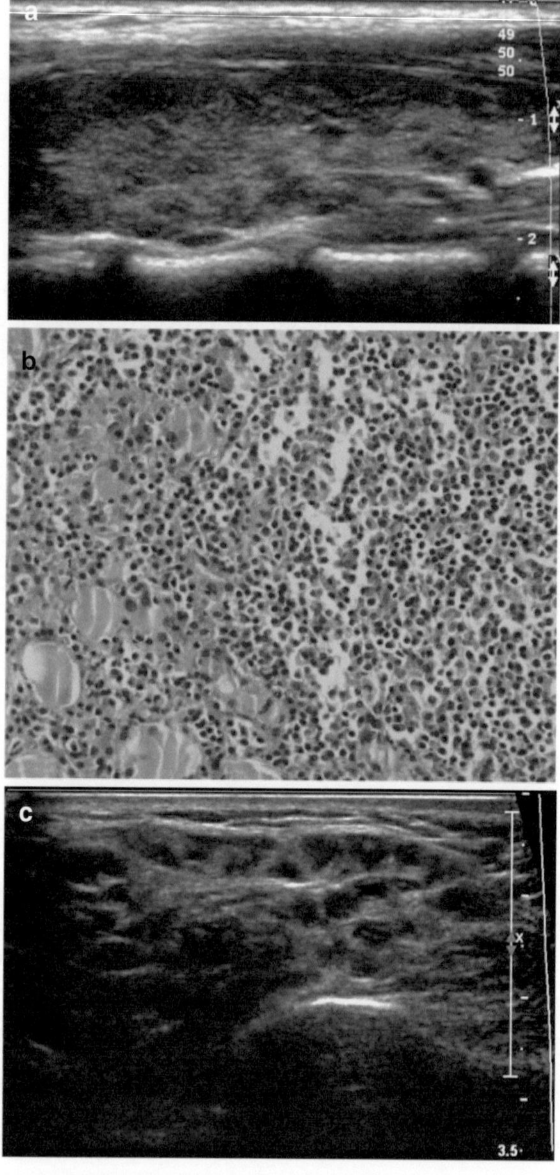

rheumatoid arthritis, or lupus erythematosus. Sjögren syndrome (SS) is another autoimmune disorder that occurs with a heightened incidence in patients with HT [17] (Fig. 10.3c). Reports of an association between ATD, particularly HT, and SS first appeared in the 1940s. Subsequently, the co-existence of SS (isolated sicca symptoms or full-blown SS) and ATD was often observed and reported [20–24]. An increased risk of SS in ATD and vice versa [22, 25] is now apparent. The incidence of ATD is nine times higher in SS than what occurs in the general population [21, 24, 26]. Several reports have indicated a prevalence of SS in ATD that varies from 3 to 32% [24, 27–29], while the prevalence of ATD in SS has been variously assessed at 3–40% [17, 30]. An incomplete symptom subset of SS may also exist in relation to ATD. These subset patients present themselves only with dry mouth. With time, many of these oral sicca patients will develop the typical symptomatology associated with SS [25, 31].

The co-existence of ATD and SS originates from the fact that they have common genetic, environmental (smoking, radiation, infection, and stress), and immuno-pathologic aspects [24, 32, 33]. Their shared features also include the susceptibility of females, they have a peak age range of 30–50 years, and they both have a predilection for the development of a MALT syndrome [25]. There is a 67-fold increased risk for a thyroid MALT lymphoma and a 44-fold increased risk for a parotid MALT lymphoma in ATD and SS, respectively [21]. In addition, they both histologically demonstrate a common periepithelial lymphocytic proliferation, a clonal B-cell expansion, and HLA class II epithelial expression [21, 22, 31, 33]. However, patients with both SS and ATD represent a milder clinical phenotype of SS, and they have a decreased incidence of lymphoma when compared to patients with only SS [24, 25, 33]. Despite the pathophysiologic similarities of ATD and SS, they are nosologically different, and their simultaneous occurrence can be interpreted as a polyautoimmunity, wherein two or more autoimmune diseases occur independently in a single patient [17].

Therapy for HT involves the use of synthetic levothyroxine as the thyroid hormone replacement. Additionally, because the clinical features of SS have been reported in a number of ATD patients, screening for SS, particularly of ATD females, is advised [31, 34, 35]. Similarly, patients with dry mouth complaints or classic SS should be evaluated for ATD. A full review of SS can be found in Chap. 7.

Acromegaly

Acromegaly, an endocrine disorder that causes multisystem organomegalies, results from excessive secretion of growth hormone (GH). Normally, the hypothalamus produces two hormones concerned with growth regulation, the growth hormone-releasing hormone (GHRH) and somatostatin. The GHRH functions to signal the pituitary gland to release GH. In turn, the released GH stimulates the liver to produce insulin-like growth factor I (IGF-I) which is the true agent involved in promoting growth [36]. Somatostatin, the other hypothalamic hormone concerned with growth, serves to regulate the release of GH by the pituitary [36]. Pituitary adenomas are the usual cause of acromegaly [37, 38] (Fig. 10.4). The increased GH produced by the adenoma will cause elevated levels of circulating IGF-I and induce the tissue overgrowths that characterize acromegaly.

Endocrinopathy acromegaly occurs equally in both genders with an incidence of three to four persons per million per year [36]. Males have a mean age of 40 years, while females with acromegaly have a reported mean age of 45 years [36]. The diagnosis of a patient's acromegaly is often delayed for 5–10 years because organ

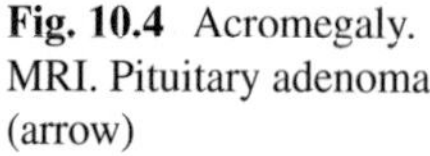

Fig. 10.4 Acromegaly. MRI. Pituitary adenoma (arrow)

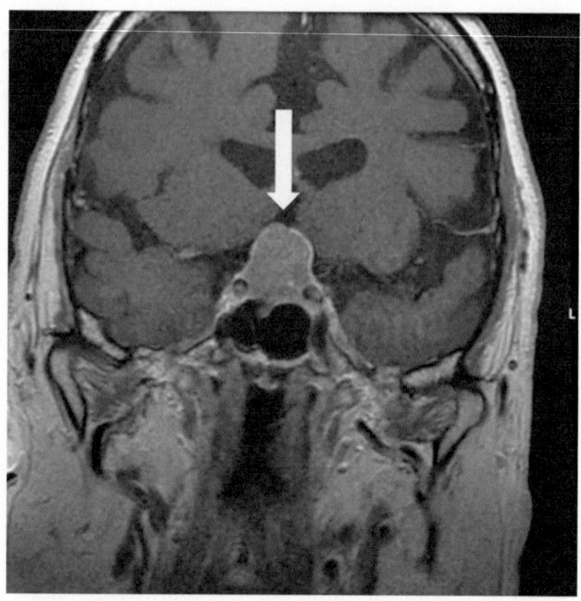

enlargement and its concurrent symptomatology are painless, slow in occurrence, and do not precipitate early medical attention. Eventually, systemic manifestations that include cardiomyopathy, hypertension, respiratory complications, neurologic disorders, diabetes, and musculoskeletal problems prompt a medical consultation.

The enlargement of multiple systemic organs and the coarsening of facial features are classic symbols of acromegaly. Sebaceous gland enlargement with hyperhidrosis and oily skin are common early signs of acromegaly [37]. The striking changes in a patient's facial appearance are what usually expedite a request for care and initiate the investigation. Thickening of the lips and nose, frontal bossing, and increased prominence of the supraorbital ridges become apparent. Orally, classic changes include mandibular prognathism, malocclusion with interdental spacing (Fig. 10.5a), and macroglossia (Fig. 10.5b) with scalloping. Sleep apnea, from craniofacial deformities and oro-pharyngeal soft tissue overgrowths, is not uncommon. Conspicuous increases in the size of the hands and feet, predominantly due to soft tissue overgrowth, also develop in acromegaly [37]. A susceptibility to neoplasia, particularly involving the colon and thyroid, suggests a routine need for a prophylactic search for the existence of a neoplasm in all acromegalic patients [39–42].

Because epiphyseal closure has already occurred in adulthood, stimulation of adult tissues by elevated levels of IGF-I causes the unique soft and hard tissue overgrowths that distort normal structural configurations and facilitate the diagnosis of acromegaly. Consequently, organ hypertrophy serves as a diagnostic linchpin. Although uncommon, salivary glands (SG) are also included as targets for the surplus circulating IGF-I. Bilateral asymptomatic submandibular gland (SMSG) enlargement has been documented in the large majority (87.5%) of acromegalics [43, 44]. The SMSG swellings are painless, normal to firm in tone when palpated,

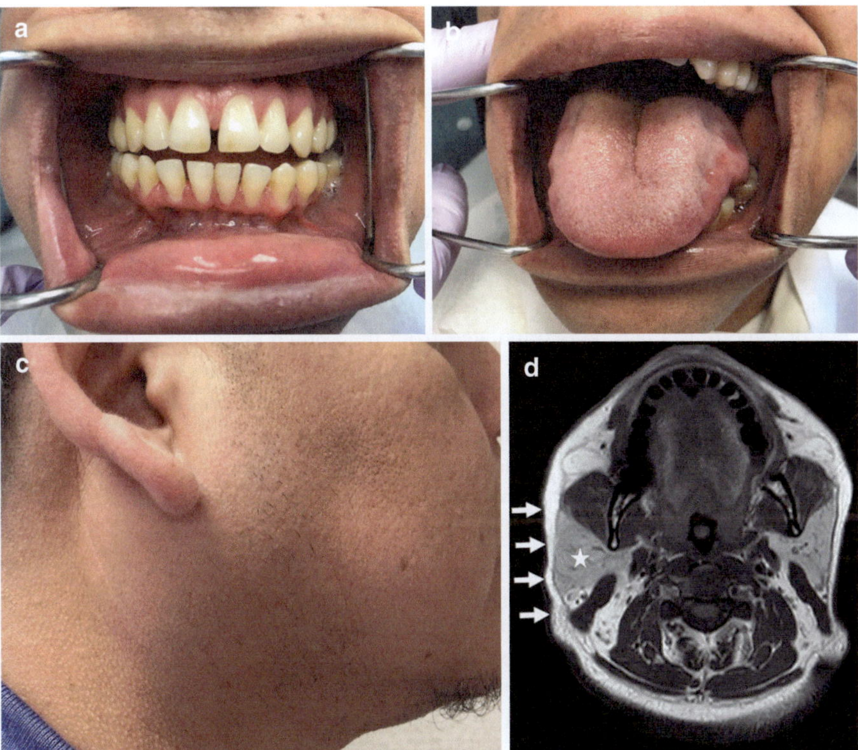

Fig. 10.5 (**a**) Acromegaly. Patient B. Open bite with interdental spacing. (**b**) Acromegaly. Patient B. Macroglossia. (**c**) Acromegaly. Patient B. Enlarged right parotid gland. (**d**) Acromegaly. Patient B. MRI. The right parotid gland (star) is larger than left parotid causing facial swelling (arrows) and asymmetry

persistent, and do not fluctuate in size when eating. Salivary flow rates from both the SMSG and PG in acromegalic patients show no abnormalities [45]. A reported histologic examination of an involved SMSG demonstrated no pathologic aberration [43] nor were any significant functional changes noted in a radioisotope study [45].

Reports of acromegalic PG enlargement were rarely found in a review of the literature [45]. However, an acromegalic patient with a parotid gland (PG) enlargement has been seen in the Salivary Gland Center (SGC) (Fig. 10.5c). The patient presented the opportunity to determine the pathophysiology behind the SG organomegaly. Does the SG enlargement represent cellular hypertrophy or cellular hyperplasia? Previous SG enlargements in acromegaly have been undocumented histologically and attributed to sialadenosis. Sialadenosis is seen in association with diabetes, alcoholism, malnutrition, bulimia, and even idiopathically. It is believed that, in sialadenosis, an autonomic demyelinating neuropathy brings about a disturbance in the PG's intracellular zymogen granule production and/or secretion [12, 46]. A cellular engorgement from granule accumulation results in an increased SG cell size—the cellular hypertrophy characteristic of sialadenosis. Consequently, the individual acinus becomes larger and joins the countless other acini in causing clinically visible PG swelling (Fig. 10.5c, d).

An MRI was performed on the acromegalic patient seen in the SGC and no pathologic changes were observed. Therefore, a fine-needle aspiration biopsy (FNAB) was performed to determine if cellular enlargement (hypertrophy) was the etiologic factor behind the parotidomegaly. A microscopic study of the tissue obtained by the FNAB testified to the presence of normal-sized acinar cells and acini [47]. Consequently, it appears that the SG enlargement in acromegaly follows a path different from the glandular hypertrophy observed in sialadenosis. Cellular hyperplasia would seem to be the cause of the pituitary-stimulated SG organomegaly. Substantiation for the concept of hyperplasia can be extrapolated from the known epithelial cell stimulating effect of an elevated circulating IGF-I. There is evidence that elevated IGF-I levels encourage epithelial proliferation, discourage apoptosis, and predilect the patient to epithelial neoplasms of the colon and thyroid [41, 42, 48–50].

Diagnosis of acromegaly is based on several clinical findings. Facial and oral alterations and thickening of the hands and feet are classic clinical features, while imaging (MRI) usually uncovers the silent pituitary adenoma that is present in 95% of patients with acromegaly [37]. Serologically, IGF-I elevations are present, and there is a failure of GH reduction with a glucose tolerance test.

Early diagnosis and treatment are essential because the complications and mortality risk associated with acromegaly are in direct proportion to the duration of exposure to the circulating excessive GH and IGF-I. Several approaches to treatment are available. Surgery to remove an existing pituitary adenoma has become the treatment of choice. Radiotherapy has been utilized to decrease the size of the adenoma prior to surgery or to control tumor remnants retained after surgery. The medication octreotide, a somatostatin analog, is used to decrease IGF-I levels by inhibiting the pituitary release of GH [51]. With treatment, some reversal of soft tissue, but not bony, overgrowth can be anticipated [50]. No treatment for the SG enlargements has been advocated. A reversal of the SG hyperplasia following medication has not been documented.

References

1. American Diabetes Association. 2. Classification and diagnosis of diabetes: *standards of medical care in diabetes-2019*. Diabetes Care. 2019;42(Suppl 1):S13–28. https://doi.org/10.2337/dc19-S002.
2. Moore PA, Guggenheimer J, Etzel KR, Weyant RJ, Orchard T. Type 1 diabetes mellitus, xerostomia, and salivary flow rates. Oral Surg Oral Med Oral Pathol Oral Radiol Endod. 2001;92(3):281–91. https://doi.org/10.1067/moe.2001.117815.
3. Hoseini A, Mirzapour A, Bijani A, Shirzad A. Salivary flow rate and xerostomia in patients with type I and II diabetes mellitus. Electron Physician. 2017;9(9):5244–9. Published 2017 Sep 25. https://doi.org/10.19082/5244.
4. Mata AD, Marques D, Rocha S, et al. Effects of diabetes mellitus on salivary secretion and its composition in the human. Mol Cell Biochem. 2004;261(1–2):137–42. https://doi.org/10.1023/b:mcbi.0000028748.40917.6f.

5. Carramolino-Cuéllar E, Lauritano D, Silvestre FJ, Carinci F, Lucchese A, Silvestre-Rangil J. Salivary flow and xerostomia in patients with type 2 diabetes. J Oral Pathol Med. 2018;47(5):526–30. https://doi.org/10.1111/jop.12712.

6. Al-Maweri SA, Altayyar MO, AlQahtani KW, et al. Xerostomia, salivary flow, and oral health status among Saudi diabetic patients: a comparative cross-sectional study. Clin Cosmet Investig Dent. 2021;13:451–8. Published 2021 Nov 5. https://doi.org/10.2147/CCIDE.S337581.

7. Stankiewicz M, Norman R. Diagnosis and management of polycystic ovary syndrome: a practical guide. Drugs. 2006;66(7):903–12. https://doi.org/10.2165/00003495-200666070-00002.

8. Sirmans SM, Pate KA. Epidemiology, diagnosis, and management of polycystic ovary syndrome. Clin Epidemiol. 2013;6:1–13. Published 2013 Dec 18. https://doi.org/10.2147/CLEP.S37559.

9. Fauser BC, Tarlatzis BC, Rebar RW, et al. Consensus on women's health aspects of polycystic ovary syndrome (PCOS): the Amsterdam ESHRE/ASRM-sponsored 3rd PCOS consensus workshop group. Fertil Steril. 2012;97(1):28–38.e25. https://doi.org/10.1016/j.fertnstert.2011.09.024.

10. Trikudanathan S. Polycystic ovarian syndrome. Med Clin North Am. 2015;99(1):221–35. https://doi.org/10.1016/j.mcna.2014.09.003.

11. Norman RJ, Wu R, Stankiewicz MT. 4: Polycystic ovary syndrome. Med J Aust. 2004;180(3):132–7. https://doi.org/10.5694/j.1326-5377.2004.tb05838.x.

12. Donath K, Seifert G. Ultrastructural studies of the parotid glands in sialadenosis. Virchows Arch A Pathol Anat Histol. 1975;365(2):119–35. https://doi.org/10.1007/BF00432384.

13. Mandic R, Teymoortash A, Kann PH, Werner JA. Sialadenosis of the major salivary glands in a patient with central diabetes insipidus—implications of aquaporin water channels in the pathomechanism of sialadenosis. Exp Clin Endocrinol Diabetes. 2005;113(4):205–7. https://doi.org/10.1055/s-2005-837555.

14. Ihrler S, Rath C, Zengel P, Kirchner T, Harrison JD, Weiler C. Pathogenesis of sialadenosis: possible role of functionally deficient myoepithelial cells. Oral Surg Oral Med Oral Pathol Oral Radiol Endod. 2010;110(2):218–23. https://doi.org/10.1016/j.tripleo.2010.03.014.

15. Bargiota A, Diamanti-Kandarakis E. The effects of old, new and emerging medicines on metabolic aberrations in PCOS. Ther Adv Endocrinol Metab. 2012;3(1):27–47. https://doi.org/10.1177/2042018812437355.

16. Simmonds MJ, Gough SC. Unravelling the genetic complexity of autoimmune thyroid disease: HLA, CTLA-4 and beyond. Clin Exp Immunol. 2004;136(1):1–10. https://doi.org/10.1111/j.1365-2249.2004.02424.x.

17. Anaya JM, Restrepo-Jiménez P, Rodríguez Y, et al. Sjögren's syndrome and autoimmune thyroid disease: two sides of the same coin. Clin Rev Allergy Immunol. 2019;56(3):362–74. https://doi.org/10.1007/s12016-018-8709-9.

18. Weetman AP. An update on the pathogenesis of Hashimoto's thyroiditis. J Endocrinol Invest. 2021;44(5):883–90. https://doi.org/10.1007/s40618-020-01477-1.

19. Caturegli P, De Remigis A, Rose NR. Hashimoto thyroiditis: clinical and diagnostic criteria. Autoimmun Rev. 2014;13(4–5):391–7. https://doi.org/10.1016/j.autrev.2014.01.007.

20. Jara LJ, Navarro C, Brito-Zerón Mdel P, García-Carrasco M, Escárcega RO, Ramos-Casals M. Thyroid disease in Sjögren's syndrome. Clin Rheumatol. 2007;26(10):1601–6. https://doi.org/10.1007/s10067-007-0638-6.

21. Lu MC, Yin WY, Tsai TY, Koo M, Lai NS. Increased risk of primary Sjögren's syndrome in female patients with thyroid disorders: a longitudinal population-based study in Taiwan. PLoS One. 2013;8(10):e77210. Published 2013 Oct 18. https://doi.org/10.1371/journal.pone.0077210.

22. Alfaris N, Curiel R, Tabbara S, Irwig MS. Autoimmune thyroid disease and Sjögren syndrome. J Clin Rheumatol. 2010;16(3):146–7. https://doi.org/10.1097/RHU.0b013e3181d52a28.

23. Robazzi TC, Adan LF. Autoimmune thyroid disease in patients with rheumatic diseases. Rev Bras Reumatol. 2012;52(3):417–30.

24. Baldini C, Ferro F, Mosca M, Fallahi P, Antonelli A. The Association of Sjögren Syndrome and Autoimmune Thyroid Disorders. Front Endocrinol (Lausanne). 2018;9:121. Published 2018 Apr 3. https://doi.org/10.3389/fendo.2018.00121.
25. Caramaschi P, Biasi D, Caimmi C, et al. The co-occurrence of Hashimoto thyroiditis in primary Sjögren's syndrome defines a subset of patients with milder clinical phenotype. Rheumatol Int. 2013;33(5):1271–5. https://doi.org/10.1007/s00296-012-2570-6.
26. Hansen BU, Ericsson UB, Henricsson V, Larsson A, Manthorpe R, Warfvinge G. Autoimmune thyroiditis and primary Sjögren's syndrome: clinical and laboratory evidence of the coexistence of the two diseases. Clin Exp Rheumatol. 1991;9(2):137–41.
27. Soy M, Guldiken S, Arikan E, Altun BU, Tugrul A. Frequency of rheumatic diseases in patients with autoimmune thyroid disease. Rheumatol Int. 2007;27(6):575–7. https://doi.org/10.1007/s00296-006-0263-8.
28. Lazúrová I, Benhatchi K, Rovenský J, et al. Autoimmune thyroid disease and autoimmune rheumatic disorders: a two-sided analysis. Ann N Y Acad Sci. 2009;1173:211–6. https://doi.org/10.1111/j.1749-6632.2009.04809.x.
29. Tektonidou MG. Presence of other autoimmune diseases in subjects with autoimmune thyroid disease. Am J Med. 2010;123(10):e23–5. https://doi.org/10.1016/j.amjmed.2010.03.030.
30. Sun X, Lu L, Li Y, Yang R, Shan L, Wang Y. Increased risk of thyroid disease in patients with Sjogren's syndrome: a systematic review and meta-analysis. PeerJ. 2019;7:e6737. Published 2019 Mar 19. https://doi.org/10.7717/peerj.6737.
31. Agha-Hosseini F, Shirzad N, Moosavi MS. Evaluation of xerostomia and salivary flow rate in Hashimoto's thyroiditis. Med Oral Patol Oral Cir Bucal. 2016;21(1):e1–5. Published 2016 Jan 1. https://doi.org/10.4317/medoral.20559.
32. Antonelli A, Ferrari SM, Corrado A, Di Domenicantonio A, Fallahi P. Autoimmune thyroid disorders. Autoimmun Rev. 2015;14(2):174–80. https://doi.org/10.1016/j.autrev.2014.10.016.
33. Jung JH, Lee CH, Son SH, et al. High prevalence of thyroid disease and role of salivary gland scintigraphy in patients with xerostomia. Nucl Med Mol Imaging. 2017;51(2):169–77. https://doi.org/10.1007/s13139-016-0455-4.
34. Biró E, Szekanecz Z, Czirják L, et al. Association of systemic and thyroid autoimmune diseases. Clin Rheumatol. 2006;25(2):240–5. https://doi.org/10.1007/s10067-005-1165-y.
35. Syed YA, Reddy BS, Ramamurthy TK, et al. Estimation of salivary parameters among autoimmune thyroiditis patients. J Clin Diagn Res. 2017;11(7):ZC01–4. https://doi.org/10.7860/JCDR/2017/26444.10128.
36. Barkan AL. New options for diagnosing and treating acromegaly. Cleve Clin J Med. 1998;65(7):343–9. https://doi.org/10.3949/ccjm.65.7.343.
37. Vilar L, Vilar CF, Lyra R, Lyra R, Naves LA. Acromegaly: clinical features at diagnosis. Pituitary. 2017;20(1):22–32. https://doi.org/10.1007/s11102-016-0772-8.
38. Melmed S, Katznelson L. Diagnosis of acromegaly. Waltham: UpToDate; 2019.
39. Cheung NW, Boyages SC. Increased incidence of neoplasia in females with acromegaly. Clin Endocrinol (Oxf). 1997;47(3):323–7. https://doi.org/10.1046/j.1365-2265.1997.2561053.x.
40. Cats A, Dullaart RP, Kleibeuker JH, et al. Increased epithelial cell proliferation in the colon of patients with acromegaly. Cancer Res. 1996;56(3):523–6.
41. dos Santos MC, Nascimento GC, Nascimento AG, et al. Thyroid cancer in patients with acromegaly: a case-control study. Pituitary. 2013;16(1):109–14. https://doi.org/10.1007/s11102-012-0383-y.
42. Dagdelen S, Cinar N, Erbas T. Increased thyroid cancer risk in acromegaly. Pituitary. 2014;17(4):299–306. https://doi.org/10.1007/s11102-013-0501-5.
43. Sober AJ, Gorden P, Roth J, AvRuskin TW. Visceromegaly in acromegaly. Evidence that clinical hepatomegaly or splenomegaly (but not sialomegaly) are manifestations of a second disease. Arch Intern Med. 1974;134(3):415–7. https://doi.org/10.1001/archinte.134.3.415.
44. Manetti L, Bogazzi F, Brogioni S, et al. Submandibular salivary gland volume is increased in patients with acromegaly. Clin Endocrinol (Oxf). 2002;57(1):97–100. https://doi.org/10.1046/j.1365-2265.2002.01576.x.

45. Thomson JA, McCrossan J, Mason DK. Salivary gland enlargement in acromegaly. Clin Endocrinol (Oxf). 1974;3(1):1–4. https://doi.org/10.1111/j.1365-2265.1974.tb03290.x.
46. Chilla R. Sialadenosis of the salivary glands of the head. Studies on the physiology and pathophysiology of parotid secretion. Adv Otorhinolaryngol. 1981;26:1–38.
47. Mandel L, Zeng Q, Silberthau KR. Parotid gland enlargement in acromegaly: a case report of this rare finding. J Oral Maxillofac Surg. 2020;78(4):564–7. https://doi.org/10.1016/j.joms.2019.12.001.
48. Rokkas T, Pistiolas D, Sechopoulos P, Margantinis G, Koukoulis G. Risk of colorectal neoplasm in patients with acromegaly: a meta-analysis. World J Gastroenterol. 2008;14(22):3484–9. https://doi.org/10.3748/wjg.14.3484.
49. Dworakowska D, Gueorguiev M, Kelly P, et al. Repeated colonoscopic screening of patients with acromegaly: 15-year experience identifies those at risk of new colonic neoplasia and allows for effective screening guidelines. Eur J Endocrinol. 2010;163(1):21–8. https://doi.org/10.1530/EJE-09-1080.
50. Abreu A, Tovar AP, Castellanos R, et al. Challenges in the diagnosis and management of acromegaly: a focus on comorbidities. Pituitary. 2016;19(4):448–57. https://doi.org/10.1007/s11102-016-0725-2.
51. Kreitschmann-Andermahr I, Kohlmann J, Kleist B, et al. Oro-dental pathologies in acromegaly. Endocrine. 2018;60(2):323–8. https://doi.org/10.1007/s12020-018-1571-y.

Chapter 11
Lymph Nodes and the Salivary Glands

Louis Mandel

Abstract Approximately 300 lymph nodes are distributed throughout the head and neck region. They lie in a close anatomic relationship with the major salivary glands (SG). Some nodes are located within the gland, predominantly within the parotid gland, while others occupy a paraglandular position around the parotid and submandibular salivary glands. Consequently because of this anatomic partnership, any disease entity, whether local or systemic, that involves the lymph nodes with the development of a primary or secondary lymphadenopathy will cause a swelling that mimics sialadenopathy.

Overview

A lymph node has been defined as an organized collection of lymphocytes, with or without germinal centers, surrounded by a capsule and associated with peripheral and central sinuses that accommodate lymphatic flow [1]. The nodes are an integral part of the body's immune system. They serve to filter the lymphatic fluid and in so doing they rid the body of waste products and pathogens.

Hundreds of lymph nodes are scattered throughout the body. In these multiple locations, the nodes and their contained lymphocytes are advantageously positioned to help in the destruction of invading viruses, bacteria, and fungi. In responding to the pathologic organisms, a lymphadenitis usually develops and is characterized by lymph node pain and swelling. Swollen lymph nodes (lymphadenopathy) also develop in relation to cancer (Figs. 11.1, 11.2, and 11.3) and diseases such as sarcoidosis, amyloidosis, and autoimmune disease. Histologically, a multiplication of lymphocytes reacting to an infectious agent are major contributors to the incidence of clinical nodal swelling.

Approximately 300 lymph nodes are located in the head and neck area. Many are in a close relationship, intraglandularly or paraglandularly, with the parotid (PG) or submandibular (SMSG) salivary glands. The intraglandular PG lymph nodes,

L. Mandel, *Clinical Management of Salivary Gland Disorders*, https://doi.org/10.1007/978-3-031-50012-1_11

Fig. 11.1 (**a**) Malignancy. Patient A. Squamous cell carcinoma. Right tonsillar area. Submandibular lymphadenopathy. (**b**) Malignancy. Patient A. Squamous cell carcinoma. Tonsillar and mouth floor area. (**c**) Malignancy. Patient A. CT scan. Enlarged submandibular lymph node (arrow)

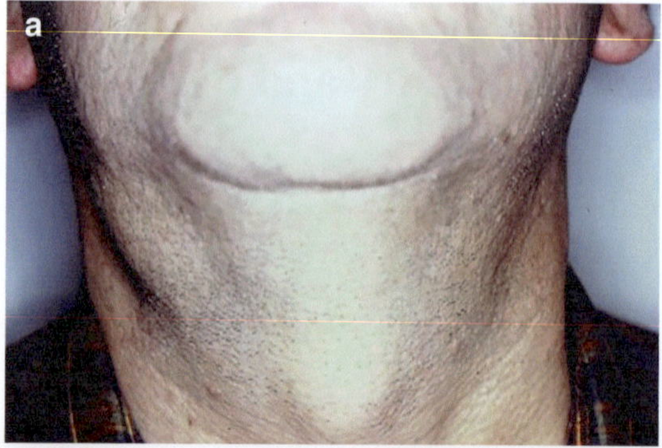

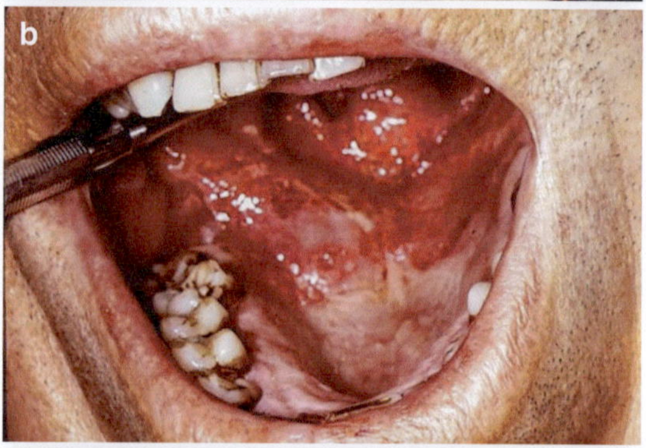

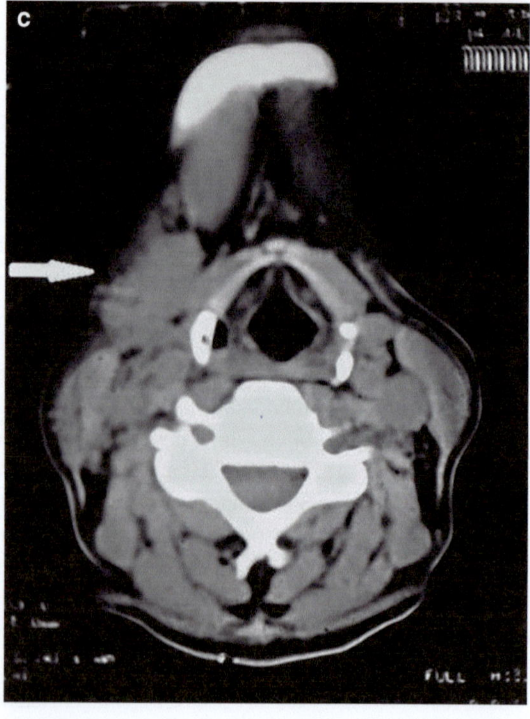

Fig. 11.2 (**a**) Malignancy.
Patient B. Gingival area
squamous cell carcinoma
(arrow). (**b**) Malignancy.
Patient B. Submandibular
lymphadenopathy

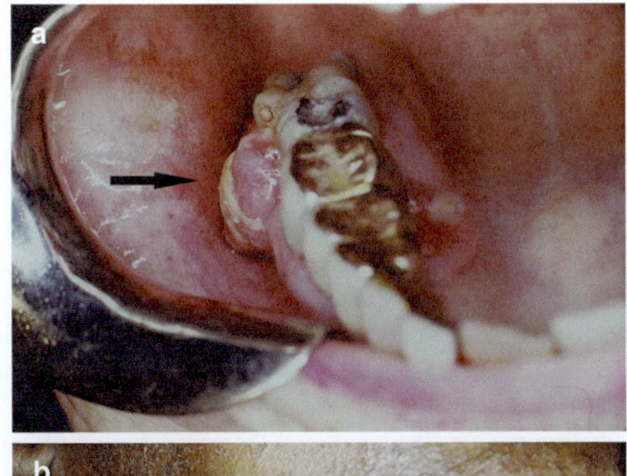

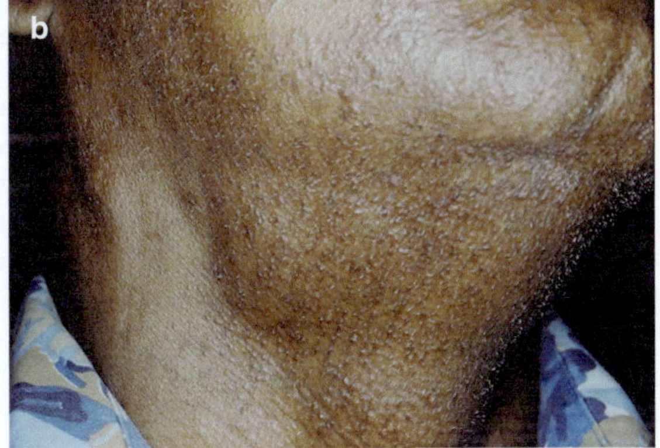

Fig. 11.3 Malignancy.
Left submandibular
lymphadenopathy
secondary to malignant
colon adenocarcinoma

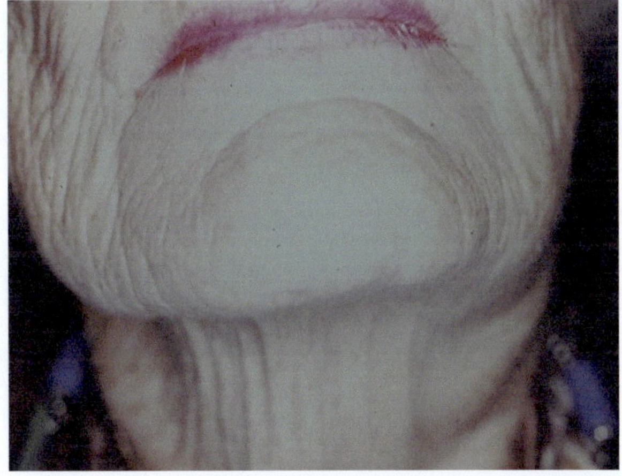

serving as part of this head/neck complex of nodes, become key elements in mimicking PG disease when they are incorporated into a systemic pathologic process
that involves lymph nodes.

The PG is artificially separated by the facial nerve into superficial and deep lobes. The superficial PG lobe has been shown to harbor between 2 and 22 nodes, while the deep lobe houses only 0–4 lymph nodes [1]. In addition, periglandular nodes on the fascial external surface of the PG and subfascial nodes are known to exist [2]. Furthermore, facial nodes on the surface of the mandibular body, buccinator nodes, and malar nodes lie in close proximity to the PG [3]. Naturally, these PG area lymph nodes, along with the intra- and periglandular PG nodes, can also become part of a pathologic systemic lymphoidal process and be interpreted as originating from PG pathology.

Lymph nodes have rarely been identified within the body of the SMSG [4–6]. The explanation for their absence in the SMSG and their presence within the PG is based on embryologic development. The lymphatic system develops after the SMSG has become encapsulated, and therefore the lymph nodes are not entrapped within the gland parenchyma. Conversely in the parotid area, the nodes establish themselves first, with the PG and its capsule subsequently forming around the developed nodes. Although lymph nodes are not found within the confines of the SMSG, many are located in the submandibular triangle in close proximity to the SMSG where they are considered part of the cervical chain of nodes. Because the SMSG is also found within the triangle, nodal disease, often metastatic in origin, that involves these submandibular nodes may imitate SMSG disease (Figs. 11.1, 11.2, and 11.3).

Clinically, it is always a challenge to differentiate a reactive from a neoplastic lymphoproliferation. A clinical examination often is not sufficient to separate these two possibilities. Histopathologically, help can be obtained by considering the overall architecture of the proliferating lymphoidal tissue as well as the cytologic features of the cells. Generally, reactive lesions maintain normal lymphoidal architecture, while neoplastic entities disrupt the architecture [7]. A fine-needle aspiration biopsy often does not supply enough material for an accurate cytologic diagnosis. A definitive diagnosis demands the microscopic study of a surgical biopsy specimen.

Castleman Disease

Castleman disease (CD), first described by Castleman and Towne in 1954 [8], is a rare benign lymphoproliferative disorder characterized by the formation of painless hyperplastic lymph nodes [9]. It is often referred to as angiofollicular lymph node hyperplasia. CD is recognized as a progressive lymphadenopathy that can appear anywhere in the lymphatic system. The lymphadenopathy has a distribution in adults of 60% in the thorax, 14% in the cervical area, 11% in the abdomen, and 4% in the axilla [10–12]. CD is rare in children, but when present, it has an increased incidence in the neck area [11, 12]. The median patient age has been reported to be 43 years [13] with a slight female predilection [14]. The etiology of CD has not been determined. However, it has been hypothesized that a chronic viral (herpesvirus-8, HIV, Epstein-Barr) or inflammatory stimulation serves to incite an immunological response that leads to the lymphocytic cellular hyperplasia associated with CD [9, 15].

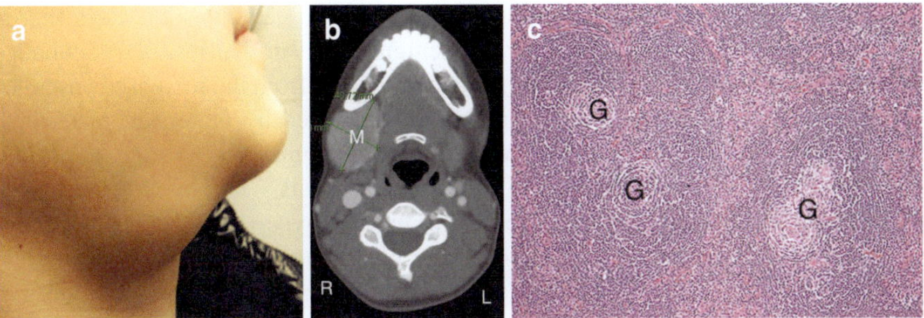

Fig. 11.4 (**a**) Castleman disease (CD). Patient C. Right submandibular swelling. (**b**) Castleman disease (CD). Patient C. CT scan depicts enhanced circumscribed submandibular mass (M). (**c**) Castleman disease. Patient C. Microscopic view of hyaline vascular CD. Lymphoid follicles contain hyalinized germinal centers (G) surrounded by concentric ring-pattern of B-cell lymphocytes

CD is classified into two clinical groups, either as a unicentric lymph node disease that tends to occur in young adults (Fig. 11.4) or a multicentric disease that typically affects middle-aged males [11]. Histopathologically, there are three recognized categories: the hyaline vascular (HV) type, the plasma cell group, and an occasional mixed variety, with 80–90% of the CD cases being HV in type [9, 15, 16]. The HV variety of CD, usually unicentric, demonstrates a benign slow asymptomatic progressive growth of either one lymph node or a localized group of nodes. Those cases of CD that occur in the head and neck area are almost always in this HV category [17]. Patients with CD of the plasma cell type tend to exhibit multicentric node involvement with aggressive growth patterns. Plasma cell group patients usually have constitutional symptoms that include fevers, sweating, fatigue, cytopenia, hyperglobulinemia and an occasional association with the POEMS (polyneuropathy, organomegaly, endocrinopathy, M-protein, skin pigmentation) syndrome. Progression to a non-Hodgkins lymphoma is a possibility in the plasma cell group [9, 18].

The parotid gland (PG) and submandibular salivary gland (SMSG) have both been victimized by CD, but the vast majority of the salivary gland cases involve the PG [16]. Lymph nodes do not become entrapped within the parenchyma of the SMSG. As previously stated, the lymphatic system develops after the SMSG has been encapsulated. Conversely, the embryologic development of the PG is such that its capsule forms after lymph node development resulting in the anatomic presence of intraglandular PG lymph nodes. The occasional involvement of the SMSG may originate from the rare presence of an intraglandular node or more likely from a periglandular lymph node that aggressively impinges upon (Fig. 11.4b) or invades the SMSG.

Clinically, parotidomegaly develops from enlargement of an intraglandular lymph node, and it is in direct proportion to the size of the lymphadenopathy. The resulting PG swelling is a circumscribed, painless, slow-growing unicentric mass that does not fluctuate in size. Diagnosis of the classic HV variety of CD is a challenge because the PG swelling is nonspecific and resembles a benign neoplasm. Conversely, the multicentricity of the CD plasma cell variety and its accompanying systemic manifestations facilitate its diagnosis.

The CT scan will reveal a solid circumscribed intraglandular PG mass that is homogeneous and has the appearance of a benign neoplasm. The lesion will enhance when contrast is used [9, 15]. The enhancement results from the increased vascularity of CD. Unfortunately, this CT appearance is shared by other benign lesions. Furthermore, a cytological examination obtained from a fine-needle aspiration biopsy (FNAB) also does not lead to a specific diagnosis. The FNAB of a HV CD nodule only shows a nondiagnostic reactive lymphoid hyperplasia [12, 17]. A definitive diagnosis can only be realized from the histologic examination of a surgical specimen. Microscopically, the HV variant is recognized by the presence of normal follicles consisting of B cells, with large mantle zones, that form characteristic onion-like concentric rings around multiple atrophic germinal centers (Fig. 11.4c). These germinal centers exhibit both an increased vascularity and a perivascular hyalinization [18]. The plasma cell type of CD is distinguished histologically by a significant plasma cell proliferation in the interfollicular region [9].

Surgical excision has proven to be the treatment of choice for unicentric CD [18, 19]. However, the treatment for multicentric CD has not been generally agreed upon, and guidelines are not available. Chemotherapy, radiotherapy, immunosuppressives, and corticosteroids have been advocated for multicentric CD patient care. Nevertheless, the most commonly practiced therapeutic approach has been a combination of chemotherapy and steroids [9, 18]. Patients with multicentric CD have a poor prognosis because there is a possibility of malignant transformation to a lymphoma. Long-term monitoring is indicated [9].

Kimura Disease

Kimura disease (KD), also known as subcutaneous angioblastic lymphoid hyperplasia with peripheral eosinophilia, is a relatively rare chronic inflammatory condition characterized by swollen lymph nodes in the head and neck. The etiology is unknown, but triggers, such as bacteria, viruses, and parasites, may act to change the immune regulation of T cells [20] and may be intimately involved in KD pathogenesis. KD is most prevalent among young adult Asians in the 20- to 30-year age category. Males dominate over females in a ratio of 3:1 [21, 22]. KD was first medically identified by Kimm in 1937 [23], but it was Kimura who in 1948 [24] described its distinctive pathological features. Consequently, he was awarded the honor of having his name used as the eponym for the disease.

Clinically, KD has a benign and self-limiting course. Patients with KD present themselves with cervicofacial swellings that originate from the presence of single or multiple dispersed subcutaneous angioblastic hyperplastic lymphoidal nodules, cervicofacial lymphadenopathies, and salivary gland swellings [22]. Unilateral, at times bilateral, parotid gland (PG) swellings can develop. Occasionally, the submandibular salivary glands are involved [21, 25–27]. Not all patients with KD have PG involvement, but its presence was noted to be as high as 60% in a review of 52 KD patients [28]. The PG swelling is benign and clinically tumor-like in its presentation. The PG tumefaction is painless, has a slow growth pattern, and has no malignant potential. The PG swelling in KD is thought to originate either from intraparotid lymphadenopathies or from a lymphoidal invasion by adjacent closely positioned positive subcutaneous lymphoidal nodules [25, 28, 29]. Despite the prevalence of KD in the cervicofacial area, multiple body parts may be involved [20]. Skin symptomatology, in the form of pruritis, pigmentation, and coarseness, is frequently present [21, 25, 26, 28]. Renal involvement, usually the nephrotic syndrome, is an associated systemic morbidity [21, 28–30] that may occur. Serologically, an eosinophilia and elevated levels of IgE are often detected and help in achieving a diagnosis. Nevertheless, a definitive diagnosis awaits histopathological evidence [22, 31].

Imaging with a CT scan will demonstrate a cervical lymphadenopathy and an enhanced, from the increased vascularity, mass-like lesion in the PG. Ultrasound will reveal multiple hypoechoic foci in the PG [25]. Neither of these imaging procedures are sufficient for the diagnosis of KD, but they can serve as adjunctive diagnostic aids.

The distinctive and diagnostic pathological features of KD mainly develop in the subcutaneous tissues and head and neck lymph nodes. Definitive recognition demands a surgical specimen. Characteristically, lymphoid tissue with germinal center hyperplasia surrounded by hyperplastic vascular structures and fibrosis is observed [22]. The germinal centers contain eosinophil infiltrates and eosinophilic microabscesses [22, 26, 28]. When the PG is involved, acinar atrophy and periductal fibrosis are also seen as components of KD's histology [22, 28].

Diagnostic confusion arises in differentiating KD from angiolymphoid hyperplasia with eosinophilia (ALHE). Although some clinical and pathologic similarities exist, major differences are present and rest in the fact that salivary gland involvement is infrequent in ALHE, males are more frequently involved in KD, and elevated IgE levels with a serologic eosinophilia are seen in KD. A review of ALHE is not indicated here because ALHE is now considered to be a benign neoplastic vasoproliferative disorder [32–35] rather than a manifestation of a lymphoproliferative disorder.

Therapy for PG involvement by KD usually involves a superficial parotidectomy and the removal of any existing extraglandular nodular masses. Surgery, along with immunosuppressive agents, has proven to be the treatment of choice [20–22, 28, 29, 31], but benign recurrence rates can be high, ranging from 14 to 44%, because of KD's unclear borders [21]. With recurrence, radiotherapy (20–30 Gy) or biological immunotherapy can become the second line of therapeutic care [20–22, 28, 29, 31]. Unfortunately, no firm consensus regarding treatment guidelines has been established owing to the relative rarity of the disease [31].

Kikuchi-Fujimoto Disease

Kikuchi-Fujimoto disease (KJ), first described in Japan in 1972 [36, 37], is an infrequently observed self-limiting histiocytic necrotizing lymphadenitis. Initially, it was described as occurring only in the Asian population [38], but the presence of KJ has now been established in all racial groups [39, 40]. Most patients are under 30 years of age, with an age range of 11–80 years and there is a female majority [39].

The etiology of KJ remains unknown. However, an idiopathic lymph nodal reaction to an injurious agent, microbial or autoimmune, has been suggested as a leading factor in its onset [40]. The diagnosis of KJ can be difficult because no criteria have been established. Unique diagnostic laboratory findings are not part of KJ's signature. Diagnosis is achieved only after the microscopic examination of an excisional biopsy of a clinically involved lymph node (LN).

Patients are seen whose symptomatology has been present for several months. Clinically, the most common symptom is the unilateral, occasionally bilateral, tender necrotizing cervical lymphadenopathy that is seen in 70–98% of KJ patients [39, 41]. Concomitant involvement of axillary and/or supraclavicular LNs may be present. Parotid gland (PG) swelling, unilateral and bilateral, has also been reported [40, 42–45]. In the PG, the pathogenesis of KJ probably originates from an intraparotid lymphadenopathy that is responsible for a clinical PG swelling and some discomfort. If the submandibular salivary gland (SMSG) appears to be involved, it can be assumed that swelling of the submandibular portion of the cervical LN chain, because it lies in close proximity to the SMSG, is mimicking SMSG pathology [46]. The SMSG rarely contains LNs. Any existing SMSG lymphocytic pathology probably originates secondarily from invading compromised paraglandular submandibular LNs.

Fever present in 36–77% [38] of patients with KJ is the second, after lymphadenopathy, most common presenting complaint. Night sweats, weight loss, skin rashes, arthralgia, and a risk of developing a lymphoma have also been reported [38, 41]. KJ should be considered in the differential diagnosis of any unexplained lymphadenopathy, particularly if fever and weight loss are present. Spontaneous resolution of KJ occurs over several months, but a low recurrence rate of 3–4% [38] has been noted.

The imaging results for KJ are nonspecific. Ultrasound of an affected node can show hypervascularity and enlargement of the node [38]. The CT scan only reveals a homogeneous large cervical node with contrast enhancement and low attenuation suggestive of necrosis [38]. With involvement of a PG intraglandular LN, the resulting lymphadenopathy scan can mimic a well-defined tumor [42].

A firm diagnosis can only be attained from a microscopic examination of a surgical specimen of an involved node. A proliferation of histiocytes, a varying amount of necrosis, karyorrhectic debris, and a paucity of neutrophils and eosinophils will be observed [38, 41, 47]. Immunohistochemistry will show histiocytes positive for myeloperoxidase and CD68, T-cells positive for CD8, and infrequent B cells [38]. These histologic findings serve to differentiate KJ from infectious causes and a frequently misdiagnosed lymphoma.

Because KJ is self-limiting with resolution within a few months, treatment can be conservative with supportive care obtained from analgesic and anti-inflammatory medications. Severe cases may require steroid and immunosuppressive therapy [38, 41, 48]. It is important to be aware that an association of KJ with systemic lupus erythematosus (SLE) has been documented. Therefore, monitoring KJ for the possible presence or eventual onset of SLE becomes part of patient management [38, 41, 42, 49–51]. Furthermore, other autoimmune diseases, including Sjögren's syndrome, can be diagnosed in an existing KJ, but the relationship is not understood [52].

References

1. McKean ME, Lee K, McGregor IA. The distribution of lymph nodes in and around the parotid gland: an anatomical study. Br J Plast Surg. 1985;38(1):1–5. https://doi.org/10.1016/0007-1226(85)90078-5.
2. Marks NJ. The anatomy of the lymph nodes of the parotid gland. Clin Otolaryngol Allied Sci. 1984;9(5):271–5. https://doi.org/10.1111/j.1365-2273.1984.tb01509.x.
3. Tirelli G, Marcuzzo AV. Lymph nodes of the perimandibular area and the hazard of the Hayes Martin maneuver in neck dissection. Otolaryngol Head Neck Surg. 2018;159(4):692–7. https://doi.org/10.1177/0194599818773084.
4. Dhiwakar M, Ronen O, Malone J, et al. Feasibility of submandibular gland preservation in neck dissection: a prospective anatomic-pathologic study. Head Neck. 2011;33(5):603–9. https://doi.org/10.1002/hed.21499.
5. Takes RP, Robbins KT, Woolgar JA, et al. Questionable necessity to remove the submandibular gland in neck dissection. Head Neck. 2011;33(5):743–5. https://doi.org/10.1002/hed.21451.
6. Soni K, Panchal V, Kathuria B, Yadav SPS, Sen R. Non-Hodgkin's lymphoma masquerading as submandibular sialadenitis. Indian J Clin Pract. 2014;25:652–4.
7. Greaves WO, Wang SA. Selected topics on lymphoid lesions in the head and neck regions. Head Neck Pathol. 2011;5(1):41–50. https://doi.org/10.1007/s12105-011-0243-5.
8. Castleman B, Towne VW. Case records of the Massachusetts General Hospital: case no. 4001. N Engl J Med. 1954;250(23):1001–5. https://doi.org/10.1056/NEJM195406102502308.
9. Xiao-Dong L, Qiu-Xu W, Wei-Xian L. Castleman disease of the parotid gland: a case report. J Oral Maxillofac Surg. 2020;78(3):400.e1–6. https://doi.org/10.1016/j.joms.2019.11.008.
10. Zhong LP, Chen GF, Zhao SF. Cervical Castleman disease in children. Br J Oral Maxillofac Surg. 2004;42(1):69–71. https://doi.org/10.1016/s0266-4356(03)00204-3.
11. Zhong LP, Wang LZ, Ji T, et al. Clinical analysis of Castleman disease (hyaline vascular type) in parotid and neck region. Oral Surg Oral Med Oral Pathol Oral Radiol Endod. 2010;109(3):432–40. https://doi.org/10.1016/j.tripleo.2009.09.025.
12. Rabinowitz MR, Levi J, Conard K, Shah UK. Castleman disease in the pediatric neck: a literature review. Otolaryngol Head Neck Surg. 2013;148(6):1028–36. https://doi.org/10.1177/0194599813479931.
13. Dispenzieri A, Armitage JO, Loe MJ, et al. The clinical spectrum of Castleman's disease. Am J Hematol. 2012;87(11):997–1002. https://doi.org/10.1002/ajh.23291.
14. Farruggia P, Trizzino A, Scibetta N, et al. Castleman's disease in childhood: report of three cases and review of the literature. Ital J Pediatr. 2011;37:50. Published 2011 Oct 20. https://doi.org/10.1186/1824-7288-37-50.
15. Abo-Alhassan F, Faras F, Bastaki J, Al-Sihan MK. Castleman disease of the parotid gland: a report of a case. Case Rep Otolaryngol. 2015;2015:265187. https://doi.org/10.1155/2015/265187.
16. Kardouni Khoozestani N, Niknami M, Ghanbarzadeh K, Ranji P. Castleman's disease intra parotid, a case report and literature review. J Dent (Shiraz). 2021;22(3):219–24. https://doi.org/10.30476/DENTJODS.2020.85683.1144.
17. Gürbüzler L, Ceylan A, Yilmaz M, Vural C. Castleman's disease of the parotid gland: a case report. Kaohsiung J Med Sci. 2010;26(8):444–7. https://doi.org/10.1016/S1607-551X(10)70071-1.
18. Cervantes CE, Correa R. Castleman disease: a rare condition with endocrine manifestations. Cureus. 2015;7(11):e380. Published 2015 Nov 17. https://doi.org/10.7759/cureus.380.
19. Guo Z, Liu C, Sun J, Zeng L, Zhang K. Castleman's disease of the left parotid gland: a case report. Int J Clin Exp Pathol. 2021;14(4):533–7. Published 2021 Apr 15.
20. Yang B, Liao H, Wang M, et al. Kimura's disease successively affecting multiple body parts: a case-based literature review. BMC Ophthalmol. 2022;22(1):154. Published 2022 Apr 2. https://doi.org/10.1186/s12886-022-02378-y.
21. Wang X, Ma Y, Wang Z. Kimura's disease. J Craniofac Surg. 2019;30(5):e415–8. https://doi.org/10.1097/SCS.0000000000005430.

22. Kok KYY, Lim ECC. Kimura's disease: a rare cause of chronic neck lymphadenopathy. J Surg Case Rep. 2021;2021(7):rjab318. Published 2021 Jul 19. https://doi.org/10.1093/jscr/rjab318.
23. Kim HT, Szeto C. Eosinophilic hyperplastic lymphogranuloma. Comparison with Mikulicz's disease. Chin Med J (Engl). 1937;23:699–700.
24. Kimura T, Yoshimura S, Ishikaura E. On the unusual granulation combined with hyperplastic changes of lymphatic tissue. Trans Soc Pathol Jpn. 1948;37:179–80.
25. Gao Y, Chen Y, Yu GY. Clinicopathologic study of parotid involvement in 21 cases of eosinophilic hyperplastic lymphogranuloma (Kimura's disease). Oral Surg Oral Med Oral Pathol Oral Radiol Endod. 2006;102(5):651–8. https://doi.org/10.1016/j.tripleo.2005.11.024.
26. Chaudhary R, Elhence P, Porwal P. Kimura's disease revisited: report of a case with a clinical and cytohistological correlation. BMJ Case Rep. 2016;2016:bcr2016214410. Published 2016 Mar 23. https://doi.org/10.1136/bcr-2016-214410.
27. Zhang R, Ban XH, Mo YX, et al. Kimura's disease: the CT and MRI characteristics in fifteen cases. Eur J Radiol. 2011;80(2):489–97. https://doi.org/10.1016/j.ejrad.2010.09.016.
28. Zhu WX, Zhang YY, Sun ZP, Gao Y, Chen Y, Yu GY. Differential diagnosis of immunoglobulin G4-related sialadenitis and Kimura's disease of the salivary gland: a comparative case series. Int J Oral Maxillofac Surg. 2021;50(7):895–905. https://doi.org/10.1016/j.ijom.2020.05.023.
29. Gupta A, Shareef M, Lade H, Ponnusamy SR, Mahajan A. Kimura's disease: a diagnostic and therapeutic challenge. Indian J Otolaryngol Head Neck Surg. 2019;71(Suppl 1):855–9. https://doi.org/10.1007/s12070-019-01601-5.
30. Muniraju M, Dechamma S. Kimura's disease: a rare cause of parotid swelling. Indian J Otolaryngol Head Neck Surg. 2019;71(Suppl 1):589–93. https://doi.org/10.1007/s12070-018-1421-5.
31. Sangwan A, Goyal A, Bhalla AS, et al. Kimura disease: a case series and systematic review of clinico-radiological features. Curr Probl Diagn Radiol. 2022;51(1):130–42. https://doi.org/10.1067/j.cpradiol.2020.10.003.
32. Ussmüller J, Donath K, Shimizu M, Bergmann I. Zur Differentialdiagnose tumoröser Raumforderungen der Gl. parotis: Angiolymphoide Hyperplasie mit Eosinophilie und Kimura's disease [Differential diagnosis of tumorous space-occupying lesions of the parotid gland: angiolymphoid hyperplasia with eosinophilia and Kimura disease]. Laryngorhinootologie. 1997;76(2):110–115. https://doi.org/10.1055/s-2007-997397.
33. Chong WS, Thomas A, Goh CL. Kimura's disease and angiolymphoid hyperplasia with eosinophilia: two disease entities in the same patient: case report and review of the literature. Int J Dermatol. 2006;45(2):139–45. https://doi.org/10.1111/j.1365-4632.2004.02361.x.
34. Sah P, Kamath A, Aramanadka C, Radhakrishnan R. Kimura's disease—An unusual presentation involving subcutaneous tissue, parotid gland and lymph node. J Oral Maxillofac Pathol. 2013;17(3):455–9. https://doi.org/10.4103/0973-029X.125220.
35. Ben Lagha I, Souissi A. Angiolymphoid hyperplasia with eosinophilia. In: StatPearls. Treasure Island: StatPearls Publishing; 2021.
36. Kikuchi M. Lymphadenitis showing focal reticulum cell hyperplasia with nuclear debris and phagocytosis. Acta Hematol Jpn. 1972;35:379–80.
37. Fujimoto Y, Kozima Y, Yamaguchi K. Cervical subacute necrotizing lymphadenitis. A new clinicopathological entity. Naika. 1972;30:920–7.
38. Masab M, Surmachevska N, Farooq H. Kikuchi disease. In: StatPearls. Treasure Island: StatPearls Publishing; 2021.
39. Bennie MJ, Bowles KM, Rankin SC. Necrotizing cervical lymphadenopathy caused by Kikuchi-Fujimoto disease. Br J Radiol. 2003;76(909):656–8. https://doi.org/10.1259/bjr/67899714.
40. Poulose V, Chiam P, Poh WT. Kikuchi's disease: a Singapore case series. Singapore Med J. 2005;46(5):229–32.
41. Rezayat T, Carroll MB, Ramsey BC, Smith A. A case of relapsing Kikuchi-Fujimoto disease. Case Rep Otolaryngol. 2013;2013:364795. https://doi.org/10.1155/2013/364795.

42. Chiang YC, Chen RM, Chao PZ, Yang TH, Lee FP. Intraparotid Kikuchi-Fujimoto disease masquerading as a parotid gland tumor. Am J Otolaryngol. 2005;26(6):408–10. https://doi.org/10.1016/j.amjoto.2005.02.020.

43. Medford A. Kikuchi's disease. Clin Med (Lond). 2007;7(2):201. https://doi.org/10.7861/clinmedicine.7-2-201.

44. Hwang JH, Yoo WH, An AR, Choi YJ. Coexistence of systemic lupus erythematosus with Kikuchi-Fujimoto disease involving the salivary gland, initially disguised as lymphoma. Rheumatology (Oxford). 2019;58(3):550–3. https://doi.org/10.1093/rheumatology/key353.

45. Kuo T, Jung SM, Wu WJ. Kikuchi's disease of intraparotid lymph nodes presenting as a parotid gland tumour with extranodal involvement of the salivary gland. Histopathology. 1996;28(2):185–7.

46. Chang C, Lin SH, Medeiros LJ, Chang KC. Kikuchi disease: an unusual case with features suggesting an infectious aetiology. Pathology. 2018;50(6):694–7. https://doi.org/10.1016/j.pathol.2018.04.005.

47. Mohanty SK, Arora R, Saha M. Kikuchi-Fujimoto disease: an overview. J Dermatol. 2002;29(1):10–4. https://doi.org/10.1111/j.1346-8138.2002.tb00157.x.

48. Nagarkar R, Adhav A. Kikuchi Fujimoto disease: a rare benign disease. SAS J Sung. 2017;3:138–40.

49. Feder HM Jr, Liu J, Rezuke WN. Kikuchi disease in Connecticut. J Pediatr. 2014;164(1):196–200.e1. https://doi.org/10.1016/j.jpeds.2013.08.041.

50. Cuglievan B, Miranda RN. Kikuchi-Fujimoto disease. Blood. 2017;129(7):917. https://doi.org/10.1182/blood-2016-08-736413.

51. Famularo G, Giustiniani MC, Marasco A, Minisola G, Nicotra GC, De Simone C. Kikuchi Fujimoto lymphadenitis: case report and literature review. Am J Hematol. 2003;74(1):60–3. https://doi.org/10.1002/ajh.10335.

52. Wiśniewska K, Pawlak-Buś K, Leszczyński P. Kikuchi-Fujimoto disease associated with primary Sjögren's syndrome—literature review based on a case report. Reumatologia. 2020;58(4):251–6. https://doi.org/10.5114/reum.2020.98438.

Chapter 12
Salivary Gland Disease in Children

Louis Mandel

Abstract As with adults who endure a wide range of salivary gland (SG) disorders, the pediatric population can be victimized by the same range of SG diseases. Sialolithiasis and ranulas represent SG disorders that demonstrate similar expressions in both adults and children. However, the young often present themselves with variations in the incidence and symptomatology of known SG abnormalities. Furthermore, there are some SG conditions that are unique to children. Mumps represent a SG disease that can affect adults, but whose occurrence is significantly higher in the young. Sjögren syndrome (SS) can occasionally develop in the pediatric population, but it manifests a symptom complex that has differences from what is seen in the more common adult SS. Juvenile recurrent parotitis, cystic fibrosis and self-limited epilepsy with centrotemporal spikes represent glandular conditions that are essentially limited to the young.

Overview

Children represent a unique element in the health spectrum of society. With some exceptions, the multiplicity of salivary gland (SG) disorders seen in adults is also present, albeit often with a decreased incidence, in children. However, there are some pathologic conditions that only involve the pediatric population. Neonatal suppurative parotitis, occurring in the newborn, represents one such example, while juvenile recurrent parotitis represents SG pathology that is limited to the young. Although children and adults are usually subject to the same SG pathologies, some conditions may present different clinical symptomatology in each patient category (Sjögren syndrome), while others that occur in both patient groups have essentially become associated with children (mumps). This chapter will review those SG pathologies that are limited to or predominantly associated with the pediatric population.

© The Author(s), under exclusive license to Springer Nature
Switzerland AG 2024
L. Mandel, *Clinical Management of Salivary Gland Disorders*,
https://doi.org/10.1007/978-3-031-50012-1_12

Another category of SG abnormalities that involves pediatric patients is the congenital/developmental group. These irregularities are reviewed separately in Chap. 3.

Mumps

Mumps is a viral disease that predominantly involves children (Fig. 12.1). To a lesser degree, adults also are affected. Because patients with this disease who were seen in the Columbia University Salivary Gland Center were all children, and because the disease is mostly associated with children, it is being listed in this chapter. More specifically, mumps is an acute contagious systemic viral disease caused by a paramyxovirus. Lifelong immunity can be expected for those individuals who become infected. At one time, it was a common infection that primarily affected children younger than 15 years of age. The introduction of a vaccine in 1964 resulted in a 99.8% reduction of documented mumps cases in the United States by the year 2001 [1].

The virus has a unique predilection for glandular and nervous tissues. The salivary glands, particularly the parotid gland (PG), central nervous system, genital organs, urinary tract, and pancreas, are some of the organ systems that are usually afflicted. A parotitis, seen in over 70% of infected patients, is the most common expression of the virus, while orchitis and central nervous system infection represent common extrasalivary gland manifestations of the virus [1, 2]. Submandibular salivary gland involvement is an occasional development.

The virus, restricted to humans, is spread by inhalation of contaminated aerosol droplets that have entered the air from the sneezing, coughing, etc. of an infected individual. With inhalation, the virus inoculates and replicates itself in the nasal or upper respiratory tracts of a non-infected person [2]. In approximately 30% of the patients, the virus will remain localized in the respiratory tract and cause only mild respiratory symptomatology or even no symptoms whatsoever [3]. More likely, active replication with viral spread from the respiratory tract to the regional lymph

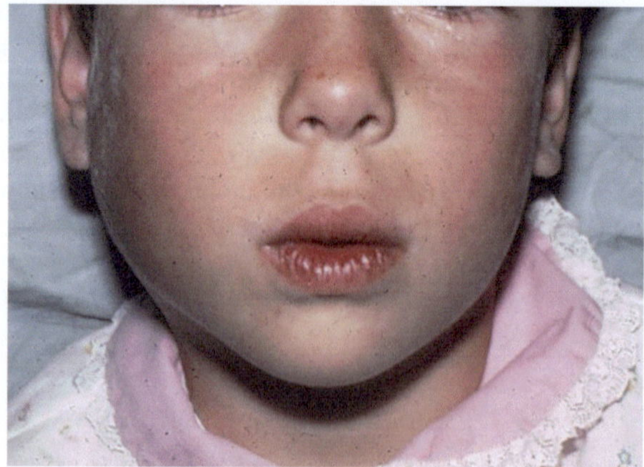

Fig. 12.1 Mumps. Right parotid swelling. (Mandel L, Chap. 9, Salivary Gland Disorders, Med Clin North Am 2014; 98:1415)

nodes occurs. Subsequently, a viremia ensues and is responsible for the virus's dissemination to the multiple organ systems [4, 5] that include the salivary glands.

Human transmission of the virus seems to occur most frequently during winter and spring months with an incubation period that varies from 15 to 24 days [6]. Prior to the development of clinical PG symptoms, a 2- to 3-day prodromal period of low-grade fever, anorexia, malaise, and headache develops [2]. Because the virus can be detected in saliva up to 7 days prior to the onset of the clinical PG swelling [7], this period of time when a diagnosis is not suspected represents an interval in which the virus is frequently dispersed to others. Infected patients are most contagious 1–2 days before onset of the symptoms of a clinical parotitis and for several days after [2]. Further compounding the problem of transmission is the fact that up to one-third of infected individuals exhibit no symptoms but nevertheless are contagious [1].

After the incubation period, PG swellings develop, peak in 2–3 days, and persist for about a week [2]. Initially, only one gland swells with contralateral PG involvement following shortly afterward, but simultaneous PG swellings can also develop clinically [8]. Bilateral PG swelling occurs in 90% of the patients with salivary gland involvement [2]. Additionally, the submandibular and sublingual salivary glands may become swollen (10%) [2] with or without the presence of a parotitis. The PG swellings are accompanied by pain, dysphagia, and a moderate trismus. Palpation of the involved glands reveals that they are tender and firm. The firm and painful swelling associated with the PG results from the viral-incited glandular inflammatory edema. As the edema increases, it meets the resistance of an unyielding fibrous PG capsule. The resulting buildup of intraglandular pressure upon sensory nerve endings is the probable cause of the patient's subjective pain. The firmness noted on palpation relates to the presence of a considerable intraglandular inflammatory infiltrate whose dissemination is also prevented by the resistant fibrous PG capsule.

Intraorally, pouting and inflammation of the PG duct orifice are usually present. Salivary flow exiting from the duct orifice tends to be diminished during the presence of the parotitis. The reduced flow apparently represents the compression effect of the glandular edema on the secreting acini and the duct system. Furthermore, a direct effect of the virus on the ductal epithelium causes duct inflammation with luminal narrowing and an additional impedance to salivary flow. With abatement of the acute infectious process, salivary flow returns to normal.

Serologically, the white blood cell and differential counts are normal while the serum amylase is elevated [2]. Microscopically, a significant PG interstitial edema is evident. An inflammatory infiltrate, consisting of lymphocytes, plasma cells, and histiocytes, is also present. Compression of the acini and ducts may be evident. Imaging, rarely necessary, reveals enlargement and enhancement of the salivary glands with fat stranding and thickening of the superficial cervical fascia [9].

A clinical diagnosis of mumps can readily be made if several salient factors are considered. Because the disease confers immunity, support for a diagnosis can be obtained from a patient with a history of never having had mumps. A recent exposure to an infected individual and a clinical picture of parotitis clinch the diagnosis. When doubt exists, laboratory testing for diagnostic antibodies and virus cultures from secretions (oral, blood, urine, or cerebrospinal fluid) can be performed for diagnostic confirmation [1].

Prevention of the disease process, by vaccinating children with the live attenuated measles-mumps-rubella (MMR) vaccine, has proven to be extremely successful. Despite this preventive approach with vaccinations, breakthrough cases of mumps have occurred and are attributed either to a waning vaccine effect or a recipient's failure to mount a sufficient antibody response [9]. No treatment is available for the management of the parotitis associated with mumps. Because the disease resolves spontaneously, treatment is directed at palliative care for each presenting symptom.

Juvenile Recurrent Parotitis

After mumps, juvenile recurrent parotitis (JRP) is the most commonly encountered childhood salivary gland disease (Figs. 12.2 and 12.3). The actual incidence of JRP has not been accurately determined. The patient incidence of JRP is difficult to establish and may not always be accurately reported because symptoms can be mild and resolve rapidly without medical attention. Furthermore, its etiology has not been satisfactorily ascertained. Presently, JRP is thought to have a multifactorial origin. Genetic factors, viral or bacterial infections, allergies, and immunological disorders have all been suggested as causative agents [10–13].

JRP is a nonsuppurative isolated inflammatory salivary gland condition that causes frequent recurrent parotid gland (PG) swellings. The submandibular and sublingual salivary glands are not involved in the disease process. For unknown reasons, the disorder spontaneously disappears with the onset of puberty. Usually the PG swellings develop unilaterally (60%), less often bilaterally (40%), and are asynchronous in their presentation [14] with a tendency for one side to be dominant [13]. JRP occurs mostly in males [11] whose first symptoms appear between 3 and 6 years of age [14–16]. At least two episodes of PG swelling occur each year [17], but as many as 5–30 episodes annually have been observed [18]. Following the subsidence of each episode of swelling, a varying asymptomatic remission period develops. Although there is a marked tendency for JRP to subside with puberty, regression may not occur until early adult life [19, 20].

Each PG swelling is sudden in onset, independent of meals, and may be accompanied by fever, pain, and malaise. The swellings last for 1–3 days, may even persist for 1–2 weeks, but resolve spontaneously. Extraoral palpation of the swollen PG reveals the gland to be firmer than normal and moderately painful. An uninvolved PG with a history of swelling reveals no abnormalities when palpated. Intraorally, during both the active and remission phases of JRP, moderately decreased salivary volumes may be noted exiting from the orifices of the PGs. Saliva milked from an exacerbated swollen gland often contains a visible tell-tale qualitative marker. Flocculations, representing mucus plugs in a background of clear saliva, will be noted. Surprisingly, salivary flow during periods of remission will be clear, and flocculations will be absent. Occasionally, a secondary infection may develop and will result in a cloudy salivary return.

Fig. 12.2 (**a**) Juvenile recurrent parotitis (JRP). Patient A (5 years old). Left parotid swelling. (**b**) JRP. Patient A. Ultrasound. Left parotid gland. Hypoechoic areas in a heterogeneous glandular background. (**c**) JRP. Patient A. Sialogram. Left parotid gland demonstrates classic sialectic pattern (circled)

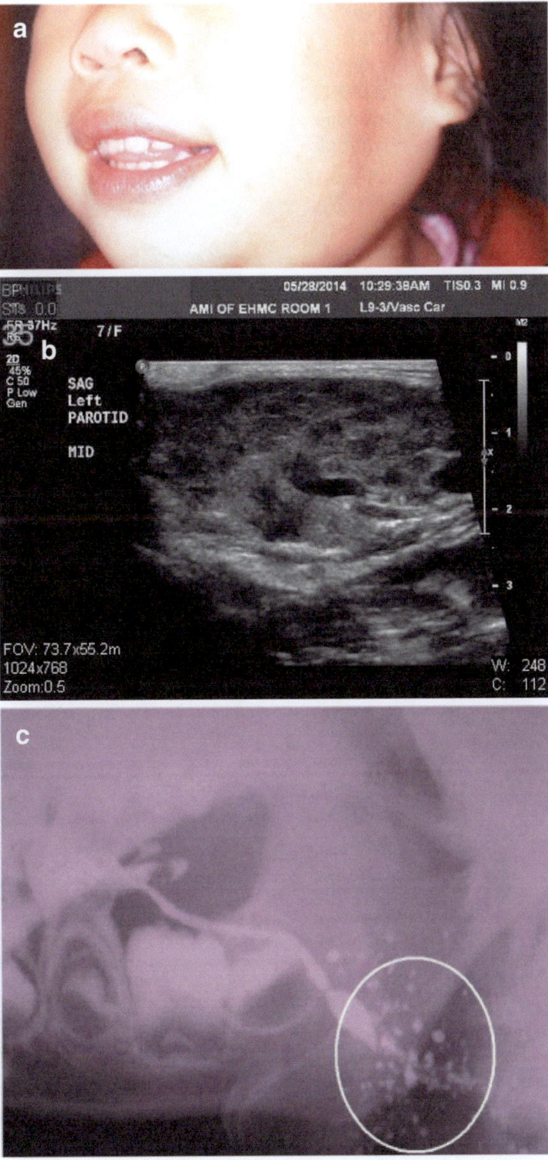

The recent introduction of sialendoscopy has added relevant diagnostic data concerning the duct system in JRP. Endoscopically, the duct walls are seen to have a whitish, rather than pink, appearance reflecting the duct's avascularity [21, 22]. Duct stricturing, along with accumulation of luminal debris, has also been observed [18]. Luminal narrowing from stricturing leads to salivary stagnation and favors the retention of inflammatory debris and the mucus flocculations seen both clinically and sialendoscopically during an acute episode.

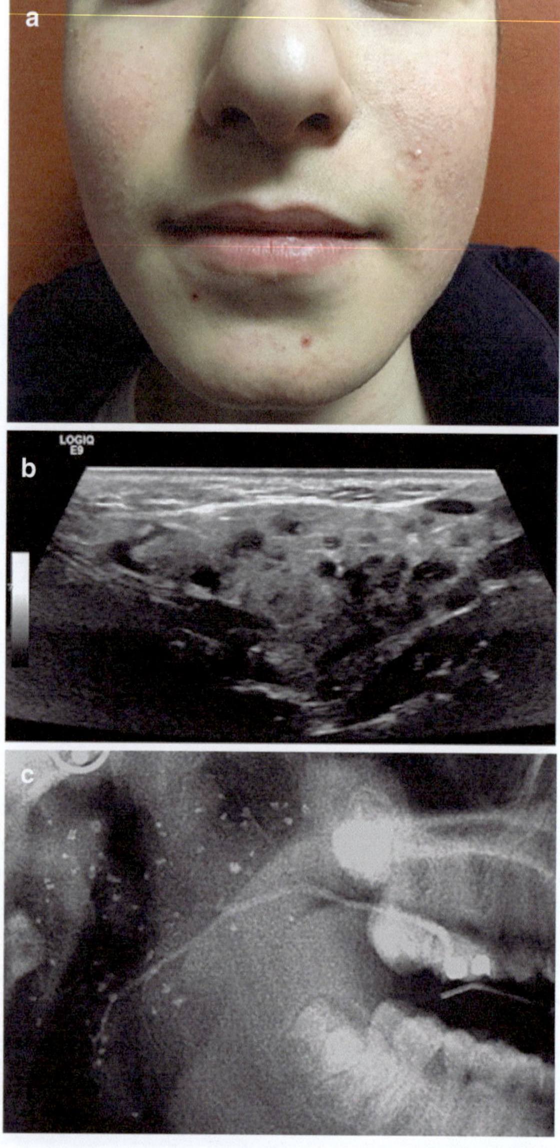

Fig. 12.3 (**a**) Juvenile recurrent parotitis (JRP). Patient B (13 years old). Left parotid swelling. (**b**) JRP. Patient B. Ultrasound left parotid gland. Multiple hypoechoic areas. (**c**) JRP. Patient B. Sialogram. Right parotid gland (asymptomatic side) demonstrates classic sialectic pattern

Histologically, JRP glandular specimens demonstrate dilation of the interlobular ducts. In addition, a periductal lymphoproliferative infiltrate is also present [23, 24]. This histologic combination is reflected in the unique pattern that is seen when JRP is imaged.

No definitive diagnostic serologic test exists for JRP. Diagnosis is based on the appropriate clinical signs, buttressed by imaging and the exclusion of other diseases. The diagnostic clinical criteria [15] established for JRP include:

1. Patient must be younger than 16 years of age
2. Recurrent unilateral or bilateral PG swellings
3. The presence of at least two episodes of PG swelling in the past 6 months

Various imaging techniques have been used to authenticate a diagnosis of JRP. Sialography has the advantage of accurately portraying duct architecture (Figs. 12.2c and 12.3c). Its drawbacks originate from the fact that it is a moderately difficult procedure that requires the use of ionizing radiation and a cooperative child. Normally, sialography of a PG duct system resembles a branching tree in wintertime. However, sialography in the presence of JRP will show sialectasis, a stippled or globular pattern also seen in Sjögren syndrome. This unique pattern represents the presence of pools of the introduced radio-opaque dye in dilated interlobular ducts. In patients with unilateral swellings, sialectasis will also be evident in the contralateral asymptomatic PG. Moreover, a very irregular "sausaged" parotid duct may occasionally be visualized and testifies to a secondary effect on the duct wall by a superimposed ascending oral infection.

A CT scan without contrast will reveal multiple, variously sized, poorly attenuated areas in both PGs. The MRI T2-weighted film demonstrates hyperintense areas that reflect accumulations of saliva in the dilated interlobular ducts. Both techniques will also reveal the increased parenchymal density associated with a parotitis. Although sialography, CT scanning, and MRI have diagnostic values, they have been replaced by ultrasonography. Because ultrasonography is a simple noninvasive procedure requiring minimal patient cooperation, it has become the diagnostic imaging procedure of choice. Multiple round hypoechoic areas will be seen scattered throughout the parenchyma of the PG (Figs. 12.2b and 12.3b). These sonolucencies are larger than the sialectic areas visualized on the sialogram because each lucency has been interpreted to represent both a dilated duct and the surrounding periductal lymphoproliferation [25]. Both histologic conditions are sonolucent and when added together will be seen as a hypoechoic area that is larger than the dilated interlobular duct depicted on the sialogram. Furthermore, heterogeneous glandular internal echoes will be seen, reflecting the inflammatory changes in the parenchyma [25].

The possible presence of mumps or juvenile Sjögren syndrome must be considered when formulating a differential diagnosis for JRP. The detailed diagnosis and therapy for both of these conditions are discussed individually elsewhere in this chapter.

Therapy for the individual PG flare-ups in JRP is conservative and palliative because spontaneous resolution usually occurs. However, massage, sialogogic agents, hydration, and good oral hygiene may hasten the process. Antibiotics are to be used only if infection is an issue. Sialendoscopy has become a key therapeutic approach utilized to avoid continued PG flare-ups [18, 23, 26]. Besides its diagnostic value, the instrument can be used therapeutically to widen the lumen in any strictured or stenosed duct. The sialendoscope also has the ability to lavage the ducts and in the process flush out debris blocking the duct lumen. Steroids or antibiotics can be incorporated as needed in the irrigating saline fluid. Remarkably high success rates with sialendoscopy, in eliminating the symptoms associated with JRP, have been obtained [15, 16]. Sialography has also been reported to have therapeutic value in the care of JRP patients [14]. The injection of the contrast solution into the duct system acts to overcome strictures, dilate ducts, and wash out debris. The value of these two treatment approaches for the glandular swellings has recently been attributed to the sole effect of the irrigation [27]. Consequently, it has been suggested that a saline irrigation alone may be sufficient for the treatment of JRP flare-ups [16, 27]. Furthermore, continued outbursts of PG swellings will cease with puberty. Therefore, palliative care alone for JRP symptomatology, combined with reassurance and watchful waiting, becomes a viable therapeutic option.

Juvenile Sjögren Syndrome

Sjögren syndrome (SS) is a chronic inflammatory autoimmune disease that mainly affects the lacrimal (LG) and salivary (SG) glands via a T-cell lymphocytic proliferation that causes acinar destruction and gland dysfunction [28, 29]. Systemically, other organs, such as the lung, kidney, thyroid, and skin, may also be involved [30]. Patients also have a heightened risk of developing a MALT lymphoma [31]. SS can be classified into two forms: primary and secondary. Primary SS patients present with only LG and SG involvement, while secondary SS will be seen in association with other systemic autoimmune diseases such as rheumatoid arthritis, lupus erythematosus, systemic sclerosis, or dermatomyositis. A detailed review of SS can be found in Chap. 7.

An American-European Consensus group has recently collaborated with the American College of Rheumatology/European League Against Rheumatism (ACR/EULAR) to establish new criteria for diagnosing primary SS [32]. The reclassification includes five objective diagnostic signs with each assigned numerical score. Heavy emphasis is placed on the serologic presence of the antibody to SS-A/Ro and the histologic demonstration of ≥ 1 immune lymphocytic foci (a focus is ≥ 50 lymphocytes) in a 4 mm^2 of labial salivary gland tissue. Included, but given less weight, are objective signs of decreased tear production, decreased salivary production, and positive ocular staining. A minimum confident SS diagnostic score demands the presence of either a positive serologic or histologic finding combined with at least one of the three other listed objective signs.

Because juvenile SS (JSS) (Fig. 12.4) presents a profile that differs moderately from adult SS, it is being listed separately and reviewed in this chapter. It has rapidly become apparent that a diagnosis of JSS cannot be accurately validated if the ACR/EULAR criteria, essentially designed for adults, are utilized [28, 29, 33]. Problems originate from the fact that JSS patients often do not have the decreased lacrimation or salivation that are hallmarks in adult SS. In a literature review of 240 JSS patients, only 46% had these sicca signs at the time of examination [29]. Hypolacrimation and hyposalivation can develop later in the course of the symptomatology associated with JSS [29, 30, 34]. Furthermore, there are no studies that demonstrate the incidence of SG lymphocytic foci in JSS [33]. Confusion arises because juveniles may have varying degrees of lymphocytic infiltration [33] that are not at a level that meets the strict definition of a focus. Moreover, children with JSS

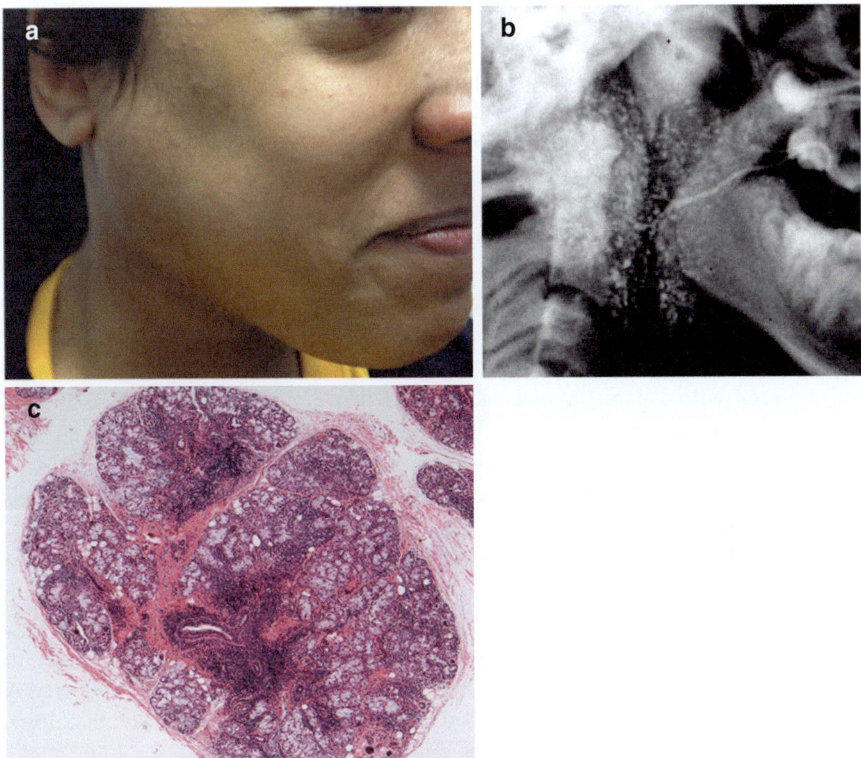

Fig. 12.4 (**a**) Juvenile Sjögren syndrome (JSS). Patient C (12 years old). Right parotid swelling. (Mandel L, J Oral Maxillofac Surg 2014;72:2485). (**b**) JSS. Patient C. Sialogram. Classic sialectic pattern associated with Sjögren syndrome is evident. (Mandel L, J Oral Maxillofac Surg 2014;72:2485). (**c**) JSS. Patient C. Labial gland. Several lymphocytic foci are present. (Mandel L, J Oral Maxillofac Surg 2014;72:2485)

have many more incidents of recurrent parotid swellings than adults. These swellings have become essential ingredients in JSS diagnosis. In contrast, the swellings are not part of the ACR/EULAR diagnostic criteria for adult SS. These variations have made it difficult to establish diagnostic standards for JSS.

JSS is not a common disease finding and its incidence has not been adequately documented. Females are more susceptible than males, and a median age of 10–12 years has been reported for JSS patients [29, 34]. Children most frequently complain of episodes of recurrent parotitis (47%) [34] which are usually bilateral [29]. Clinical involvement of the submandibular salivary gland does not seem to be an issue. Arthralgias are not an uncommon associated complaint [34, 35] in the presence of a history of recurrent parotitis. As in adult SS, JSS patients may have other associated autoimmune diseases [29, 34], but few such cases have been reported [36].

Making a diagnosis of JSS is problematic because of its infrequent occurrence and because its presenting symptomatology differs from that seen in adults. The diagnosis of JSS is usually attained from a patient's clinical history of recurrent parotid swellings and arthralgia [34]. As in adult SS, serologic testing for anti-SSA/Ro, volume studies of lacrimation and salivation, histologic findings, and the possible co-existence of another autoimmune entity may play roles in establishing or negating a JSS diagnosis. However, a recurrent parotitis and a positive serology have been considered sufficient evidence for diagnosis [34].

Imaging also can play a significant role in JSS diagnosis. Sialography (Fig. 12.4b) usually will show the classic pattern of sialectasis (dilated interlobular ducts) in both parotid glands (PG) even if the PG clinical swellings are consistently unilateral in their presentation. Scintigraphy will reveal dysfunction of any involved salivary gland. A CT scan will image multiple lucent areas in the PG, while an MRI (T2 weighted) will reveal many saliva-containing dilated hyperintense interlobular ducts. Because of its simplicity and ready availability, ultrasonography has become the standard imaging procedure utilized to establish the existence and the extent of JSS's involvement of the salivary glands. Multiple hypoechoic areas, varying in size, will be seen with a parenchymal background that is nonhomogeneous in at least three of the four major glands [28, 36]. The hypoechoic areas represent both duct ectasia and the periductal lymphoproliferation characteristically seen in SS patients.

Differentiating JSS from JRP is essential and can be difficult because of their obvious similarities. Both conditions involve unilateral/bilateral recurrent swellings of the PG in youngsters. Additionally, imaging will reflect the presence of sialectasis in both JSS and JRP. Difficulties with differential diagnosis also develop because ultrasound exhibits similar hypoechoic areas in both glandular diseases. Differentiation is facilitated with the knowledge that JSS is observed mostly in females while JRP more often occurs in young boys and disappears with puberty. A clinical diagnosis of JSS can be clinched by the presence of a diagnostic histology, the eventual development of sicca signs, and a positive serology. No serologic markers for JRP have been demonstrated.

No acceptable treatment regimen for JSS has been established. Anti-inflammatories, corticosteroids, cyclophosphamide, and methotrexate have been administered with minimal success [28, 35]. Treatment is essentially symptomatic and aimed when necessary at increasing or replacing secretions with sialogogues, mouth washes, and artificial saliva/tears. However, such therapy for JSS is often not required because the signs and symptoms of decreased secretions are infrequent developments in children. Hydroxychloroquine, an immunomodulator, is widely prescribed for this systemic condition, but it has demonstrated limited success. Its value may rest in the care of any existing arthralgia. The biologics rituximab, etanercept, or infliximab have also been advocated [37]. Treatment of individual PG swellings has met with some success when sialendoscopy has been used. The sialendoscope serves to dilate the duct lumen and simultaneously flush out luminal debris that is blocking any decreased salivary flow [38]. Some diminution in subjective PG symptomatology can be anticipated.

Cystic Fibrosis

Cystic fibrosis (CF) is an inherited autosomal recessive genetic disease, mainly affecting Caucasian children and young adults, that may have a fatal outcome. It has a prevalence rate of 1:3500 in the United States [39]. CF results from a mutation of the CFTR gene that causes an increased viscosity in all exocrine gland secretions along with difficulty in mucus secretion clearance [39]. The sweat glands, respiratory tract, and pancreas are the secreting organs most frequently involved.

The secretions from the sweat glands in CF contain a very high salt content which persists throughout life such that it is utilized as a key diagnostic test for CF. Sweat chloride concentrations of $\geq$60 mEq/L are considered the diagnostic gold standard [39, 40]. Besides a positive sweat test, a conclusive diagnosis of CF includes detection of the CFTR gene mutation.

The viscous secretions that develop in the respiratory tract along with difficulty in its clearance lead to pulmonary obstructive disease, probably the most morbid aspect of CF. Respiratory alterations are reported to be present in 80% of CF infants and preschoolers [41]. Before antibiotics, few CF children survived beyond 2 years of age [39] because of the concomitant respiratory infections. To inhibit the progression to pulmonary infection, the airway must be kept free of the secretions via constant physical therapy procedures (bronchodilators) and enzymes to combat the viscosity of the secretions. Maintenance of a clear airway discourages disease progression. Because the respiratory tract inadequately clears itself of the thick mucus secretions, CF patients face increased mortality rates from constant respiratory infections with progressive lung disease. Effective antibiotics are available and serve as major agents in the control of infection associated with CF symptomatology. Pancreatic insufficiency, after the respiratory tract and sweat gland involvements, represents the third diagnostic feature that is classically manifest in CF. Insufficient pancreatic enzymes lead to malabsorption of lipids and the fat-soluble vitamins (A, D, E, K). Therefore, upkeep of the patient's nutritional state is a significant component of CF therapy. Presently, new therapies are being developed whose purpose is to correct the pathologic variants in the CFTR gene [39].

As can be expected in CF, the alterations in the exocrine secreting glands will affect the salivary glands (SG). Gross anatomic changes in the SG have not been reported to occur in relation to CF. Instead, substantial alterations in the chemical constituents of saliva develop. Among the major SG, the parotid gland (PG), a serous gland, is least affected. However, sialochemical changes in the submandibular salivary gland (SMSG) saliva have been reported. They include increased chloride and sodium levels such that SMSG saliva has been suggested as an alternative to sweat testing for CF [40, 42, 43]. Calcium levels in the SMSG are also elevated [44–46], but surprisingly no increased incidence of sialolithiasis has been reported. Additionally, the SMSG flow rate has been reported to be decreased in CF [42, 44, 45]. Clinically, it seems that CF has its SG effects on both the quality and quantity of the SMSG secretions.

Chest radiographs and CT scanning are imaging procedures used to aid in the diagnosis of CF. Radiographs will reveal the extent of respiratory disease's progression to bronchiectasis. The CT scan is used when detailed knowledge of the lung disease is required [39].

Histologic evidence of SG changes in CF has been reported. The microscopic examination of the SMSG reveals dilated acini and ducts filled with inspissated mucus [42]. These duct plugs serve to incite a chronic inflammatory infiltrate [42]. The serous parotid gland is histologically normal [44].

Treatment of CF involves both the medical profession and the family. Their focus must be directed toward keeping the airway clear of secretory obstruction via physical therapy and pharmacologic agents. Because CF patients are prone to respiratory infection, appropriate antibiotic therapy is indicated for any existing respiratory infection. Furthermore, because of the malnutritional state associated with the pancreatic insufficiency seen in CF, it is imperative to maintain optimal nutrition for CF patients [39].

Neonatal Acute Suppurative Parotitis

Neonatal acute suppurative parotitis (NAP) is an uncommon infectious parotid gland (PG) condition that involves the newborn. It has a reported prevalence of 3.8–14/10,000 premature newborns [43, 47, 48], while its incidence in full-term babies is 1/100,000 [43]. Submandibular salivary gland involvement has not been reported [49].

In NAP, *Staphylococcus aureus* is the usual organism that infects the PG, but other gram-positive, gram-negative, and anaerobic bacteria have been identified as causative agents. Etiologically, an ascending retrograde duct infection, originating from the oral flora and facilitated by a dehydration incited decreased salivary flow, is thought to be the primary means for the development of NAP. Hematogenous dissemination of bacteria into the PG has been suggested as another possible pathway for NAP occurrence [47, 49, 50]. Risk factors that pave the way for the onset of NAP include premature birth, dehydration, immunosuppression, and inadequate breastfeeding [43, 49, 50].

NAP should be suspected in a neonate with a facial swelling who demonstrates incessant crying and a reluctance to feed [48]. A unilateral, occasionally bilateral, swollen PG is present [47, 50]. The other cardinal signs of inflammation (pain, erythema, warmth) will also be evident. A fever may or may not be present [48]. Pus will usually be observed draining intraorally from the parotid duct orifice [47]. Serologic findings are commensurate with acute infection and include leukocytosis and an elevated sedimentation rate [43, 49, 51].

A confident diagnosis of NAP can be obtained from its clinical signs and symptoms. Substantiation can be derived from an ultrasound study. An enlarged PG with edema, increased vascularity, and hypoechoic abscessed areas will be evident [49, 50].

Therapy of NAP involves hydration and antibiotics tailored to the culpable organism that has been recovered from pus or even blood when there is hematogenous spread [48]. A rapid therapeutic response can be anticipated with fever subsiding in 24 h and PG swelling dissipating in 3–5 days [49]. The parotid duct acts as a natural drainage pathway and promotes the gland's rapid response to therapy. Occasionally, drainage from the parotid duct is not present in NAP, and supportive therapy with hydration and antibiotics does not eliminate the problem. In such a circumstance, surgical intervention is mandated [43, 49].

Self-limited Epilepsy with Centrotemporal Spikes

Self-limited epilepsy with centrotemporal spikes (SLECTS) is an idiopathic age-specific benign epileptic syndrome that was previously known as benign epilepsy of childhood with centrotemporal spikes [52, 53]. SLECTS accounts for 15–20% of epilepsy syndromes seen in children [53] (Fig. 12.5). Children, 1–14 years of age, often with a familial history and a slight male dominance, present with histories of focal seizures that last for 1–3 min. Most seizures develop during sleep and are accompanied by hypersalivation. These episodes spontaneously disappear with the onset of puberty. In addition to the focal seizures, the cardinal features of SLECTS [54, 55] include:

1. Hypersalivation with drooling
2. Unilateral facial sensorimotor symptoms characterized by paresthesias involving the tongue, lips, gums, and inner cheeks
3. Oropharyngeal and laryngeal manifestations
4. Speech arrest

Significant aid in achieving a diagnosis can be obtained when an electroencephalogram demonstrates characteristic high-voltage sharp waves that originate from the brain's centrotemporal region and are activated by drowsiness and sleep [53]. Although these spikes are seen in other neurologic conditions, their presence serves to authenticate a diagnosis when added to the known cardinal features of SLECTS.

Because of its benign course and spontaneous resolution, treatment often is not necessary. When required, successful SLECTS treatment can be achieved with a regimen of antiseizure medications that may include carbamazepine, valproic acid, or clobazam [56].

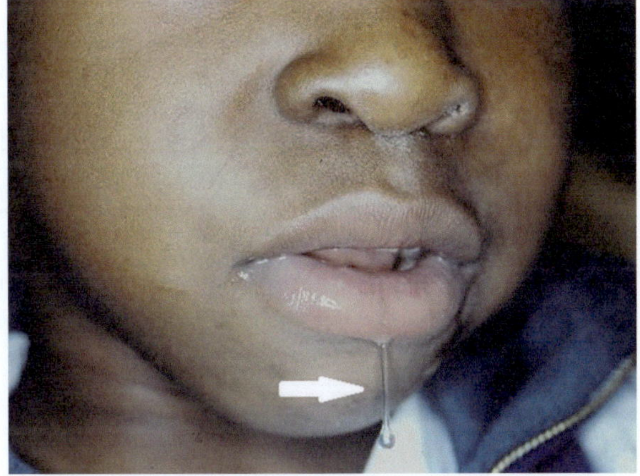

Fig. 12.5 Self-limited epilepsy with centrotemporal spikes (SLECTS) associated with increased salivation and drooling in an 11-year-old male (arrow)

Kawasaki Disease

Kawasaki disease (KD) is considered an acute self-limiting febrile disease that is characterized by a systemic vasculitis of small and medium caliber vessels [57]. KD develops almost exclusively in children under 5 years of age [58], with males dominating in a ratio of 1.5:1 [59]. It occurs when a genetically predisposed individual is exposed to some unknown trigger [57, 60]. The suggestion has been made that infectious or environmental agents that cause an inflammatory cascade may be etiologically responsible [59, 61].

A diagnosis of KD is based on the presence of a fever, for at least 5 days, that does not respond to antibiotic therapy [59] and includes at least four of the following five major clinical features [58, 59, 61]:

1. Conjunctival congestion
2. Oropharyngeal mucositis (strawberry tongue, lip fissuring)
3. Cervical lymphadenopathy
4. Rash, primarily truncal
5. Swelling and/or erythema of hands and/or feet

Most patients (65%) that present themselves with KD have oropharyngeal symptoms in association with a cervical lymphadenopathy [62]. Additionally cardiac, liver, and pancreatic involvement often are present, but usually subclinical in their manifestations [59, 60].

Salivary gland symptomatology associated with KD can occur. Unilateral, at times bilateral, parotitis may even serve as a presenting sign of KD [59, 61, 63]. In most cases, the parotid gland (PG) sialadenitis subsides with antibiotic therapy, but the accompanying fever persists and eventually other pathognomonic signs of KD appear [59, 61, 63, 64]. The submandibular and sublingual salivary glands do not develop symptomatology associated with KD.

A computerized tomographic scan will reveal an enhanced and enlarged PG. Intraparotid lymph node enlargement may also be noted [64].

Histologically, an autopsy study of KD patients revealed that 81% of the PG specimens demonstrated a periductal and interacinar infiltration of lymphocytes and mononuclear cells [61]. In addition, an intrasalivary gland arteritis in 39% of the KD patients has also been observed [65].

Antibiotic therapy is used for the treatment of the presenting parotitis. Control of the unrelenting fever and the inflammatory sequelae of KD is often accomplished with the administration of intravenous gamma globulin [58, 61, 64]. Infliximab is advocated as a second-line therapy for those patients who have an inadequate response to the gamma globulin [60].

Neonatal Drooling

Drooling in the newborn is not to be interpreted as a pathologic problem. Rather, it represents an ongoing progressive physiologic muscular development that is incomplete in the neonatal infant. The drooling can be considered a normal condition up to the age of 30 months [66]. At the age of 30 months, the oral motor musculature has developed sufficiently to control the problem. Continued drooling beyond the age of 4 years indicates a need for an investigation [67] as to the possible coexistence of a systemic neurodegenerative condition.

A further review of neonatal/infant drooling can be found in Chap. 2.

References

1. Davison P, Morris J. Mumps. In: StatPearls. Treasure Island: StatPearls Publishing; 2021.
2. Hviid A, Rubin S, Mühlemann K. Mumps. Lancet. 2008;371(9616):932–44. https://doi.org/10.1016/S0140-6736(08)60419-5.
3. Kessler AT, Bhatt AA. Review of the major and minor salivary glands, part 1: anatomy, infectious, and inflammatory processes. J Clin Imaging Sci. 2018;8:47. Published 2018 Nov 15. https://doi.org/10.4103/jcis.JCIS_45_18.
4. Centers for Disease Control and Prevention (CDC). Exposure to mumps during air travel—United States, April 2006 [published correction appears in MMWR Morb Mortal Wkly Rep. 2006 Apr 21;55(15):434]. MMWR Morb Mortal Wkly Rep. 2006;55(14):401–2.
5. Centers for Disease Control and Prevention (CDC). Updated recommendations for isolation of persons with mumps. MMWR Morb Mortal Wkly Rep. 2008;57(40):1103–5.
6. Richardson M, Elliman D, Maguire H, Simpson J, Nicoll A. Evidence base of incubation periods, periods of infectiousness and exclusion policies for the control of communicable diseases in schools and preschools [published correction appears in Pediatr Infect Dis J 2001 Jul;20(7):653]. Pediatr Infect Dis J. 2001;20(4):380–91. https://doi.org/10.1097/00006454-200104000-00004.
7. Connell AR, Connell J, Leahy TR, Hassan J. Mumps outbreaks in vaccinated populations—is it time to re-assess the clinical efficacy of vaccines? Front Immunol. 2020;11:2089. Published 2020 Sep 18. https://doi.org/10.3389/fimmu.2020.02089.
8. Katz SL, Gershon AA, Hotez PJ. Infectious disease of children. New York: Mosby Year Book; 1998. p. 280–9.
9. Zenk J, Iro H, Klintworth N, Lell M. Diagnostic imaging in sialadenitis. Oral Maxillofac Surg Clin North Am. 2009;21(3):275–92. https://doi.org/10.1016/j.coms.2009.04.005.
10. Ericson S, Zetterlund B, Ohman J. Recurrent parotitis and sialectasis in childhood. Clinical, radiologic, immunologic, bacteriologic, and histologic study. Ann Otol Rhinol Laryngol. 1991;100(7):527–35. https://doi.org/10.1177/000348949110000702.
11. Iro H, Zenk J. Salivary gland diseases in children. GMS Curr Top Otorhinolaryngol Head Neck Surg. 2014;13:Doc06. Published 2014 Dec 1. https://doi.org/10.3205/cto000109.
12. Singh P, Gupta D. Juvenile recurrent parotitis. Indian J Pediatr. 2019;86(8):749. https://doi.org/10.1007/s12098-019-02901-y.
13. Iordanis K, Panagiotis D, Angelos C, et al. Unilateral sialendoscopy for juvenile recurrent parotitis: what happens to the other side? Laryngoscope. 2021;131(6):1404–9. https://doi.org/10.1002/lary.29187.

14. Tucci FM, Roma R, Bianchi A, De Vincentiis GC, Bianchi PM. Juvenile recurrent parotitis: diagnostic and therapeutic effectiveness of sialography. Retrospective study on 110 children. Int J Pediatr Otorhinolaryngol. 2019;124:179–84. https://doi.org/10.1016/j.ijporl.2019.06.007.

15. Garavello W, Redaelli M, Galluzzi F, Pignataro L. Juvenile recurrent parotitis: a systematic review of treatment studies. Int J Pediatr Otorhinolaryngol. 2018;112:151–7. https://doi.org/10.1016/j.ijporl.2018.07.002.

16. Berta E, Angel G, Lagarde F, Fonlupt B, Noyelles L, Bettega G. Role of sialendoscopy in juvenile recurrent parotitis (JRP). Eur Ann Otorhinolaryngol Head Neck Dis. 2017;134(6):405–7. https://doi.org/10.1016/j.anorl.2017.06.004.

17. Hackett AM, Baranano CF, Reed M, Duvvuri U, Smith RJ, Mehta D. Sialoendoscopy for the treatment of pediatric salivary gland disorders. Arch Otolaryngol Head Neck Surg. 2012;138(10):912–5. https://doi.org/10.1001/2013.jamaoto.244.

18. Wood J, Toll EC, Hall F, Mahadevan M. Juvenile recurrent parotitis: review and proposed management algorithm. Int J Pediatr Otorhinolaryngol. 2021;142:110617. https://doi.org/10.1016/j.ijporl.2021.110617.

19. Geterud A, Lindvall AM, Nylén O. Follow-up study of recurrent parotitis in children. Ann Otol Rhinol Laryngol. 1988;97(4 Pt 1):341–6. https://doi.org/10.1177/000348948809700403.

20. Park JW. Recurrent parotitis in childhood. Clin Pediatr (Phila). 1992;31(4):254–5. https://doi.org/10.1177/000992289203100415.

21. Canzi P, Occhini A, Pagella F, Marchal F, Benazzo M. Sialendoscopy in juvenile recurrent parotitis: a review of the literature. Acta Otorhinolaryngol Ital. 2013;33(6):367–73.

22. Schneider H, Koch M, Künzel J, et al. Juvenile recurrent parotitis: a retrospective comparison of sialendoscopy versus conservative therapy. Laryngoscope. 2014;124(2):451–5. https://doi.org/10.1002/lary.24291.

23. Papadopoulou-Alataki E, Dogantzis P, Chatziavramidis A, et al. Juvenile recurrent parotitis: the role of sialendoscopy. Int J Inflam. 2019;2019:7278907. Published 2019 Sep 29. https://doi.org/10.1155/2019/7278907.

24. Katz P, Hartl DM, Guerre A. Treatment of juvenile recurrent parotitis. Otolaryngol Clin North Am. 2009;42(6):1087. https://doi.org/10.1016/j.otc.2009.09.002.

25. Nozaki H, Harasawa A, Hara H, Kohno A, Shigeta A. Ultrasonographic features of recurrent parotitis in childhood. Pediatr Radiol. 1994;24(2):98–100. https://doi.org/10.1007/BF02020162.

26. Erkul E, Gillespie MB. Sialendoscopy for non-stone disorders: the current evidence. Laryngoscope Investig Otolaryngol. 2016;1(5):140–5. Published 2016 Sep 7. https://doi.org/10.1002/lio2.33.

27. Geisthoff UW, Droege F, Schulze C, et al. Treatment of juvenile recurrent parotitis with irrigation therapy without anesthesia [published online ahead of print, 2021 Jun 12]. Eur Arch Otorrinolaringol. 2022;279(1):493–9. https://doi.org/10.1007/s00405-021-06928-w.

28. Aburiziza AJ. Primary juvenile Sjögren's syndrome in a 3-year-old pediatric female patient: diagnostic role of salivary gland ultrasonography: case report. Open Access Rheumatol. 2020;12:73–8. Published 2020 May 29. https://doi.org/10.2147/OARRR.S248977.

29. Marino A, Romano M, Giani T, et al. Childhood Sjogren's syndrome: an Italian case series and a literature review-based cohort. Semin Arthritis Rheum. 2021;51(4):903–10. https://doi.org/10.1016/j.semarthrit.2020.11.004.

30. Yokogawa N, Lieberman SM, Sherry DD, Vivino FB. Features of childhood Sjögren's syndrome in comparison to adult Sjögren's syndrome: considerations in establishing child-specific diagnostic criteria. Clin Exp Rheumatol. 2016;34(2):343–51.

31. Váróczy L, Gergely L, Zeher M, Szegedi G, Illés A. Malignant lymphoma-associated autoimmune diseases—a descriptive epidemiological study. Rheumatol Int. 2002;22(6):233–7. https://doi.org/10.1007/s00296-002-0229-4.

32. Shiboski CH, Shiboski SC, Seror R, et al. 2016 American College of Rheumatology/European League Against Rheumatism classification criteria for primary Sjögren's syndrome: a consen-

sus and data-driven methodology involving three international patient cohorts. Ann Rheum Dis. 2017;76(1):9–16. https://doi.org/10.1136/annrheumdis-2016-210571.

33. Schiffer BL, Stern SM, Park AH. Sjögren's syndrome in children with recurrent parotitis. Int J Pediatr Otorhinolaryngol. 2020;129:109768. https://doi.org/10.1016/j.ijporl.2019.109768.

34. Basiaga ML, Stern SM, Mehta JJ, et al. Childhood Sjögren syndrome: features of an international cohort and application of the 2016 ACR/EULAR classification criteria. Rheumatology (Oxford). 2021;60(7):3144–55. https://doi.org/10.1093/rheumatology/keaa757.

35. Cimaz R, Casadei A, Rose C, et al. Primary Sjögren syndrome in the paediatric age: a multicentre survey. Eur J Pediatr. 2003;162(10):661–5. https://doi.org/10.1007/s00431-003-1277-9.

36. Krumrey-Langkammerer M, Haas JP. Salivary gland ultrasound in the diagnostic workup of juvenile Sjögren's syndrome and mixed connective tissue disease. Pediatr Rheumatol Online J. 2020;18(1):44. Published 2020 Jun 9. https://doi.org/10.1186/s12969-020-00437-6.

37. Doolan G, Faizal NM, Foley C, et al. Treatment strategies for Sjögren's syndrome with childhood onset: a systematic review of the literature [published online ahead of print, 2021 Jul 20]. Rheumatology (Oxford). 2021;keab579. https://doi.org/10.1093/rheumatology/keab579.

38. Nahlieli O, Shacham R, Shlesinger M, Eliav E. Juvenile recurrent parotitis: a new method of diagnosis and treatment. Pediatrics. 2004;114(1):9–12. https://doi.org/10.1542/peds.114.1.9.

39. López-Valdez JA, Aguilar-Alonso LA, Gándara-Quezada V, et al. Cystic fibrosis: current concepts. Fibrosis quística: conceptos actuales. Bol Med Hosp Infant Mex. 2021;78(6):584–96. https://doi.org/10.24875/BMHIM.20000372.

40. Gonçalves AC, Marson FAL, Mendonça RMH, et al. Chloride and sodium ion concentrations in saliva and sweat as a method to diagnose cystic fibrosis. J Pediatr (Rio J). 2019;95(4):443–50. https://doi.org/10.1016/j.jped.2018.04.005.

41. Accurso FJ, Sontag MK, Wagener JS. Complications associated with symptomatic diagnosis in infants with cystic fibrosis. J Pediatr. 2005;147(3 Suppl):S37–41. https://doi.org/10.1016/j.jpeds.2005.08.034.

42. Tandler B. Salivary gland changes in disease. J Dent Res. 1987;66(2):398–406. https://doi.org/10.1177/00220345870660020301.

43. Hadizadeh T, Uwaifo OO. Neonatal acute suppurative parotitis. Clin Pediatr (Phila). 2020;59(11):1019–21. https://doi.org/10.1177/0009922820927478.

44. Davis PB. Pathophysiology of cystic fibrosis with emphasis on salivary gland involvement. J Dent Res. 1987;66 Spec No:667–71. https://doi.org/10.1177/00220345870660S210.

45. da Silva Modesto KB, de Godói Simões JB, de Souza AF, et al. Salivary flow rate and biochemical composition analysis in stimulated whole saliva of children with cystic fibrosis. Arch Oral Biol. 2015;60(11):1650–4. https://doi.org/10.1016/j.archoralbio.2015.08.007.

46. El Khoury J, Haber E, Nasr M, Hokayem N. Botulinum neurotoxin A for parotid enlargement in cystic fibrosis: the first case report [published correction appears in J Oral Maxillofac Surg. 2017 Jan;75(1):227]. J Oral Maxillofac Surg. 2016;74(9):1771–3. https://doi.org/10.1016/j.joms.2016.03.038.

47. Avcu G, Belet N, Karli A, Sensoy G. Acute suppurative parotitis in a 33-day-old patient. J Trop Pediatr. 2015;61(3):218–21. https://doi.org/10.1093/tropej/fmv012.

48. Khan N, Abdullah A, Zafar F. Neonatal parotitis: a case report. J Pak Med Assoc. 2021;71(6):1682–5. https://doi.org/10.47391/JPMA.04-550.

49. Kolekar S, Chincholi TS, Kshirsagar A, Porwal N. Acute neonatal parotid abscess: a rare case report. Afr J Paediatr Surg. 2016;13(4):199–201. https://doi.org/10.4103/0189-6725.194675.

50. Ismail EA, Seoudi TM, Al-Amir M, Al-Esnawy AA. Neonatal suppurative parotitis over the last 4 decades: report of three new cases and review. Pediatr Int. 2013;55(1):60–4. https://doi.org/10.1111/j.1442-200X.2012.03738.x.

51. Dias Costa F, Ramos Andrade D, Cunha FI, Fernandes A. Group B streptococcal neonatal parotitis. BMJ Case Rep. 2015;2015:bcr2014209115. Published 2015 Jun 10. https://doi.org/10.1136/bcr-2014-209115.

52. Scheffer IE, Berkovic S, Capovilla G, et al. ILAE classification of the epilepsies: position paper of the ILAE Commission for Classification and Terminology. Epilepsia. 2017;58(4):512–21. https://doi.org/10.1111/epi.13709.
53. Galicchio S, Espeche A, Cersosimo R, et al. Self-limited epilepsy with centro-temporal spikes: a study of 46 patients with unusual clinical manifestations. Epilepsy Res. 2021;169:106507. https://doi.org/10.1016/j.eplepsyres.2020.106507.
54. Demirbilek V, Bureau M, Cokar O, Panayiotopoulos C. Chapter 13. Self-limited focal epilepsies in childhood. In: Bureau M, Genton P, Dravet C, Delgado-Escueta A, Guerrini R, Tassinari C, Won T, editors. Epileptic syndromes in infancy, childhood and adolescence. 6th ed. John Libby Eurotext. pp. 219–260.
55. Colamaria V, Sgrò V, Caraballo R, et al. Status epilepticus in benign rolandic epilepsy manifesting as anterior operculum syndrome. Epilepsia. 1991;32(3):329–34. https://doi.org/10.1111/j.1528-1157.1991.tb04659.x.
56. Espeche A, Galicchio S, Cersósimo R, et al. Self-limited epilepsy of childhood with affective seizures: a well-defined epileptic syndrome? Epilepsy Behav. 2021;117:107885. https://doi.org/10.1016/j.yebeh.2021.107885.
57. Hara T, Furuno K, Yamamura K, et al. Assessment of pediatric admissions for Kawasaki disease or infectious disease during the COVID-19 state of emergency in Japan [published correction appears in JAMA Netw Open. 2021 May 3;4(5):e2114112]. JAMA Netw Open. 2021;4(4):e214475. Published 2021 Apr 1. https://doi.org/10.1001/jamanetworkopen.2021.4475.
58. Rowley AH, Gonzalez-Crussi F, Shulman ST. Kawasaki syndrome. Curr Probl Pediatr. 1991;21(9):387–405. https://doi.org/10.1016/0045-9380(91)90008-9.
59. Scardina GA, Fucà G, Carini F, et al. Oral necrotizing microvasculitis in a patient affected by Kawasaki disease. Med Oral Patol Oral Cir Bucal. 2007;12(8):E560–4. Published 2007 Dec 1.
60. Botti M, Costagliola G, Consolini R. Typical Kawasaki disease presenting with pancreatitis and bilateral parotid gland involvement: a case report and literature review. Front Pediatr. 2018;6:90. Published 2018 Apr 11. https://doi.org/10.3389/fped.2018.00090.
61. Li Y, Yang Q, Yu X, Qiao H. A case of Kawasaki disease presenting with parotitis: a case report and literature review. Medicine (Baltimore). 2019;98(22):e15817. https://doi.org/10.1097/MD.0000000000015817.
62. Parra-García GD, Callejas-Rubio JL, Ríos-Fernández R, Sainz-Quevedo M, Ortego-Centeno N. Otolaryngologic manifestations of systemic vasculitis. Acta Otorrinolaringol Esp. 2012;63(4):303–10. https://doi.org/10.1016/j.otorri.2011.09.002.
63. Do HJ, Baek JG, Kim HJ, et al. Kawasaki disease presenting as parotitis in a 3-month-old infant. Korean Circ J. 2009;39(11):502–4. https://doi.org/10.4070/kcj.2009.39.11.502.
64. Yokoyama K. Parotitis as an initial symptom of Kawasaki disease. Case Rep Pediatr. 2017;2017:5937276. https://doi.org/10.1155/2017/5937276.
65. Amano S, Hazama F, Kubagawa H, Tasaka K, Haebara H, Hamashima Y. General pathology of Kawasaki disease. On the morphological alterations corresponding to the clinical manifestations. Acta Pathol Jpn. 1980;30(5):681–94.
66. Morales Chávez MC, Nualart Grollmus ZC, Silvestre-Donat FJ. Clinical prevalence of drooling in infant cerebral palsy. Med Oral Patol Oral Cir Bucal. 2008;13(1):E22–6. Published 2008 Jan 1.
67. Blasco PA, Allaire JH. Drooling in the developmentally disabled: management practices and recommendations. Consortium on drooling. Dev Med Child Neurol. 1992;34(10):849–62.

Chapter 13
Radiation

Louis Mandel

Abstract Radiation in the form of external beam radiation is a key element in the therapeutic toolbox utilized for the treatment of cancer. Because of the anatomic location of the major salivary glands, they often are in the path of the destructive radiation beam being utilized in the therapy of head and neck malignancies. A radiation sialadenitis develops whose primary sign is hyposalivation with associated oral pain and problems with mastication and swallowing.

Radioactive iodine (^{131}I) is used as a key element in the treatment of differentiated thyroid cancer. Unfortunately, the administration of radioactive iodine has an adverse effect on iodine avid tissues, most frequently the salivary glands. Sialadenitis with obstructive symptomatology often develops from the effects of ^{131}I radioactivity. Hyposalivation becomes an issue when high ^{131}I doses are administered.

Overview

Radiotherapy utilizes ionizing radiation to destroy cancer cells. This therapeutic effect of radiation is derived from its ability to damage cellular DNA which in turn leads to death of the cancer cell. The response of the malignant cells to radiation varies in direct relation to the susceptibility of individual cell types and in direct proportion to the intensity of the radiation. Some tumors are relatively radiosensitive and their cells are readily killed by mild radiation doses, while other cell types are more resistant to radiation and require higher doses of radiation. Lymphomas can be categorized as being radiosensitive, while salivary gland epithelial tumors are more resistant to the effects of radiation and need higher therapeutic doses of radiation. Tumor type, size, location, and stage dictate the exact approach of radiation to treatment.

The major thrust of radiotherapy is aimed at tumor eradication. However, it has also been used to shrink a tumor prior to surgery and in so doing make surgery more

L. Mandel, *Clinical Management of Salivary Gland Disorders*, https://doi.org/10.1007/978-3-031-50012-1_13

successful. It has also been utilized for the treatment of neoplastic recurrences and even for palliative care whose goal is to enhance the quality of life.

Radiotherapy is often used along with surgery, chemotherapy, and immunotherapy in the treatment of malignant neoplasms. A dominant objective feature of therapy is the sparing of normal tissues through which the radiation beam must pass as it travels to its target. To avoid damage to surrounding normal tissues, several low-dosage radiation beams are directed at the cancerous growth from different angles such that the tumor receives a lethal radiation dose when the beams converge while negating significant damage to the traversed adjacent normal tissues.

Inevitably, when malignancies in the head and neck area are radiated, the surrounding normal anatomic structures suffer collateral damage. The injuries occur in varying degrees and are dependent upon the intensity of radiation to which the structure has been exposed and obviously is determined by the technique of radiotherapy that is being utilized. Salivary glands are often in the "line of fire" when radiation is directed at head and neck malignancies that are in close proximity to the glands. Consequently, hyposalivation is a common comorbidity that develops following salivary gland injury from radiation.

External Beam Irradiation

By representing 5–10% of all body malignancies [1], head and neck cancer (HNC) has obtained the dubious distinction of being the sixth most common cancer in the world [2]. The squamous cell carcinoma (SCC) is considered the most prevalent malignancy in the head and neck area and is reported to represent 90% of all HNC [2]. A major therapeutic approach for SCC's care, besides surgery, chemotherapy, and immunotherapy, involves radiotherapy (RT). More than 50,000 patients with HNC are treated with RT each year [3].

Because of their anatomic proximity to most HNC, the salivary glands inevitably are exposed to irradiation during RT of these malignancies. Unfortunately, the salivary glands are sensitive to radiation. The parotid gland (PG) and the submandibular salivary gland (SMSG) are often in the direct path of the RT beam. The radiation-sensitive PG serous cells, with their aqueous secretions, are readily destroyed by the ionizing radiation, while mucous cells in the SMSG demonstrate a modicum of resistance to the RT [4–7]. A thick sticky saliva develops as the proportion of mucus secretion produced by the SMSG's mucous cells and other (sublingual, minor) salivary glands becomes proportionately more dominant over the serous PG secretions. Besides altering salivary quality, the destructive effects of RT result in a dose-related hyposalivation (Fig. 13.1a). Consequently, there is a loss of saliva's lubricating, buffering, and antimicrobial powers. Other oral complications (Figs. 13.1b–d) subsequent to the RT include problems with swallowing, mucositis, dysgeusia, oral burning, atrophic or fissured tongue, increased incidence of dental caries, candidiasis, osteoradionecrosis, and a trismus that results from a radiation-induced fibrosis of the muscles of mastication [8]. The decreased salivary flow also

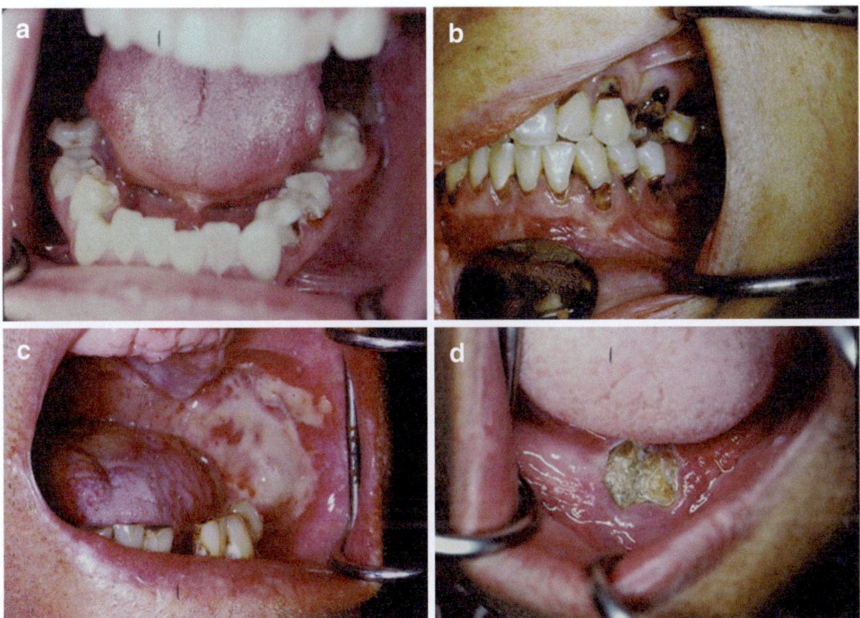

Fig. 13.1 (**a**) Radiation. Hyposalivation has caused carious breakdown of teeth following cancericidal radiation for parotid carcinoma. (**b**) Radiation. Rampant dental caries subsequent to radiotherapy for tongue carcinoma. (**c**) Radiation. Mucositis secondary to radiotherapy for tonsillar area squamous cell carcinoma. (**d**) Radiation. Osteoradionecrosis following cancericidal radiation for mouth floor carcinoma

favors an ascending salivary ductal infection from the oral cavity. Therefore, superimposition of the symptomatology associated with chronic parotitis (CP) can be initiated as a secondary complication. A review of chronic parotitis can be found in Chap. 5.

Historically, clinicians determined RT fields using standard radiographic films for tumor location and configuration and bony landmarks [9]. The following RT resulted in radiation sialadenitis with objective hyposalivation and subjective xerostomia becoming serious issues. In order to avoid the ensuing salivary gland injury, new radiation techniques have evolved. These advances have brought about the introduction of intensity-modulated radiotherapy (IMRT). IMRT has made it possible to concentrate multiple radiation beams, originating from different angles, on the targeted facial-cervical region, and in so doing minimize the dosage received by salivary gland tissue located adjacent to the objective tumor target. This RT procedure has now become the standard of care for the treatment of HNC.

In addition to the SCC, the nasopharyngeal carcinoma (NPC) represents another head and neck malignancy wherein RT has commonly been deployed for treatment. Therapeutic radiation for the NPC presents special challenges because of this malignancy's centrally positioned anatomic location as well as its proximity to the brain stem and spinal cord. Given these conditions, effective IMRT therapy demands an approach that inevitably exposes the PG/SMSG to increased radiation. In addition, associated metastatic lymph nodes may also require RT and may have a close anatomic relation with the salivary glands. Therefore, the IMRT directed at these nodes can cause significant gland damage [6].

An effective cancericidal radiation dose involves the administration of 50–70 Gy to the HNC target in daily fractions of 1.8–2 Gy over a 6- to 7-week period [4, 10]. Damage to an adjacent salivary gland is dependent upon dose, time interval of each fraction, and the portion of the salivary gland that is in the field of irradiation [4]. Again because of the proximity of the PG/SMSG to the cancer target, some spillover of the radiation will occur, albeit less with the IMRT technique. Exposure to 40 Gy will cause extensive, but not complete, damage to PG function [11, 12]. A moderate recovery of salivary flow has been observed with the passage of time [13, 14]. Significant glandular destruction occurs when an individual salivary gland is exposed to RT dosages in the 50–70 Gy range. Some degree of hyposalivation will become evident with an exposure to 10 Gy [4] and will result in a 50–57% decrease in salivary flow [4, 7, 15]. Of great importance is the fact that glands receiving a mean dose below or equal to a threshold (24 Gy for unstimulated PG saliva and 26 Gy for stimulated PG saliva) show substantial recovery of salivary flow. After an initial loss, salivary flow rate rebounds and continues to improve with time [13, 16–18].

The mechanism for the irradiation-induced damage to the salivary gland remains an enigma. However, it has been suggested from studies on rhesus monkeys that the lethal effect of RT occurs via two different mechanisms. Acute degeneration occurs when serous cells undergo death through apoptosis at low radiation dosages, while a late necrosis is dose dependent and reflects a lack of acinar stem cell repopulation that results from cellular DNA injury [5, 6, 13, 19]. Although the gland's acini are primarily afflicted, the ducts usually remain intact.

Bethanechol, a cholinergic agonist with minimal side effects, has been advocated as a pre-radiation treatment [20]. When prescribed prior to IMRT, post-therapeutic patients had higher whole unstimulated and stimulated salivary rates than patients who did not receive bethanechol. Obviously if feasible, employing the application of lower doses of IMRT to adjacent salivary glands results in less gland damage. Furthermore, the practitioner should be aware that the concomitant use of chemotherapy is reported to increase the intensity of irradiated gland hyposalivation [21]. Treatment of the oral conditions resulting from RT's effect on the salivary glands includes a variety of palliative procedures. The sialogogues, pilocarpine or cevimeline, can be prescribed along with the adjunctive use of sugarless chewing gum or sour candy to stimulate any residual surviving salivary parenchyma. Aggressive fluoride therapy is required to control the extensive dental caries that will develop from a significant loss of saliva. Artificial saliva, moisturizers, and lubricant mouthwashes are available commercially to ameliorate the subjective discomfort associated with a dry mouth and/or mucositis. Candidiasis can be treated with antifungals. Oral hygiene must be scrupulously maintained and dehydration should be avoided.

Radioactive Iodine (^{131}I)

Thyroid cancer has proven to be a not uncommon endocrine malignancy. An estimated 52,000 new cases were reported in the United States in 2019 [22]. The increasing use of ultrasound to detect small, nonpalpable malignant thyroid nodules will cause this incidence to increase. Over 90% of these thyroid cancers are differentiated thyroid cancers (DTC), usually papillary or follicular carcinomas [23]. Thyroid cancer is a malignancy of the relatively young, mostly women in the fifth decade of their life. Standard care for DTC involves total or subtotal thyroidectomy followed by the oral ingestion of radioactive iodine (RAI) in the form of ^{131}I. As part of their normal metabolic activity, the benign and malignant thyroid cells absorb and concentrate the RAI. Because it is radioactive, the ^{131}I will eradicate postsurgical remnants of benign and/or malignant thyroid tissue. The resulting ablation facilitates postoperative surveillance via an increased ability to monitor alterations in serum thyroglobulin. This therapeutic approach, thyroidectomy followed by ^{131}I thyroid ablation, has proven to be very effective therapeutically and for monitoring.

Simultaneous with its destructive effect on thyroid tissue, RAI can cause adverse reactions in other iodine avid tissues, most frequently the salivary glands (SG). Sialadenitis is a common result when RAI doses of 75–100 mCi are administered therapeutically [24] (Figs. 13.2 and 13.3). Within 24–48 h, SG pain and swelling develop in 50% of the recipients [25], usually involving the parotid gland (PG), often bilaterally. The ^{131}I causes a vasculitis with endothelial wall injury and an increased vascular permeability. The consequent escape of fluid and cells from the vascular channels causes a rapid onset of a clinical SG swelling. The inflammatory swelling is transient, subsiding in a few days, and coincides with the immediate post-ingestion period of increased patient radioactivity which in the past required patient isolation.

Renal and salivary excretory activity rapidly comes into play and functions to lower serum ^{131}I levels. Within a short period, the vascular endothelial wall re-establishes its normal permeability gradient and integrity. Abnormal extravasation ends and the intraglandular inflammatory elements recede. Pain and swelling subside and the patient usually enters a symptom-free period which may be transient or permanent.

Following this early SG reaction, manifestations of duct obstruction and parenchymal damage tend to occur months later if ablation RAI doses of ≥75 mCi have been administered (Figs. 13.4 and 13.5). The sodium iodide symporter molecule, the transporter of ^{131}I into the saliva, resides in the basolateral membrane of the duct cells [26]. The high concentration of RAI in the duct wall, caused by the symporter molecule, damages the DNA of the duct's stem cells, and along with irradiation's direct effect on the duct cell's plasma membrane, cell death and scarring are the inescapable consequences. Duct fibrosis and luminal stricturing represent the end game of this irradiation-induced inflammation. Further narrowing of the lumen results from the ductal shedding of inflammatory debris that acts to obstruct the duct lumen (Fig. 13.6). Salivary flow is impeded and the salivary retention causes

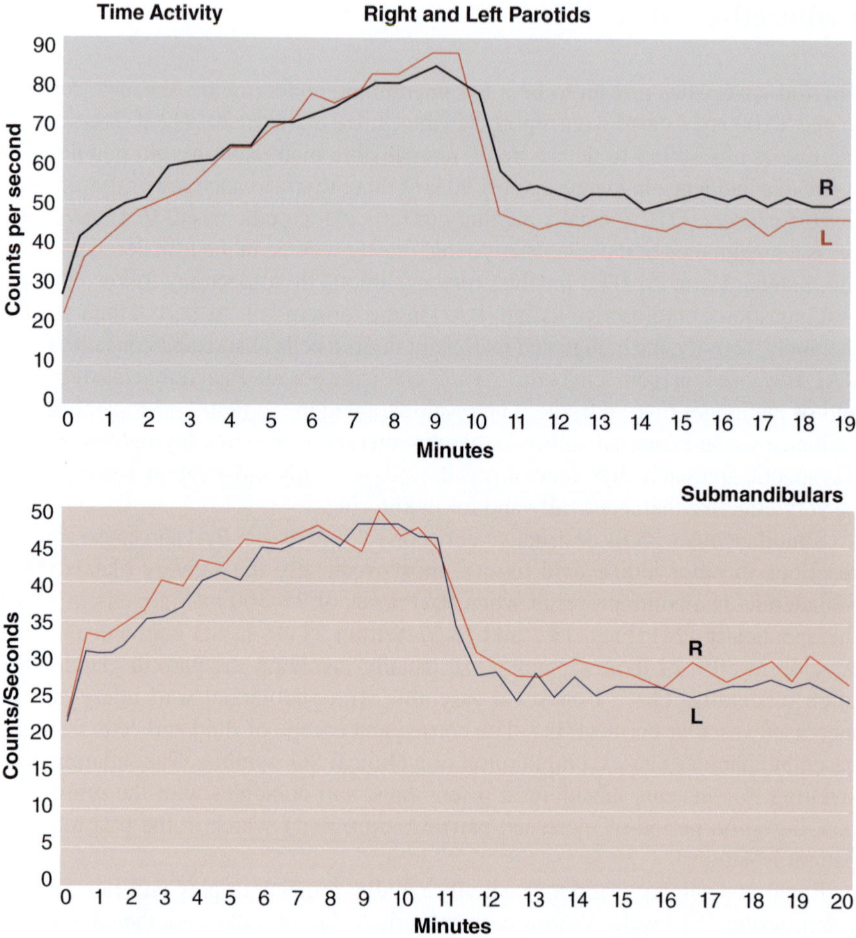

Fig. 13.2 Radioactive iodine (RAI). Scintiscan taken 5 months after patient received 30 mCi ^{131}I. Normal technetium pertechnetate (TPT) uptake by the parotid and submandibular glands. Stimulation (lemon candy) at 10-min mark demonstrates normal secretion by all salivary glands. (Mandel L, Chapter 9, Shifrin AL, Endocrine Emergencies 2022)

swelling and pain that is accentuated during eating when salivary stimulation is heightened. As many as 44% of patients will develop symptoms of obstructive sialadenitis months after having been exposed to RAI ablation [27].

Both PGs and both submandibular salivary glands (SMSGs) are injured by the ^{131}I radioactivity. However, they are asymmetrically involved, with any combination of 1–4 PGs/SMSGs demonstrating varying degrees of ductal and/or parenchymal damage. Reports of injury to the sublingual salivary gland are not available. Clinical symptomatology of glandular damage is more often observed in the PGs than the SMSGs. The explanation may rest in the fact that the SMSG has a higher proportion of striated ducts than the PG. These relatively more numerous striated ducts contain

Fig. 13.3 (**a**) Radioactive iodine. Patient A. Left parotid swelling following administration of 75 mCi ^{131}I 11 months previously (Mandel L, Chapter 9, Shifrin AL, Endocrine Emergencies 2022). (**b**) Radioactive iodine. Patient A. CT scan demonstrates left parotid sialadenitis (Mandel L, Chapter 9, Shifrin AL, Endocrine Emergencies 2022). (**c**) Radioactive iodine. Patient A. Scintiscan. Right parotid with normal pickup and secretion. Left parotid graph reveals delayed TPT pickup and failure to secrete at a 10-min mark. (Mandel L, Chapter 9, Shifrin AL, Endocrine Emergencies 2022)

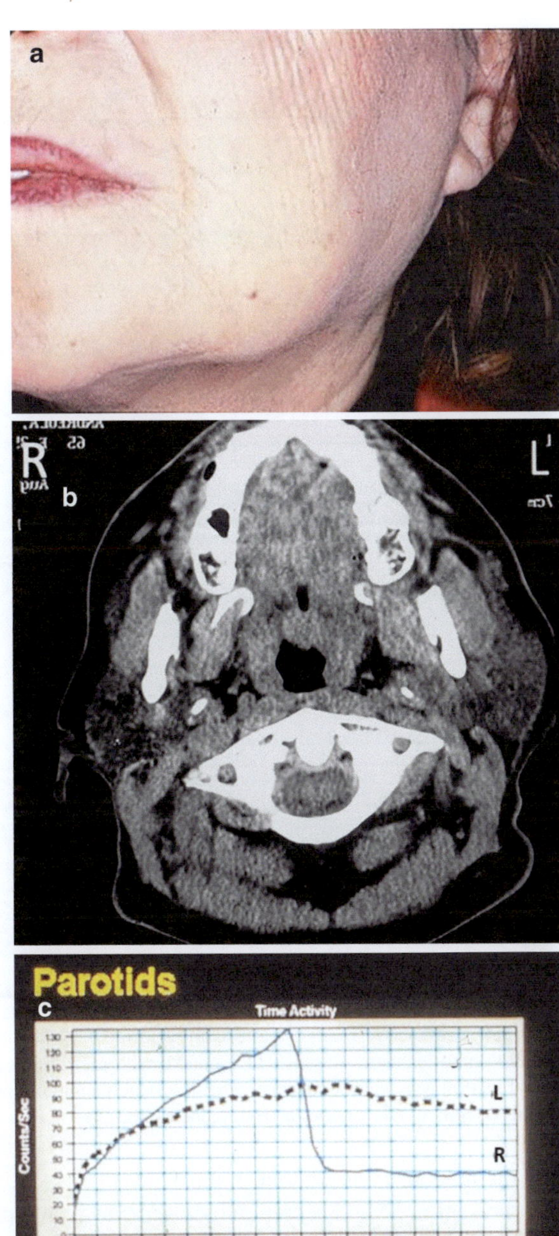

the iodine transport molecule that will allow a higher rate of ^{131}I clearance through the SMSG than that which occurs in the PG. This rapid SMSG transit for ^{131}I decreases the exposure time available for radiation injury. Furthermore, serous cells, predominantly located in the PGs, are more susceptible to the effects of radiation

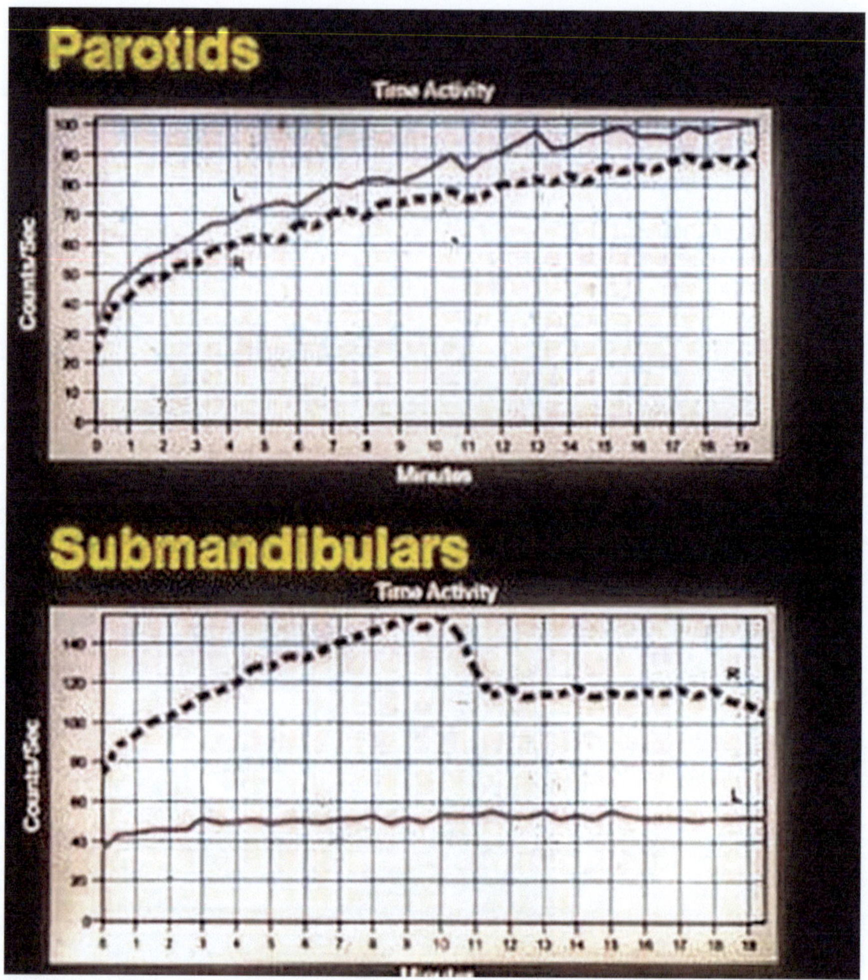

Fig. 13.4 Radioactive iodine. Scintiscan performed 7 months after patient received 150 mCi [131]I. Both parotids show sluggish TPT uptake with a failure to secrete. The right submandibular gland function is essentially normal, whereas the left submandibular shows no activity (Mandel L, Chapter 9, Shifrin AL, Endocrine Emergencies 2022)

than the mucous cells present in the SMSG [1, 4, 5]. Additionally, the mucus element present in SMSG secretion may serve as a protective asset against radiation.

Although the SG swellings are exacerbated during periods of salivary stimulation, they usually subside after eating because the luminal obstruction is not complete, and saliva slowly passes through the narrowed lumen. Salivary flow is also aided when soft intraluminal plugs, formed by the inflammatory exudate, are spontaneously expelled with the aid of attending hydrostatic salivary pressure. Some symptom amelioration now occurs, but the SG inflammation, initiated by the ^{131}I-induced duct obstruction with the retained saliva, can persist for varying periods, with remission intervals that can last from weeks to months.

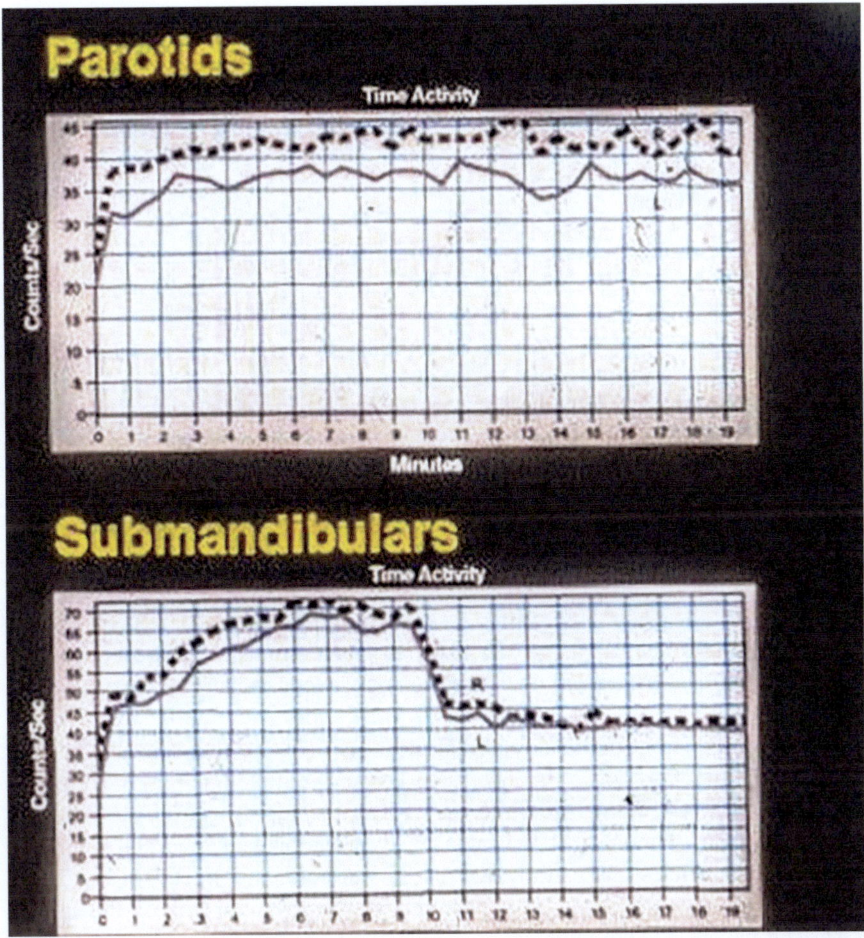

Fig. 13.5 Radioactive iodine. Scintiscan performed 12 months after patient received cumulative dose of more than 500 mCi ^{131}I. Both parotids are not functioning, while both submandibular glands show normal activity

Persistent glandular symptomatology from obstruction can lead to the development of a long-standing chronic sialadenitis. Chronic obstructive sialadenitis is also reported to occur in as many as two-thirds of the patients who have received ^{131}I doses of 100–150 mCi [28]. Unsurprisingly, damage to the SGs is in direct proportion to the administered ^{131}I dosage [27–29]. With time, symptoms resolve in most patients with only 5% of patients reporting problems when seen 7 years after RAI treatment [30]. It would seem that the active inflammatory process has subsided, and although some duct stricturing is present, the narrowed scarred lumen is apparently wide enough to accommodate salivary demand and eliminate subjective complaints.

In the presence of thyroid cancer metastasis or recurrence, high or repeated ^{131}I dosages are required. Hyposalivation will then become evident when the dose

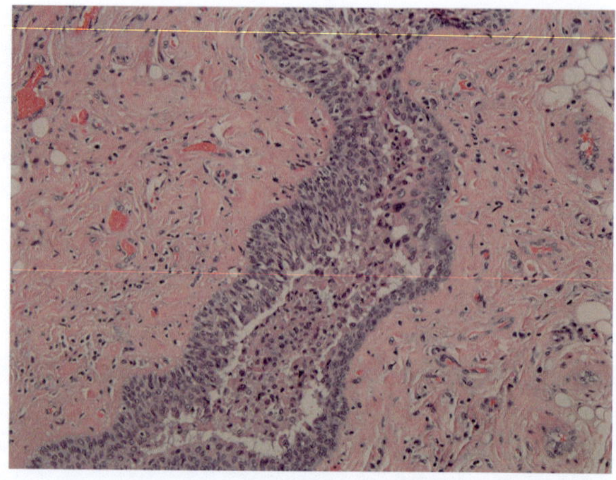

Fig. 13.6 Radioactive iodine effect on submandibular gland duct. Duct lumen obstructed by inflammatory debris. Epithelial metaplasia of duct wall is present. Patient had been treated 8 months previously with 75 mCi [131]I

range approaches 300 mCi. This high level of RAI is sufficient to initiate a significant loss of parenchymal acini [5, 29, 31]. Gross SG parenchymal destruction with eradication of salivary production can be anticipated when total levels of administered ^{131}I reach 500 mCi. Obstructive symptoms will not be present because parenchymal salivary production has been eliminated. However, a superimposed secondary ascending duct infection may occur because of the absence of salivary lavage.

The takeaway from the data regarding dosages indicates that salivary function decreases in direct proportion to increasing levels of radioiodine [32, 33]. Besides sialadenitis, adverse effects from the use of RAI include dysgeusia, nasolacrimal duct obstruction, pulmonary fibrosis, gonadal dysfunction, leukemia, and secondary primary malignancies that can involve the SGs or colorectal tract [34–36]. These numerous adverse problems have encouraged the reassessment of the use of RAI. The papers of Schlumberger et al. [37] and Mallick et al. [38] have given impetus to the present trend to use lower doses of ^{131}I for ablation. A meaningful decrease in the incidence and severity of complications, particularly in the occurrence of sialadenitis, has resulted. Published reports have indicated that successful ^{131}I ablation can be achieved with 30 mCi and can be used to treat the low-risk patient. Furthermore, American Thyroid Association guidelines state that the use of ^{131}I is not justified in all DTC patients, and its use in low-risk disease (no local tumor invasion, no metastasis, no aggressive histology) can be completely avoided [39].

Treatment of the anticipated adverse effects of ^{131}I on the SG begins in the immediate post-^{131}I period. Sour lemon candy and cholinergic drugs have been advocated to increase salivation and speed up the transit time of ^{131}I through the SG. However, it is counterargued that sour candy or medication stimulation will bring an increased blood flow with increased amounts of ^{131}I into the SG. Alternatively, recombinant thyroid-stimulating hormone can be administered prior to ablation because it is generally accepted that it allows for a more rapid renal clearance of ^{131}I, and in so doing it will decrease SG RAI exposure [27].

Fig. 13.7 Radioactive iodine. Method for parotid gland massage (Mandel L, Chapter 9, Shifrin AL, Endocrine Emergencies 2022)

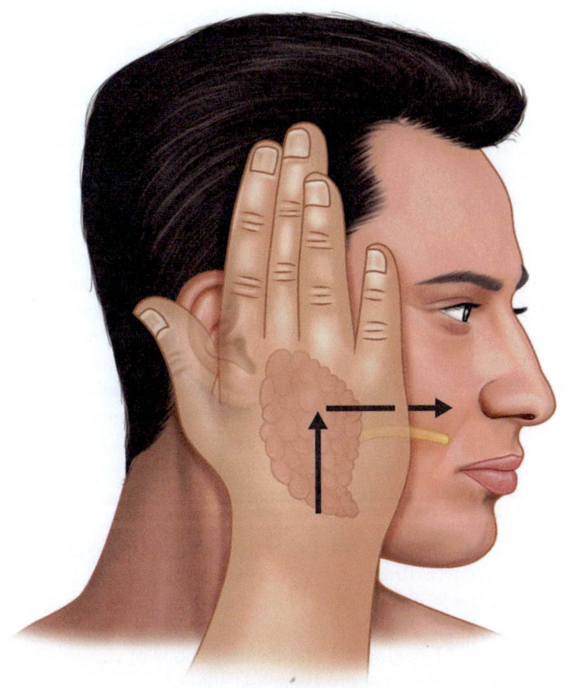

Following ^{131}I administration, aggressive PG massage is helpful in reducing SG dysfunction [25] (Fig. 13.7). Sialendoscopy has proven to be beneficial in alleviating the SG symptomatology [40] that results from the onset of obstructive symptomatology. Sialendoscopy has the ability to open a luminal pathway because the instrument can break up strictures while its lavaging ability can flush out obstructing luminal debris. Sialogogic agents can also be used to encourage salivary flushing and prevent salivary stagnation and accumulation of luminal debris. Dehydration must be avoided by maintaining an acceptable daily fluid intake. If residual SG parenchyma is present, some saliva is being produced and cholinergic agents can be utilized to ameliorate any existing dry mouth symptomatology. Commercially prepared artificial saliva, oral lubricants, and mouthwashes are of some value. Fluoride therapy should be instituted in anticipation of an increase in dental caries resulting from hyposalivation.

References

1. Teng F, Fan W, Luo Y, et al. Reducing xerostomia by comprehensive protection of salivary glands in intensity-modulated radiation therapy with helical tomotherapy technique for head-and-neck cancer patients: a prospective observational study. Biomed Res Int. 2019;2019:2401743. Published 2019 Jul 14. https://doi.org/10.1155/2019/2401743.

 2. Deboni AL, Giordani AJ, Lopes NN, et al. Long-term oral effects in patients treated with radiochemotherapy for head and neck cancer. Support Care Cancer. 2012;20(11):2903–11. https://doi.org/10.1007/s00520-012-1418-7.
 3. Randall K, Stevens J, Yepes JF, et al. Analysis of factors influencing the development of xerostomia during intensity-modulated radiotherapy. Oral Surg Oral Med Oral Pathol Oral Radiol. 2013;115(6):772–9. https://doi.org/10.1016/j.oooo.2013.01.006.
 4. Garg AK, Malo M. Manifestations and treatment of xerostomia and associated oral effects secondary to head and neck radiation therapy. J Am Dent Assoc. 1997;128(8):1128–33. https://doi.org/10.14219/jada.archive.1997.0371.
 5. Nagler RM. The enigmatic mechanism of irradiation-induced damage to the major salivary glands. Oral Dis. 2002;8(3):141–6. https://doi.org/10.1034/j.1601-0825.2002.02838.x.
 6. Mohammadi N, Seyyednejhad F, Alizadeh Oskoee P, Savadi Oskoee S, Mofidi N. Evaluation of radiation-induced xerostomia in patients with nasopharyngeal carcinomas. J Dent Res Dent Clin Dent Prospects. 2007;1(2):65–70. https://doi.org/10.5681/joddd.2007.011.
 7. Baharudin A, Khairuddin A, Nizam A, Samsuddin AR. Evaluation of irradiated salivary gland function in patients with head and neck tumours treated with radiotherapy. J Laryngol Otol. 2009;123(1):108–13. https://doi.org/10.1017/S0022215108002466.
 8. Lalla RV, Treister N, Sollecito T, et al. Oral complications at 6 months after radiation therapy for head and neck cancer. Oral Dis. 2017;23(8):1134–43. https://doi.org/10.1111/odi.12710.
 9. Eisbruch A. Reducing xerostomia by IMRT: what may, and may not, be achieved. J Clin Oncol. 2007;25(31):4863–4. https://doi.org/10.1200/JCO.2007.13.4874.
10. Schulz RE, Bonzanini LIL, Ortigara GB, et al. Prevalence of hyposalivation and associated factors in survivors of head and neck cancer treated with radiotherapy. J Appl Oral Sci. 2021;29:e20200854. Published 2021 Apr 19. https://doi.org/10.1590/1678-7757-2020-0854.
11. Carl W. Managing the oral manifestations of cancer therapy, part I: head-and-neck radiation therapy. Compendium. 1988;9(4):306–18.
12. Marucci L, Marzi S, Sperduti I, et al. Influence of intensity-modulated radiation therapy technique on xerostomia and related quality of life in patients treated with intensity-modulated radiation therapy for nasopharyngeal cancer. Head Neck. 2012;34(3):328–35. https://doi.org/10.1002/hed.21736.
13. Eisbruch A, Ten Haken RK, Kim HM, Marsh LH, Ship JA. Dose, volume, and function relationships in parotid salivary glands following conformal and intensity-modulated irradiation of head and neck cancer. Int J Radiat Oncol Biol Phys. 1999;45(3):577–87. https://doi.org/10.1016/s0360-3016(99)00247-3.
14. Hey J, Setz J, Gerlach R, et al. Parotid gland-recovery after radiotherapy in the head and neck region—36 months follow-up of a prospective clinical study. Radiat Oncol. 2011;6:125. Published 2011 Sep 27.
15. Dreizen S, Daly TE, Drane JB, Brown LR. Oral complications of cancer radiotherapy. Postgrad Med. 1977;61(2):85–92. https://doi.org/10.1080/00325481.1977.11712115.
16. Lal P, Nautiyal V, Verma M, Yadav R, Maria Das KJ, Kumar S. Objective and subjective assessment of xerostomia in patients of locally advanced head-and-neck cancers treated by intensity-modulated radiotherapy. J Cancer Res Ther. 2018;14(6):1196–201. https://doi.org/10.4103/jcrt.JCRT_200_17.
17. Eisbruch A, Kim HM, Terrell JE, Marsh LH, Dawson LA, Ship JA. Xerostomia and its predictors following parotid-sparing irradiation of head-and-neck cancer. Int J Radiat Oncol Biol Phys. 2001;50(3):695–704. https://doi.org/10.1016/s0360-3016(01)01512-7.
18. Wang X, Eisbruch A. IMRT for head and neck cancer: reducing xerostomia and dysphagia. J Radiat Res. 2016;57 Suppl 1(Suppl 1):i69–75. https://doi.org/10.1093/jrr/rrw047.
19. Möller P, Perrier M, Ozsahin M, Monnier P. A prospective study of salivary gland function in patients undergoing radiotherapy for squamous cell carcinoma of the oropharynx. Oral Surg Oral Med Oral Pathol Oral Radiol Endod. 2004;97(2):173–89. https://doi.org/10.1016/s1079-2104(03)00473-6.

20. Jaguar GC, Lima EN, Kowalski LP, et al. Double blind randomized prospective trial of bethanechol in the prevention of radiation-induced salivary gland dysfunction in head and neck cancer patients. Radiother Oncol. 2015;115(2):253–6. https://doi.org/10.1016/j.radonc.2015.03.017.

21. Rades D, Warwas B, Gerull K, Pries R, Leichtle A, Bruchhage KL, Hakim SG, Schild SE, Cremers F. Prognostic factors for complete recovery from xerostomia after radiotherapy of head-and-neck cancers. In Vivo. 2022;36(4):1795–800. https://doi.org/10.21873/invivo.12894. PMID: 35738613; PMCID: PMC9301398.

22. Siegel RL, Miller KD, Jemal A. Cancer statistics, 2019. CA Cancer J Clin. 2019;69(1):7–34. https://doi.org/10.3322/caac.21551.

23. Sunavala-Dossabhoy G. Radioactive iodine: an unappreciated threat to salivary gland function. Oral Dis. 2018;24(1–2):198–201. https://doi.org/10.1111/odi.12774.

24. Doi SA, Woodhouse NJ, Thalib L, Onitilo A. Ablation of the thyroid remnant and I-131 dose in differentiated thyroid cancer: a meta-analysis revisited. Clin Med Res. 2007;5(2):87–90. https://doi.org/10.3121/cmr.2007.763.

25. Son SH, Lee CH, Jung JH, et al. The preventive effect of parotid gland massage on salivary gland dysfunction during high-dose radioactive iodine therapy for differentiated thyroid cancer: a randomized clinical trial. Clin Nucl Med. 2019;44(8):625–33. https://doi.org/10.1097/RLU.0000000000002602.

26. Caglar M, Tuncel M, Alpar R. Scintigraphic evaluation of salivary gland dysfunction in patients with thyroid cancer after radioiodine treatment. Clin Nucl Med. 2002;27(11):767–71. https://doi.org/10.1097/00003072-200211000-00003.

27. An YS, Yoon JK, Lee SJ, Song HS, Yoon SH, Jo KS. Symptomatic late-onset sialadenitis after radioiodine therapy in thyroid cancer. Ann Nucl Med. 2013;27(4):386–91. https://doi.org/10.1007/s12149-013-0697-5.

28. Jeong SY, Kim HW, Lee SW, Ahn BC, Lee J. Salivary gland function 5 years after radioactive iodine ablation in patients with differentiated thyroid cancer: direct comparison of pre- and postablation scintigraphies and their relation to xerostomia symptoms. Thyroid. 2013;23(5):609–16. https://doi.org/10.1089/thy.2012.0106.

29. Raza H, Khan AU, Hameed A, Khan A. Quantitative evaluation of salivary gland dysfunction after radioiodine therapy using salivary gland scintigraphy. Nucl Med Commun. 2006;27(6):495–9. https://doi.org/10.1097/00006231-200606000-00004.

30. Grewal RK, Larson SM, Pentlow CE, et al. Salivary gland side effects commonly develop several weeks after initial radioactive iodine ablation. J Nucl Med. 2009;50(10):1605–10. https://doi.org/10.2967/jnumed.108.061382.

31. Konings AW, Coppes RP, Vissink A. On the mechanism of salivary gland radiosensitivity [published correction appears in Int J Radiat Oncol Biol Phys. 2006 Jan 1;64(1):330]. Int J Radiat Oncol Biol Phys. 2005;62(4):1187–94. https://doi.org/10.1016/j.ijrobp.2004.12.051.

32. Sánchez Barrueco A, González Galán F, Alcalá Rueda I, et al. Incidence and risk factors for radioactive iodine-induced sialadenitis. Acta Otolaryngol. 2020;140(11):959–62. https://doi.org/10.1080/00016489.2020.1802507.

33. Kim JW, Kim JM, Choi ME, Kim SK, Kim YM, Choi JS. Does salivary function decrease in proportion to radioiodine dose? Laryngoscope. 2020;130(9):2173–8. https://doi.org/10.1002/lary.28342.

34. Kloos RT, Duvuuri V, Jhiang SM, Cahill KV, Foster JA, Burns JA. Nasolacrimal drainage system obstruction from radioactive iodine therapy for thyroid carcinoma. J Clin Endocrinol Metab. 2002;87(12):5817–20. https://doi.org/10.1210/jc.2002-020210.

35. Lee SL. Complications of radioactive iodine treatment of thyroid carcinoma. J Natl Compr Cancer Netw. 2010;8(11):1277–87. https://doi.org/10.6004/jnccn.2010.0094.

36. Rubino C, de Vathaire F, Dottorini ME, et al. Second primary malignancies in thyroid cancer patients. Br J Cancer. 2003;89(9):1638–44. https://doi.org/10.1038/sj.bjc.6601319.

37. Schlumberger M, Catargi B, Borget I, et al. Strategies of radioiodine ablation in patients with low-risk thyroid cancer. N Engl J Med. 2012;366(18):1663–73. https://doi.org/10.1056/NEJMoa1108586.
38. Mallick U, Harmer C, Yap B, et al. Ablation with low-dose radioiodine and thyrotropin alfa in thyroid cancer. N Engl J Med. 2012;366(18):1674–85. https://doi.org/10.1056/NEJMoa1109589.
39. Haugen BR, Alexander EK, Bible KC, et al. 2015 American Thyroid Association management guidelines for adult patients with thyroid nodules and differentiated thyroid cancer: the American Thyroid Association guidelines task force on thyroid nodules and differentiated thyroid cancer. Thyroid. 2016;26(1):1–133. https://doi.org/10.1089/thy.2015.0020.
40. Bhayani MK, Acharya V, Kongkiatkamon S, et al. Sialendoscopy for patients with radioiodine-induced sialadenitis and xerostomia. Thyroid. 2015;25(7):834–8. https://doi.org/10.1089/thy.2014.0572.

Chapter 14
Mumps-like Salivary Gland Swellings

Louis Mandel

Abstract There is a group of abnormal salivary gland swellings (pneumoparotid, anesthesia mumps, iodide mumps) that to some extent have similarities to the signs and symptoms of mumps. The liberty of classifying them into one category, for want of a better option, has been taken. Sudden onset of unilateral or bilateral salivary gland swellings function as their hallmark. As with mumps, the parotid gland is usually involved unilaterally or bilaterally, but submandibular gland swellings can also occur. The group's limited similarity to mumps is also derived from the fact that treatment is essentially palliative because spontaneous resolution can be anticipated. However a significant difference from mumps symptomatology is that pain is not a significant factor.

Introduction

There are several conditions involving the salivary glands (SG), unilaterally and bilaterally, that have a cursory resemblance to mumps. Pneumoparotid, anesthesia mumps, and iodide mumps are SG abnormalities that seem to belong in this category. Sudden onset of SG swelling with rapid and spontaneous resolutions are characteristic elements of these entities. Problems with infection are usually not part of their symptom complex. Suppuration is not present, and the pain associated with mumps is absent or moderate. Because these SG swellings are self-limiting and transient in nature, treatment need only be supportive. Following the acute episode of SG swelling and its resolution, no permanent pathologic changes have been reported except in patients who have maintained constant and prolonged periods of increased intraoral pressure, as in habit-incited pneumoparotid. In these patients, secondary infection can develop from the continued forced retrograde insufflation of bacteria into the SG ductal system.

L. Mandel, *Clinical Management of Salivary Gland Disorders*,
https://doi.org/10.1007/978-3-031-50012-1_14

Pneumoparotid

Pneumoparotid, the retrograde entry of air through the parotid orifice and into the parotid salivary ducts, has been observed to cause unilateral or bilateral parotid gland (PG) swellings. The condition occurs only in the presence of a significantly increased intraoral pressure. Normally, the intraoral pressure is 2–3 mmHg, but it can be forced to reach levels of 140–150 mmHg [1]. Wind instrument players and glass blowers are individuals who have an occupational hazard. They have the ability to increase intraoral pressure by consciously and strenuously blowing up their cheeks, and in the process, they become susceptible to the development of pneumoparotid. Pneumoparotid can also occur from persistent coughing, with the use of the continuous positive air pressure (CPAP) unit for sleep apnea (Fig. 14.1) and during dental treatment with air pressurized dental instruments. However, the most frequent cause is a self-induction habit (Fig. 14.2) by people with/without psychologic disorders [2]. Of interest is the fact that soldiers have been known to self-induce pneumoparotid by vigorously blowing into a bottle and in so doing increasing their intraoral pressure. In turn, this activity leads to the development of PG

Fig. 14.1 (a) Pneumoparotid. Patient A being treated for sleep apnea with CPAP. Left parotid swelling present upon awakening. (b) Pneumoparotid. Patient A. Aerated foamy saliva exiting parotid duct orifice

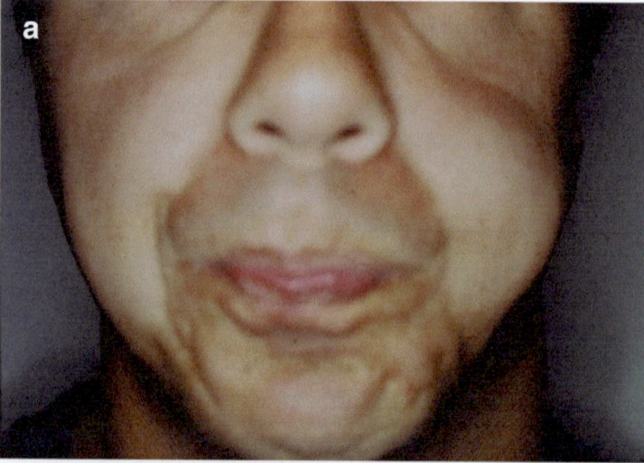

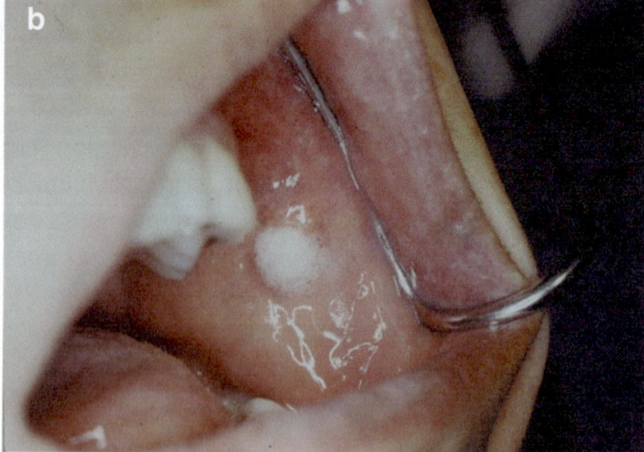

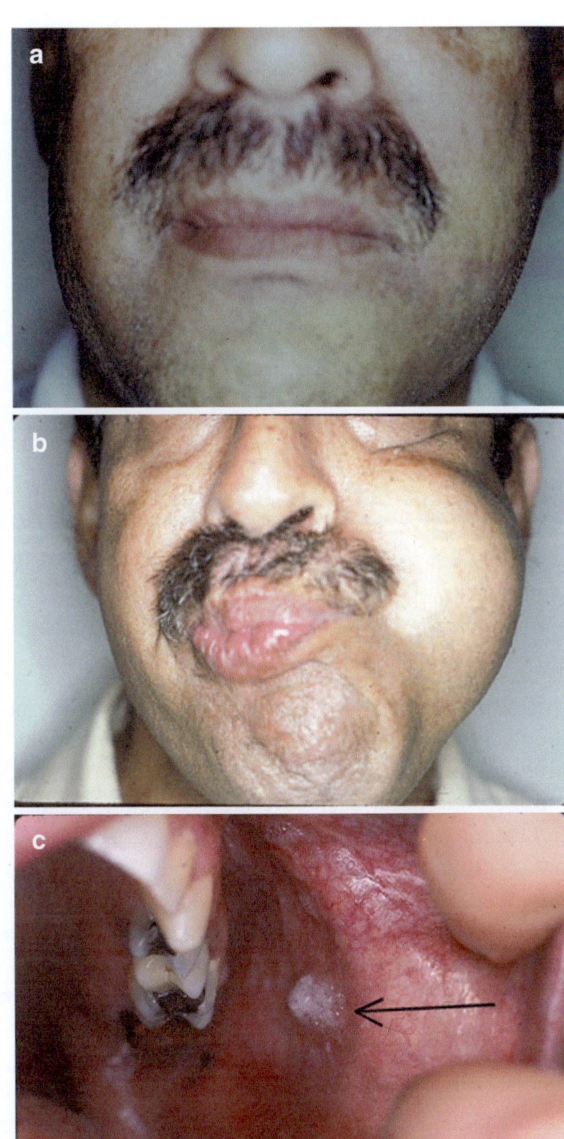

Fig. 14.2 (**a**) Pneumoparotid. Patient B. Left parotid swelling following chronic cheek blowing habit (Mandel L, et al. Oral Surg Oral Med Oral Pathol 1991;72:22). (**b**) Pneumoparotid. Patient B. Cheek blowing habit (left) (Mandel L, et al. Oral Surg Oral Med Oral Pathol 1991;72:22). (**c**) Pneumoparotid. Patient B. Aerated foamy saliva exiting parotid duct orifice (arrow) (Mandel L, et al. Oral Surg Oral Med Oral Pathol 1991;72:22)

swellings that mimic mumps [2]. Consequently, they could avoid a disagreeable assignment because of their "medical problem."

The anatomic design of the parotid duct orifice, as it exits intraorally on the buccal papilla (Fig. 14.3) adjacent to the maxillary molar area, normally discourages air reflux via several mechanisms [2]. The diameter of the duct orifice is narrower than the duct itself, thus hindering retrograde air movement. Moreover, the orifice is slit-shaped and surrounded by redundant mucosal tissue which seals the orifice when

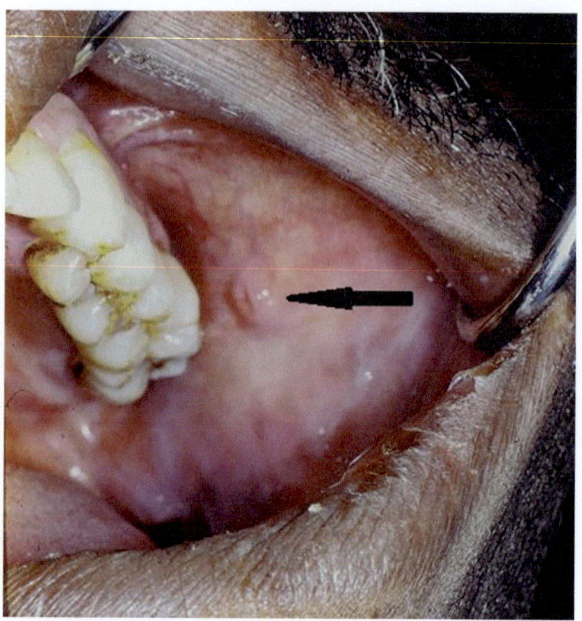

Fig. 14.3 Parotid duct orifice on buccal papilla (arrow)

the intraoral pressure is elevated. Furthermore, the normal anatomic angulation of the duct favors its squeezing and closure by the buccinator muscle. The increased oral pressure also serves to compress the parotid duct as it traverses the masseter muscle's lateral surface. Nevertheless, significant increases in intraoral pressure distort the musculature around the orifice so that the entry of air into the parotid duct is not totally inhibited. The presence of anatomic abnormalities, a patulous duct, and a weak buccinator muscle further encourage ductal air invasion [3].

Following initial and continued episodes of increased intraoral pressure in a vulnerable patient, PG swelling from the retrograde duct entry of air rapidly becomes visible. The swelling follows the general anatomic outline of the PG, but it may extend to involve the cervical area. Pain may or may not be present. The PG swelling may last from hours to a few days, but spontaneous resolution can be expected. Occasionally, air escapes the confines of the PG. A subcutaneous emphysema or pneumomediastinum can develop because of acinar rupture and because the limiting PG capsule is incomplete in the superior medial part of the PG [2]. There are two objective signs whose presence acts to clinch a clinical diagnosis of pneumoparotid. Palpation of the swelling will elicit a crackling sensation, reflecting the presence of air in the PG apparatus. Second, saliva should be expressed by manually pressuring the PG extraorally and observing saliva's quality as it exits intraorally through the duct orifice. A frothy bubbly salivary return (Figs. 14.1b and 14.2c) will be seen rather than the clear aqueous flow normally observed. This unique salivary pathognomonic feature represents the forced mixture of refluxed air and saliva within the limiting confines of the duct lumen.

Imaging techniques have proven to be key factors in diagnosis. Standard CT scanning and CT sialography are most helpful [4, 5] because the air in the PG and the ductal system will clearly be observed. Furthermore, inflammatory changes associated with any existing secondary parotitis will be reflected by an increased size and density of the infected PG. Parapharyngeal, retropharyngeal, subcutaneous, and mediastinal emphysema may also be imaged if air escapes through the PG's incomplete capsule in the superior medial aspect of the gland [2].

Sialography can depict the status of the duct system. Initially, no duct changes are present because pathologic changes have not had the opportunity to evolve. However, radiolucencies within the duct may be seen. They represent pockets of air previously forced into the duct and trapped there by the injection of the sialographic dye. If the problem of increased oral pressure is maintained over time, the major duct and eventually the secondary duct system will develop dilations from air distension. The duct's irregularity can then be accentuated by the onset of a secondary infection, referred to as pneumoparotitis, with duct stricturing originating from the effects of the constant aeration-incited inflammation and/or reflux into the duct by the abundant invasive oral bacteria. The symptomatology of a PG emphysema is now complicated by the presence of a superimposed secondary PG infection, and a "sausaged" duct outline will become evident sialographically reflecting the presence of a pneumoparotitis. The secondary parotitis, with its accompanying pain and suppuration, serves to confuse the path to an accurate pneumoparotid clinical diagnosis. Plain radiographs will show air in the ductal system. Ultrasound can function as a key diagnostic aid because it will depict multiple hyperechoic areas that correspond to the air in the gland.

Pneumoparotid requires a minimal treatment approach because spontaneous resolution can be anticipated. Observation with palliative care is the primary option. Antibiotics may be prescribed prophylactically in an attempt to prevent a secondary infection or therapeutically to treat an existing pneumoparotitis. To avoid an inevitable superimposed infection from continuation of the cause, a conscious effort to stop any unintentional habit must be attempted, but success is difficult to attain. Behavioral modification and psychologic care may be required. Parotidectomy is performed only when a secondary chronic PG infection has caused serious glandular destruction.

Anesthesia Mumps

Anesthesia mumps (AM), the acute onset of a unilateral or bilateral transient swelling of a noninfected parotid gland (PG) following general anesthesia, is not an uncommon entity. The submandibular salivary gland is rarely involved. AM has a reported incidence of 0.16–0.2% following general anesthesia [6] with no age or sex predilection.

Unilateral occasionally bilateral PG swellings, lasting from several minutes to several days, are the commonly recognized presenting signs that are usually observed in the recovery room during the immediate postoperative period. Spontaneous resolution without complications can be anticipated. As a rule, AM occurs in a wide age range of postoperative patients and is accompanied by only moderate discomfort. It has been recognized postoperatively following a variety of procedures that include bronchoscopy, orthopedic surgery, neurosurgery, spinal surgery, colon surgery, and endoscopy.

Two distinct etiologic AM categories have been recognized. They can be separated by ascertaining whether the swelling is related to a tissue emphysema or some as yet unknown circumstance. In the first group, retrograde air insufflation into the PG is appreciated when glandular palpation causes a sensation of crepitation and a frothy saliva is observed exiting from the PG intraoral duct orifice. The etiology, signs, and symptoms associated with this AM group are identical to those observed in patients with pneumoparotid. The difference rests in the methodology of AM's onset. Patients undergoing general anesthesia often are subjected to significant elevations of the intraoral air pressure caused by the positive pressure from face mask ventilation. Furthermore, the coughing, sneezing, bucking, and straining that frequently accompany the general anesthetic procedure or develop during the immediate postoperative period will increase the intraoral air pressure. In addition, neuromuscular blocking medications used in conjunction with general anesthesia result in muscle relaxation and facilitate AM's onset [7]. Muscle tone surrounding the parotid duct orifice decreases with the use of these agents. The resulting flaccid duct orifice presents a diminished impediment to the entry of intraoral air, whose pressure has been increased, into the gland's ductal system. A diagnosis of pneumoparotid, initiated by events associated with general anesthesia, can now be made when it is substantiated by crepitation from palpation of the involved swelling and the expression of frothy saliva at the duct orifice.

It must be emphasized that not all AM patients will demonstrate the classic signs and symptomatology associated with pneumoparotid. These patients may not have had a general anesthetic for their operative procedure. They represent the second etiologic category of AM. Retrograde air entry into the PG will not be present as evidenced by the absence of crepitation. The origin of this variety of AM has not been definitively determined. However, a hypothesis has been suggested. Endotracheal intubation may act to stimulate parasympathetic receptors in the pharyngeal wall [8, 9]. The parasympathetics will cause a PG hypersalivation. In turn, the increased salivary flow may be impeded by a compressed parotid duct. The duct compression can originate from a prolonged rotated head position, with the face turned to one side, and/or from the tight fitting with adhesives of airway devices to the side of the face during the operative procedure [10]. Salivary flow is impeded and its retention is thought to be the cause of the PG swelling. Relieving the duct compression following the termination of the operative procedure results in an unobstructive salivary flow and subsidence of the PG swelling.

Imaging of the PG in AM can clearly differentiate the two varieties of AM. Air insufflation into the PG will readily be diagnosed in the first variety with imaging via ultrasound, radiography, or CT scanning. If the problem is not the first group's forced entry of air into the gland, the CT scan or ultrasound will display enlarged glands with an increased density (the second group), and no air invasion or abnormal pathologic signs will be seen [11].

Because spontaneous resolution of the PG swelling occurs within minutes or days, treatment is essentially supportive. Warm compresses may be applied and analgesics can be prescribed for any pain that is present. Reassurance and observation are major treatment options that are always available to the practitioner.

Iodide Mumps

Iodide mumps (IM) was first described in 1956 as occurring in a kidney-impaired patient undergoing intravenous pyelography [12]. The condition is characterized by swelling of the salivary glands (SG) that follows the intravascular injection of an ionic or nonionic iodine-containing contrast agent that is being used for imaging. IM is a relatively uncommon adverse reaction that involves the SG bilaterally (86%), although unilateral involvement (14%) is not infrequent [13]. Bilateral submandibular salivary gland (SMSG) swellings are more commonly seen than either parotid gland or sublingual salivary gland swellings. Following the intravascular introduction of the contrast, SG swellings develop within a few minutes or occur as long as 5 days post-injection [14]. Pain may be an issue. Fortunately, rapid spontaneous remission of the IM swellings can be anticipated, usually within 2–3 days. No long-term consequences have been observed.

Although the literature reports IM as a rare finding, its incidence is probably higher than the indicated rarity because patients do not tend to report transient swellings that cause only slight discomfort. However, its incidence has been reported to vary between 1 and 2% following the use of contrast [15]. Diagnosis is based on the clinical history of the patient having undergone the administration of an iodine-containing contrast solution and the development of subsequent SG swellings.

The exact mechanism for the onset of IM has not been established. In most patients, the injected dose of contrast-containing iodide is usually not high enough to cause IM. It has been hypothesized that the SG reaction in IM is an idiosyncratic response to the iodide in the contrast solution [14, 16]. Alternatively, it has been suggested that the SG swellings are a toxic response to the iodide. Normally, the injected contrast iodide in the circulating plasma is trapped by the SG and concentrated in the ductal system. This results in a concentration of iodide in the SG that is 100 times higher than the plasma level [15]. The SG ductal cells contain the sodium-iodide symporter, which is the molecule that transports iodide into the saliva. In the process of transporting the increased plasma iodide, the duct epithelium becomes inflamed and thickens at the expense of the lumen. The gland swells because of the salivary retention that results from the decrease in duct luminal width [15]. With the eventual clearance of the iodide, the inflammatory ductal response subsides, the lumen returns to its normal dimension, salivary retention ends, and the SG swelling recedes.

Impaired kidney function, if present, is a contributing factor because approximately 97% of circulating iodide is eliminated through the kidney [17]. Therefore, if contrast is used in a patient with a damaged kidney, the circulating iodide will be retained at higher than normal levels for longer time periods. The SG ductal system then becomes subject to the increased toxicity caused by its exposure to prolonged and higher concentrations of circulating iodide.

Objective evidence regarding the presence of IM can be obtained from ultrasound findings [18]. Diffuse homogeneous bilateral swellings of the SG and tubular hypoechoic areas, representing obstructed dilated ducts, are consistently seen. Additionally, a Doppler study will reveal an increased glandular vascularity [15].

Histologic study, whether obtained from a surgical or fine-needle aspiration biopsy, reveals normal glandular tissue. Edematous infiltrations are evident, but there are no signs of an inflammatory infiltrate [15].

Because of the spontaneous resolution of the SG swellings within a few days, supportive therapy is the treatment approach of choice. Analgesics can be prescribed if indicated. Corticosteroids, antihistamines, and anti-inflammatory agents have been administered as preventive measures and postoperatively as therapeutic medications [13]. In both situations, the results have been questionable. Dialysis may be of value for IM treatment if renal dysfunction is an issue [19].

References

1. Luaces R, Ferreras J, Patiño B, Garcia-Rozado A, Vázquez I, López-Cedrún JL. Pneumoparotid: a case report and review of the literature. J Oral Maxillofac Surg. 2008;66(2):362–5. https://doi.org/10.1016/j.joms.2006.10.007.
2. Gazia F, Freni F, Galletti C, et al. Pneumoparotid and pneumoparotitis: a literary review. Int J Environ Res Public Health. 2020;17(11):3936. Published 2020 Jun 2. https://doi.org/10.3390/ijerph17113936.
3. Han S, Isaacson G. Recurrent pneumoparotid: cause and treatment. Otolaryngol Head Neck Surg. 2004;131(5):758–61. https://doi.org/10.1016/j.otohns.2004.04.035.
4. Alcalde RE, Ueyama Y, Lim DJ, Matsumura T. Pneumoparotid: report of a case. J Oral Maxillofac Surg. 1998;56(5):676–80. https://doi.org/10.1016/s0278-2391(98)90473-6.
5. McGreevy AE, O'Kane AM, McCaul D, Basha SI. Pneumoparotitis: a case report. Head Neck. 2013;35(2):E55–9. https://doi.org/10.1002/hed.21873.
6. Rosique MJ, Rosique RG, Costa IR, Lara BR, Figueiredo JL, Ribeiro DG. Parotitis after epidural anesthesia in plastic surgery: report of three cases. Aesthetic Plast Surg. 2013;37(4):838–42. https://doi.org/10.1007/s00266-013-0112-6.
7. Kwon SY, Kang YJ, Seo KH, Kim Y. Acute unilateral anesthesia mumps after hysteroscopic surgery under general anesthesia: a case report. Korean J Anesthesiol. 2015;68(3):300–3. https://doi.org/10.4097/kjae.2015.68.3.300.
8. Asghar A, Karam K, Rashid S. A case of anesthesia mumps after sacral laminectomy under general anesthesia. Saudi J Anaesth. 2015;9(3):332–3. https://doi.org/10.4103/1658-354X.154743.
9. Montazeri N, Darabi MH, Hessami K, et al. A case of bilateral anesthesia mumps after cesarean section under spinal anesthesia: a rare case and literature review. Case Rep Obstet Gynecol. 2022;2022:5004358. Published 2022 Oct 4. https://doi.org/10.1155/2022/5004358.
10. Adachi YU, Matsuda N. Is it fluid or air causing anesthesia mumps? J Anesth. 2012;26(4):638–9. https://doi.org/10.1007/s00540-012-1387-5.
11. Bahadur S, Fayyaz M, Mehboob S. Salivary gland swelling developing after endoscopy: "anesthesia mumps". Gastrointest Endosc. 2006;63(2):345–7. https://doi.org/10.1016/j.gie.2005.09.008.
12. Sussman RM, Miller J. Iodide mumps after intravenous urography. N Engl J Med. 1956;255(9):433–4.

13. Zhang G, Li Y, Zhang R, et al. Acute submandibular swelling complicating arteriography with iodide contrast: a case report and literature review. Medicine (Baltimore). 2015;94(33):e1380. https://doi.org/10.1097/MD.0000000000001380.
14. Park SJ, Hong HS, Lee HK, Joh JH, Cha JG, Kim HC. Ultrasound findings of iodide mumps. Br J Radiol. 2005;78(926):164–5.
15. Jiao A, Farsad K, McVinnie DW, Jahangiri Y, Morrison JJ. Characterization of iodide-induced sialadenitis: meta-analysis of the published case reports in the medical literature. Acad Radiol. 2020;27(3):428–35.
16. Drori A, Yosha-Orpaz L. Case 277: iodide mumps. Radiology. 2020;295(2):490–4.
17. Zhang G, Li T, Wang H, Liu J. The pathogenesis of iodide mumps: a case report. Medicine (Baltimore). 2017;96(47):e8881.
18. Greco S, Centenaro R, Lavecchia G, Rossi F. Iodide mumps: sonographic appearance. J Clin Ultrasound. 2010;38(8):438–9.
19. Bohora S, Harikrishnan S, Tharakan J. Iodide mumps. Int J Cardiol. 2008;130(1):82–3.

Chapter 15
Iatrogenic Duct Injury

Louis Mandel

Abstract The salivary production of the major salivary glands finds its way into the oral cavity via each gland's unique ductal system. These ducts occupy an anatomic area that is subject to a wide variety of surgical procedures. Iatrogenic damage to a salivary duct often proves to be an unexpected complication when neighboring surgery is being performed. A not uncommon problem that develops with a sialoadenectomy is the secondary occurrence of a sialocele or a salivary fistula following duct damage. Sublingual duct injury from an adjacent mouth floor procedure can result in the formation of a ranula. Parotid duct obstruction with salivary retention can be a sequel to rhytidectomy or even as a secondary complication following parotid or submandibular sialolithectomy.

Iatrogenic Duct Injury

Overview of Salivary Ducts

Parotid Duct

The parotid duct (PD), also known as Stensen duct, was named after Niels Stensen, a Danish pioneer in anatomy [1]. He described the PD as first forming after receiving tributaries from the deep lobe of the parotid gland (PG). Subsequently, several ductules from the PG's superficial lobe join the PD which then exits the anterior portion of the PG. Upon emerging from the gland, the duct generally follows a course direction that corresponds approximately to a line drawn from the tragus of the ear to the vertical midpoint of the upper lip [2, 3].

The PD takes a path along the lateral surface of the masseter muscle where it is in close proximity to the buccal branches of the facial nerve and the transverse facial artery. Upon reaching the anterior border of the masseter muscle, the duct bends

L. Mandel, *Clinical Management of Salivary Gland Disorders*,
https://doi.org/10.1007/978-3-031-50012-1_15

medially and penetrates or runs along the surface of the buccal fat pad [4]. The PD now pierces the buccinator muscle and courses for a short distance obliquely forward between the buccinator muscle and the oral mucous membrane [5] as it approaches its orifice. The PD has its intraoral exit on the buccal papilla adjacent to the maxillary second molar (Fig. 14.3). Of interest is the fact that the PD may be doubled with two parotid ducts occasionally being observed emptying the PG [1, 6]. The PD's length has been reported to measure 4–7 cm with an internal luminal width that varies between 0.5 and 1.6 mm [1, 5]. Its ostium represents the narrowest section of the duct.

As the PD crosses the masseter muscle, it receives a duct from the separately positioned and superiorly located, but not always present, accessory PG (APG). The incidence for the presence of the APG has been reported to vary between 21 and 70% [6]. Besides considering the location of the APG, the practitioner should be aware that it is in this area that the PD is very superficially placed in relation to the external face. Here, the PD lies just below the skin surface [1]. This shallow situation makes the duct quite vulnerable to extraoral trauma.

Submandibular Duct

The submandibular duct (SMD), also known as Wharton duct, arises from the superficial lobe of the submandibular salivary gland. This lobe is positioned inferior to the mandible in the submandibular triangle. The duct moves superiorly to the posterior border of the mylohyoid muscle (MM) where it makes a right angle bend (the genu of the duct). The SMD duct now enters the oral cavity, receives a branch from the orally positioned deep submandibular lobe, and runs horizontally forward in the sublingual space lateral to the hyoglossus and genioglossal muscles and medial to the insertion of the MM. The duct terminates anteriorly at its ostium on the caruncle located adjacent to the lingual frenum (Fig. 15.1). Occasionally, a doubling of the SMD will be observed [7, 8].

Fig. 15.1 Caruncle mouth floor (arrow)

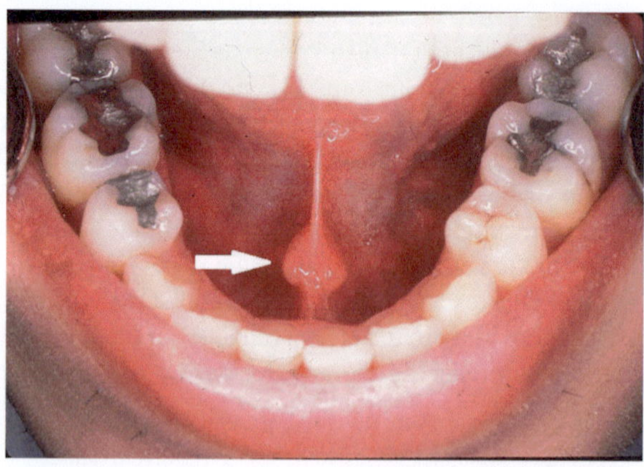

Posteriorly, in the region of the mandibular third molar, the duct has a close relationship with the lingual nerve (LN). Classically, the LN moves from a lateral location to cross under the SMD as the nerve travels medially to innervate the tongue. Variations of this anatomic relationship exist with the lingual nerve occasionally crossing the SMD superiorly rather than making its usual inferior crossing [8]. The SMD also has a varying relationship with the major duct of the sublingual salivary gland (SLSG), the not always present duct of Bartholin (BD). Most frequently the BD, when present, empties into the distal segment of the SMD (Fig. 17.2). At times, the BD will empty through its own ostium situated on the caruncle adjacent to the SMD orifice [7].

The length of the SMD is approximately 5 cm while its width is reported to be 1.5 mm [8, 9]. Its passage in the sublingual space on the oral surface of the MM is in close proximity to the medial surface of the SLSG whose position is roughly identified by the mouth floor's elevated sublingual fold. As the SMD moves anteriorly in the mouth floor, it becomes more superficial in relation to the oral mucosa. The extended length of the SMD, as it superficially traverses the mouth floor, makes it susceptible to oral traumatic insult.

Sublingual Salivary Gland Ducts (Ducts of Rivinus, Bartholin Duct)

Anatomically, the sublingual space (SLS) occupies the floor of the mouth. The SLS is a fascial space whose base is limited by the mylohyoid muscle (MM), while it is confined superiorly by the mouth floor mucosa and tongue. The lingual surface of the mandible serves as the anterior and lateral borders of the SLS, while the base of the tongue and its musculature limit the SLS posteriorly. Key anatomic inhabitants of the SLS include structures associated with the salivary apparatus, the lingual nerve and vessels, and the hypoglossal and glossopharyngeal nerves. Salivary structures harbored in the SLS include the deep lobe of the submandibular salivary gland (SMSG), the submandibular duct (Wharton duct), and the sublingual salivary gland (SLSG) with its ducts of Rivinus and, its not always present major duct, the duct of Bartholin (BD).

The SLSG, the smallest of the major salivary glands, is located in the mouth floor just beneath the mucosa of the sublingual fold. The generally accepted anatomic concept is that the gland consists of 8–20 lobes linked together by connective tissue bands [10]. The secretions of the lobes of the SLSG empty into the mouth via multiple ducts of Rivinus. These ducts, originating from individual lobes, open directly above on the mucosa of the sublingual fold. Occasionally, a BD is present, anteriorly positioned, and when present it transmits secretions from the SLSG that empty into the anterior segment of the submandibular duct or exit independently through its own ostium on the sublingual caruncle [10–12], a papilla located just lateral to the lingual frenum.

Iatrogenic Parotid Duct Injury

Parotid Duct Injury

Parotidectomy: Sialocele/Salivary Fistula

The salivary gland most frequently associated with a sialocele is the parotid gland (PG). A PG sialocele is defined as a leakage of ductal saliva that accumulates without proper drainage in the subcutaneous tissues around the PG and/or the parotid duct (PD), frequently following a parotidectomy. Most often, parotidectomies are performed because of the presence of a neoplasm, usually in the PG's superficial lobe. Tumors of the PG comprise 2% of the head and neck tumors with 75–80% of these PG tumors being benign [13]. Surgical trauma, particularly to the PD, from a therapeutic parotidectomy for these PG neoplasms is a known common cause for sialocele formation [14]. However, sialoceles can also develop following facial trauma (Fig. 15.2), infection, and a variety of facial surgical procedures [15]. External trauma usually spares the submandibular salivary gland because the gland is somewhat sheltered by its anatomic location in the submandibular triangle where it receives mandibular protection.

The sialocele tends to make its presence known 1–2 weeks after the causative event [16]. It is also possible for a salivary fistula (SF) to develop when the leaking salivary fluid, associated with the sialocele, is not successfully contained and drains onto an epithelial surface. Postoperatively, an SF can also evolve without the preexisting presence of a sialocele (Fig. 15.2). Sialoceles and/or SF have variously been reported to occur in 5–39% of patients following a superficial lobe parotidectomy [17–19] for tumor therapy. Risk factors for increased occurrences of sialocele/SF include tumor size, pathology, need for nodal dissection, and tumor location. The incidence of sialocele/SF is increased when surgery involves the middle or inferior segment of the PG's superficial lobe, unfortunately an area where most PG tumors are located [18, 19].

The sialocele may appear as an immediate or late complication following the causative PG surgery. Clinically, the PG sialocele will manifest itself as a salivary fluid accumulation in the preauricular region. Diagnosis is facilitated by massaging the PG and observing whether the pressure has caused the PG to express saliva into the surgically created fluid field. There is no fever; the swelling is usually painless, soft, and cyst-like when palpated; and the overlying skin is not erythematous. Fluid aspirated from the sialocele will be clear, reflecting the physical appearance of normal saliva. When analyzed, the fluid will testify to the presence of salivary amylase. Early treatment of the sialocele is advised to prevent the possibility of an onset of sepsis or the development of a complicating SF [14, 16]. With sepsis, inflammatory signs such as erythema, elevated skin and body temperatures, and pain can become concerning issues.

Imaging can be helpful in localizing the area of gland/duct damage and revealing the extent of a sialocele/SF. Sialography offers an excellent means of visualizing the

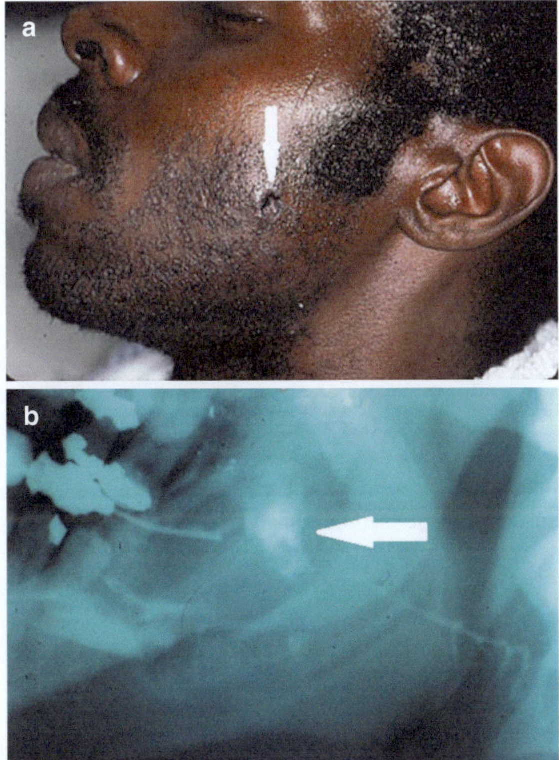

Fig. 15.2 (**a**) Salivary fistula (arrow) following gunshot wound to face. Patient A. (**b**) Salivary fistula. Patient A. Parotid sialogram demonstrates dye extravasation (arrow) at point of duct rupture

injured ductal structures (Fig. 15.2), but the procedure is invasive and can present difficulties in its performance. A CT scan of the sialocele will reveal a simple or multilocular smooth bordered cyst-like mass that has a lower density than the surrounding tissues. MRI sialography represents another acceptable diagnostic imaging procedure. Ultrasonography is helpful in that it will readily image the fluid containing cyst-like lesion.

In order to avoid an increased incidence of sialocele/SF complications following the total removal of the PG's superficial lobe, an alternative therapeutic and more conservative surgical approach has been advocated. A partial rather than the total excision of the PG's superficial lobe has been suggested. However, the results are in question. Wong et al. [20] found no difference in the incidence of sialocele/SF following complete PG superficial lobectomy when contrasted with a partial superficial lobectomy. Other studies found surprising increases in sialocele/SF complications after partial superficial lobectomy when compared to complete superficial lobectomy [17, 18, 21]. The explanation for this increased incidence may be derived from the fact that more PG parenchyma is retained after a partial superficial lobectomy, and its secretions are available to increase the conditions that cause the sialocele/SF [22].

No consensus guidelines regarding treatment of an established sialocele are available [14]. In a study of 398 post-parotidectomy patients, no difference in sialocele development was observed whether or not a drain was preventively placed as part of the surgical procedure [19]. Treatment of an established sialocele depends on whether the sialocele is an immediate or late complication. However, the practitioner should be aware that spontaneous sialocele resolution within 6 months can be expected [16–18, 22]. Surgically identifying and suturing a damaged duct's remnants and the insertion of a stent during the perioperative period can be difficult, but if the procedure is successful, it will prevent the onset of a sialocele or SF [23]. A sialocele that has developed as an early complication of PG surgery can be treated via an intraoral surgical approach to the fluid collection and the placement of a catheter that extends from the sialocele to the buccal mucosa. A new intraoral salivary ostium will develop to facilitate salivary drainage [16].

A sialocele that appears as a late surgical complication can be managed therapeutically via a conservative approach. Conservative therapy requires aspiration of the trapped secretions followed by a compression dressing for a patient for whom anti-sialogogic medications (glycopyrrolate, atropine, scopolamine) have been prescribed. Repetition of the procedure may be necessary if the initial response is poor. Botulinum toxin and even low-dosage radiotherapy have been added to this treatment regimen [19].

Treatment of a SF depends on the time of its appearance in relation to the injurious event. When an SF develops as an immediate complication after the injury, surgical intervention is indicated. There are three basic pathways to the prevention/treatment of a SF [24]. Initially, in the early stage after trauma, surgical exploration with debridement, duct anastomosis, and suturing of the PG capsule is advised [25]. If duct anastomosis is unsuccessful, a new salivary channel can be constructed by surgically placing a drain that extends from the point of leakage to the buccal mucosa of the oral cavity. Late SF development is best treated via a nonsurgical third approach that involves aspiration of any accumulated fluid followed by external compression dressings and supplemented with anticholinergic medications and even botulinum toxin.

Extraoral Trauma

External facial trauma commonly involves the parotid duct/parotid gland (PD/PG). The injury from sharp penetrating trauma usually originates from an automobile accident or knife. Often, the end result of any such damage to glandular integrity is the development of a sialocele and/or salivary fistula. The clinical recognition of these complications and their treatment has been reviewed in the previous section titled "Parotidectomy."

Facial Rhytidectomy

Safe and successful rhytidectomy requires an appreciation of the anatomy of the superficial musculoaponeurotic sheath (SMAS) and the parotid-masseteric fascia (PMF). The SMAS represents the facial continuation of the superficial cervical fascia, while the PMF is the extension of the superficial layer of the deep cervical fascia onto the parotid-masseteric surface. Restoring facial contour that has changed with age requires surgical mobilization of SMAS via blunt and sharp dissections.

The surgical dissection of SMAS usually begins by incising SMAS over the zygomatic arch. Adequate SMAS flap development requires its mobilization as far forward as the nasolabial fold [26]. Posteriorly, in the region of the parotid gland (PG), the SMAS is intimately involved with the PMF. Surgical separation of these two fascial layers, without perforating the thin PMF, is required to achieve a satisfactory facial result. The procedure is difficult and demands precision and caution because the PG, its major duct, and branches of the facial nerve lie immediately below the very thin PMF. Therefore, in order to avoid glandular complications, a precise superficial surgical dissection must be performed in the posterior region when organizing a SMAS flap. More anteriorly, a distinct anatomic plane, facilitating separation, exists between the SMAS and PMF layers. The problem with surgical trauma to vital structures beneath the thin PMF is compounded when surgeons switch from a superficial SMAS dissection to a deeper plane. This sub-SMAS approach is used to enhance the surgical outcome which can best be accomplished with a thicker, more vascularized flap. With a surgically mobilized flap that extends anteriorly from the nasolabial fold and posteriorly from the posterior aspect of the PG, the SMAS flap can now be manually manipulated. Essentially, it is retracted posterosuperiorly until its retraction creates the desired cosmetic effect on the facial features. Unfortunately, the resulting tension may have a deleterious compression effect on the PD (Fig. 15.3).

Injuries to the PD following this facial plastic surgical procedure are not uncommon and can be manifest in two different ways. Sialoceles with/without drainage from the posterior dissection site have been reported [15, 27–29] and probably result from poor anatomic recognition of the intimacy of SMAS and PMF. Deliberate or inadvertent deep dissection can lead to PMF perforation with surgical trauma to the underlying PD and sialocele formation where the duct crosses the masseter muscle [26]. Following sialocele treatment and healing, stricturing of the surgically injured PD may present problems relating to salivary obstruction. Alternatively, a second mechanism of PD damage from rhytidectomy may be a result of luminal narrowing from stretching and excessive compression exerted by a repositioned SMAS on the PD as the duct bends around the anterior border of the masseter muscle (Fig. 15.3) [27, 30] or as the duct traverses the lateral surface of this muscle. As a consequence of PD luminal width reduction, salivary retention and swelling

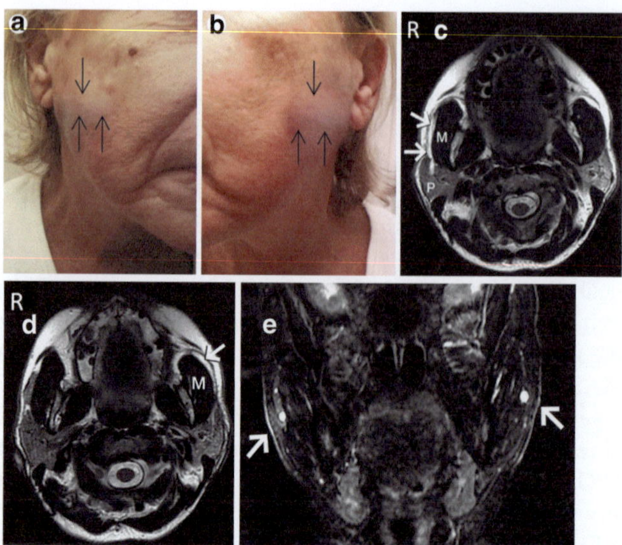

Fig. 15.3 (**a**) Rhytidectomy. Patient A. Right parotid duct swelling (arrows) (Mandel L, et al. J Oral Maxillofac Surg 2012;70:449). (**b**) Rhytidectomy. Patient A. Left parotid duct swelling (arrows) (Mandel L, et al. J Oral Maxillofac Surg 2012;70:449). (**c**) Rhytidectomy. Patient A. MRI. Note dilated right parotid duct (arrows) exiting parotid gland (P) and onto surface of masseter muscle (M) (Mandel L, et al. J Oral Maxillofac Surg 2012;70:449). (**d**) Rhytidectomy. Patient A. MRI. Note dilated left parotid duct (arrow) at another level as it bends around anterior border of masseter muscle (M) (Mandel L, et al. J Oral Maxillofac Surg 2012;70:449). (**e**) Rhytidectomy. Patient A. MRI. Dilated right and left parotid ducts (arrows) along lateral surface of masseter muscles (Mandel L, et al. J Oral Maxillofac Surg 2012;70:449)

develop in the PD in tandem with any increase in salivary demand. The swelling is noted facially along the course of the PD and can even involve the PG [31]. The swelling tends to be transient because the retained saliva can gradually seep through the narrowed lumen when salivary demand decreases. Manual pressure upon the swelling will hasten the evacuation of the retained saliva.

If a sialocele has developed, treatment is indicated as per the discussion of sialocele in the previous section. The status of the partially obstructed PD caused by SMAS compression can be improved with a variety of procedures. Stenting [32, 33], balloon sialoplasty [34], and sialendoscopic procedures [32, 33, 35] have been advocated therapeutically. Widening of the narrowed duct lumen is the objective whose purpose is to expedite an unimpeded salivary flow. A return to normal salivary flow discourages salivary retention and ascending bacterial infection.

Imaging via sialography offers the best means of visualizing the constricted duct lumen and the resulting duct dilation from obstruction with salivary retention. MRI sialography will also succeed in identifying the problem.

Iatrogenic Submandibular Duct Injury

Submandibular Duct Injury: Mouth Floor Surgery

Salivary duct blockage from scarring with luminal stricture formation inevitably causes salivary gland obstructive symptomatology. Such a scenario is often a sequel to mouth floor surgery that may inadvertently involve the area of the submandibular gland duct (SMD) orifice in the anterior mouth floor [36, 37]. Wound healing with scarring and stricturing of the SMD orifice and its surrounding tissues can be expected. The obstructive stricture will cause repeated episodes of submandibular salivary gland (SMSG) swelling, most evident during the periods of increased salivary demand associated with eating. Chronic obstruction leads to gland parenchymal degeneration, while the simultaneously associated salivary retention and stagnation favor an orally ascending bacterial invasion. Bacterial sialadenitis with acinar destruction are possible end results. To prevent the SMSG's downward spiral originating from the strictured SMD orifice, surgical intervention is mandated. The location of the stricture in the more anterior (distal) portion of the duct, where the duct is relatively superficially placed and accessible, offers the opportunity to create a new orifice posteriorly (proximally). Consequently, the area of SMD obstruction will be by-passed.

Therapeutic surgery for the orifice narrowing requires an anteroposterior linear incision in the mucosa of the mouth floor's cuspid-bicuspid area (Fig. 15.4a). The incision is made parallel and just medial to the height of the sublingual fold. Via blunt dissection, the body of the SMD can be freed from its partial embrace by the medial aspect of the sublingual salivary gland (Fig. 15.4b). With the duct isolated, a longitudinal incision is made into its superior wall posterior to the strictured orifice. This results in a filleted duct whose wings are then sutured to the adjacent mouth floor mucosa (Fig. 15.4c). The residual anterior duct segment and its orifice with the surrounding caruncular tissue should be excised. The mouth floor mucosa, anterior to the filleted duct, is sutured. Healing is rapid and a newly created patent SMD orifice will be present in the cuspid-bicuspid region of the mouth floor.

More frequently, iatrogenic stricturing of the SMD involves the more proximal segments of the duct, the so-called body of the SMD. Duct stricturing can develop following trauma from accidental slippage of a dental instrument during a dental procedure, or even from any soft tissue surgical procedure performed in the mouth floor that is adjacent to the SMD. Success in by-passing a proximal stricture is dependent on the stricture's location. Success rates decrease with strictures that are posteriorly positioned.

Submandibular Duct Injury: Sialolithectomy

SMD sialolithectomy can also be a precipitating factor in SMD injury and stricturing. Ductal inflammation, scarring, and stricturing can result from both the irritating effect of the sialolith on the duct wall and the healing following the surgical duct

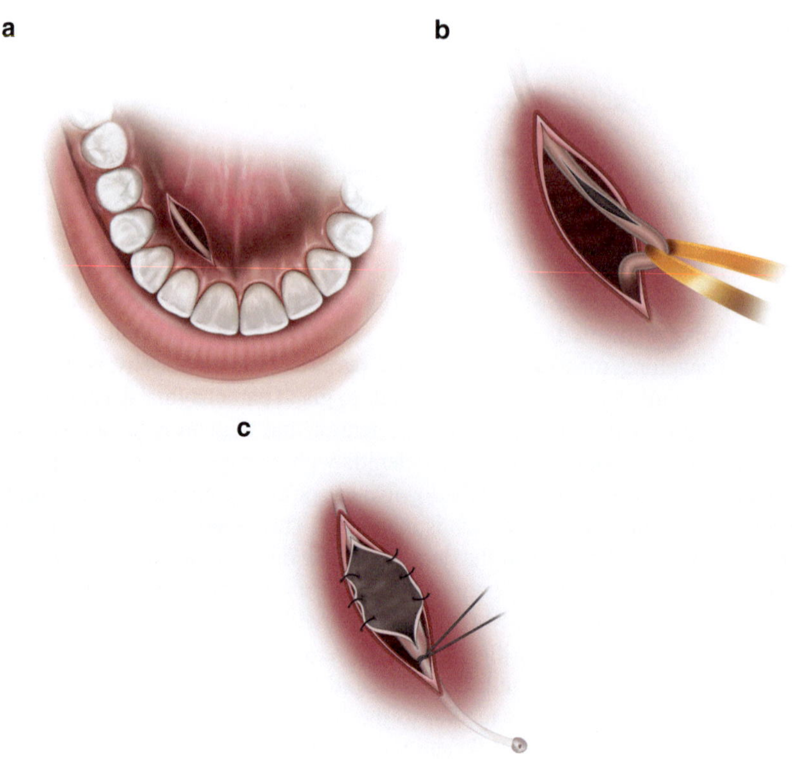

Fig. 15.4 (**a**) Surgical bypass submandibular duct. Incision medial to sublingual fold (Mandel L, et al. Oral Surg Oral Med Oral Pathol Oral Radiol Endod 1999;88:532). (**b**) Surgical bypass submandibular duct. Duct exposed and retracted (Mandel L, et al. Oral Surg Oral Med Oral Pathol Oral Radiol Endod 1999;88:532). (**c**) Surgical bypass. Filleted submandibular duct sutured to adjacent mucosa (Mandel L, et al. Oral Surg Oral Med Oral Pathol Oral Radiol Endod 1999;88:532)

trauma associated with the sialolith's removal. Furthermore, the disruption of a duct of Rivinus or a duct of Bartholin can occur during SMD sialolithectomy. Such an adverse event can lead to ranula formation [38].

A stricture's location proximal to the orifice but distal to the hilar area of the duct favors an initial treatment approach via sialendoscopy [39]. The sialendoscope's ability to overcome the stricture and widen the duct makes it the treatment of choice when the body of the SMD is involved. If sialendoscopy is not successful, surgical duct bypass surgery can be attempted as described. The bypass procedure is only feasible if the stricture is located such that a posteriorly placed new duct opening can be created. Obviously, accessibility and visibility impede success in the more proximal portions of the SMD.

Iatrogenic Sublingual Duct Injury

Sublingual Duct Injury

Secondary to Submandibular Duct Surgery

Injury to the salivary gland structures located in the sublingual space usually is iatrogenic in origin. It is important to be aware that surgical mobilization of the submandibular duct (SMD) depends upon a knowledge of the SMD's relation to the sublingual salivary gland (SLSG) and its ductal system. Procedures such as SMD sialolithectomy or SMD repositioning require an awareness that the SMD lies in very close proximity to the SLSG. In freeing the SMD from its cradling by the SLSG, the surgery and the lateral retraction of the SLSG cause trauma to the gland. The consequent injury to the SLSG and its ductal structures may lead to a ruptured duct, salivary leakage, and the development of a ranula [11].

Implant Insertion

Sublingual duct injury may also be a result of mandibular implant insertion. Implants have a very high success rate and are widely used by the dental profession. However, a caveat comes with their placement. The practitioner must constantly be aware of the surrounding anatomy and the need for accurate implant positioning. Impingement by the implant upon adjacent vital structures must be avoided (Fig. 15.5). Knowledge of the anatomic configuration of the mandible must be incorporated into successful mandibular implant placement. Lingual cortical perforation by a misdirected mandibular implant will impinge upon adjacent mouth floor soft tissues (Fig. 15.5c, d) [40]. The SLSG has a close anatomic relationship with the sublingual fossa on the lingual aspect of the mandible. The gland and its ductal system can be victimized by trauma generated by the inferior tip of a lingually malposed mandibular implant that has perforated into the sublingual fossa (Fig. 15.5d). The problem is accentuated when the SLSG apparatus rubs against the perforated implant as the gland moves in harmony with the mouth floor during speech and deglutition. SLSG duct rupture with escaping secretions can occur to form a ranula.

SLSG duct damage from sialolithectomy, submandibular duct repositioning, and mandibular implant surgery are known complications. However, a variety of soft tissue mouth floor surgical procedures also can inadvertently compromise an adjacent SLSG duct and cause a ranula. Furthermore, slippage of a dental instrument during dental care can lacerate the mouth floor and a SLSG duct. Ranula development may be the end result.

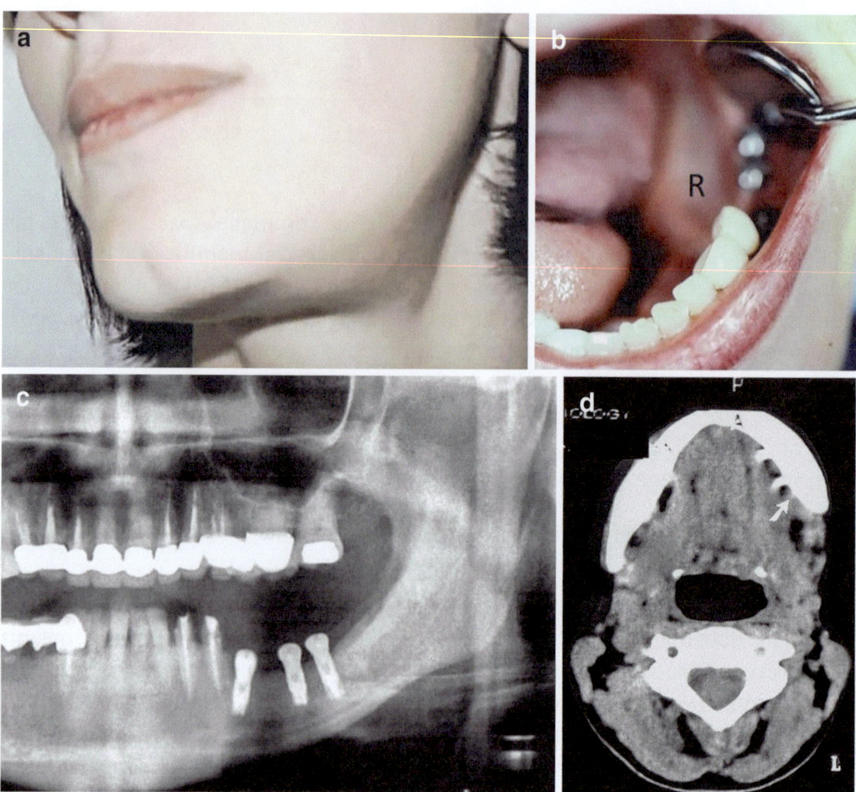

Fig. 15.5 (**a**) Plunging ranula following implant placement. Patient B. Extraoral view (Mandel L, J Oral Maxillofac Surg 2008;66:1743). (**b**) Plunging ranula following implant placement (R). Patient B. Intraoral view (Mandel L, J Oral Maxillofac Surg 2008;66:1743). (**c**) Plunging ranula. Implant placement. Patient B. Panoramic radiograph reveals three implants (Mandel L, J Oral Maxillofac Surg 2008;66:1743). (**d**) Plunging ranula following implant placement. Patient B. CT scan demonstrates cortical perforation by two anterior implants. Posterior third implant is barely visible (arrow) (Mandel L, J Oral Maxillofac Surg 2008;66:1743)

References

1. Stringer MD, Mirjalili SA, Meredith SJ, Muirhead JC. Redefining the surface anatomy of the parotid duct: an in vivo ultrasound study. Plast Reconstr Surg. 2012;130(5):1032–7. https://doi.org/10.1097/PRS.0b013e318267d610.
2. Steinberg MJ, Herréra AF. Management of parotid duct injuries. Oral Surg Oral Med Oral Pathol Oral Radiol Endod. 2005;99(2):136–41. https://doi.org/10.1016/j.tripleo.2004.05.001.
3. Uzmansel D, Elvan Ö, Aktekin M. Precise localization of parotid duct: a cadaveric study. Anat Sci Int. 2022;97(1):59–64. https://doi.org/10.1007/s12565-021-00626-7.
4. Hwang K, Cho HJ, Battuvshin D, Chung IH, Hwang SH. Interrelated buccal fat pad with facial buccal branches and parotid duct. J Craniofac Surg. 2005;16(4):658–60. https://doi.org/10.1097/01.scs.0000157019.35407.55.

5. Zenk J, Hosemann WG, Iro H. Diameters of the main excretory ducts of the adult human submandibular and parotid gland: a histologic study. Oral Surg Oral Med Oral Pathol Oral Radiol Endod. 1998;85(5):576–80. https://doi.org/10.1016/s1079-2104(98)90294-3.
6. Heidmann E, Baatjes KJ, Correia J. Anatomy of the parotid duct: assessing variations of the parotid gland drainage pattern. Transl Res Anat. 2021;25:100152.
7. Zhang L, Xu H, Cai ZG, et al. Clinical and anatomic study on the ducts of the submandibular and sublingual glands. J Oral Maxillofac Surg. 2010;68(3):606–10. https://doi.org/10.1016/j.joms.2009.03.068.
8. Günenç Beşer C, Erçakmak B, Ilgaz HB, Vatansever A, Sargon MF. Revisiting the relationship between the submandibular duct, lingual nerve and hypoglossal nerve. Folia Morphol (Warsz). 2018;77(3):521–6. https://doi.org/10.5603/FM.a2018.0010.
9. Grewal JS, Jamal Z, Ryan J. Anatomy, head and neck, submandibular gland. In: StatPearls. Treasure Island: StatPearls Publishing; 2021.
10. Castelli WA, Huelke DF, Celis A. Some basic anatomic features in paralingual space surgery. Oral Surg Oral Med Oral Pathol. 1969;27(5):613–21. https://doi.org/10.1016/0030-4220(69)90093-0.
11. Chen CJ, Guo P, Chen XY. Recurrent sublingual ranula or saliva leakage from the submandibular gland? Anatomical consideration of the ductal system of the sublingual gland. J Oral Maxillofac Surg. 2015;73(4):675.e1–7. https://doi.org/10.1016/j.joms.2014.10.012.
12. Moss-Salentijn L, Hendricks-Klyvert M. A bilateral, superficial location of human sublingual glands: report of a case. J Oral Maxillofac Surg. 1987;45(11):983–6. https://doi.org/10.1016/0278-2391(87)90456-3.
13. Ruohoalho J, Mäkitie AA, Aro K, et al. Complications after surgery for benign parotid gland neoplasms: a prospective cohort study. Head Neck. 2017;39(1):170–6. https://doi.org/10.1002/hed.24496.
14. Maharaj S, Mungul S, Laher A. Botulinum toxin A is an effective therapeutic tool for the management of parotid sialocele and fistula: a systematic review. Laryngoscope Investig Otolaryngol. 2020;5(1):37–45. Published 2020 Jan 23. https://doi.org/10.1002/lio2.350.
15. Lawson GA 3rd, Kreymerman P, Nahai F. An unusual complication following rhytidectomy: iatrogenic parotid injury resulting in parotid fistula/sialocele [published correction appears in Aesthet Surg J. 2012 Nov;32(8):1040. Kreyerman, Peter [corrected to Kreymerman, Peter]]. Aesthet Surg J. 2012;32(7):814–21. https://doi.org/10.1177/1090820X12455798.
16. Donoso T, Domancic S, Argandoña J. Delayed treatment of parotid sialocele: a functional approach and review. J Oral Maxillofac Surg. 2015;73(2):284–90. https://doi.org/10.1016/j.joms.2014.08.039.
17. Witt RL. The incidence and management of siaolocele after parotidectomy. Otolaryngol Head Neck Surg. 2009;140(6):871–4. https://doi.org/10.1016/j.otohns.2009.01.021.
18. Britt CJ, Stein AP, Gessert T, Pflum Z, Saha S, Hartig GK. Factors influencing sialocele or salivary fistula formation postparotidectomy. Head Neck. 2017;39(2):387–91. https://doi.org/10.1002/hed.24564.
19. Kinberg EC, Garneau JC, Eljazzar R, et al. Postparotidectomy sialocele: 6-year review of underlying factors. Head Neck. 2022;44(3):745–8. https://doi.org/10.1002/hed.26969.
20. Wong WK, Shetty S. The extent of surgery for benign parotid pathology and its influence on complications: a prospective cohort analysis. Am J Otolaryngol. 2018;39(2):162–6. https://doi.org/10.1016/j.amjoto.2017.11.015.
21. Iftikhar H, Dhanani R, Awan S, Zahid N, Momin SNA. Factors associated with drain output in patients undergoing to parotidectomy. Int Arch Otorhinolaryngol. 2020;24(2):e211–4. https://doi.org/10.1055/s-0039-1698781.
22. Torre-León C, Canario Q, Garratón M. A novel approach in the treatment of a post-traumatic sialocele. Otolaryngol Head Neck Surg. 2013;148(3):529–30. https://doi.org/10.1177/0194599812470435.

23. Chung CM, Wee SJ, Lim H, Cho SH, Lee JW. Early management of parotid gland injury with oral nortriptyline and closed drain. Arch Craniofac Surg. 2020;21(4):253–6. https://doi.org/10.7181/acfs.2019.00773.
24. Rahpeyma A, Khajehahmadi S. Delayed management of parotid sialocele: role for two-week intraoral drainage. Curr Med Sci. 2022;42(4):902–4. https://doi.org/10.1007/s11596-022-2619-z. Epub 2022 Aug 13. PMID: 35963951.
25. Lazaridou M, Iliopoulos C, Antoniades K, Tilaveridis I, Dimitrakopoulos I, Lazaridis N. Salivary gland trauma: a review of diagnosis and treatment. Craniomaxillofac Trauma Reconstr. 2012;5(4):189–96. https://doi.org/10.1055/s-0032-1313356.
26. Marten TJ. Facelift. Planning and technique. Clin Plast Surg. 1997;24(2):269–308.
27. Barron R, Margulis A, Icekson M, Zeltser R, Eldad A, Nahlieli O. Iatrogenic parotid sialocele following rhytidectomy: diagnosis and treatment. Plast Reconstr Surg. 2001;108(6):1782–6. https://doi.org/10.1097/00006534-200111000-00055.
28. Moyer JS, Baker SR. Complications of rhytidectomy. Facial Plast Surg Clin North Am. 2005;13(3):469–78. https://doi.org/10.1016/j.fsc.2005.04.005.
29. Crimp C, Hand M, Chesnut C. Identification and management of postoperative sialoceles in dermatologic surgery. Dermatol Surg. 2021;47(8):1163–5. https://doi.org/10.1097/DSS.0000000000003123.
30. Nahlieli O, Abramson A, Shacham R, Puterman MB, Baruchin AM. Endoscopic treatment of salivary gland injuries due to facial rejuvenation procedures. Laryngoscope. 2008;150:763.
31. Mandel L, Silver AJ. Bilateral parotid duct obstruction after rhytidectomies: case report. J Oral Maxillofac Surg. 2012;70(2):449–52. https://doi.org/10.1016/j.joms.2011.02.0.
32. Dumpis J, Feldmane L. Experimental microsurgery of salivary ducts in dogs. J Craniomaxillofac Surg. 2001;29(1):56–62. https://doi.org/10.1054/jcms.2000.0190.
33. Nahlieli O, Shacham R, Yoffe B, Eliav E. Diagnosis and treatment of strictures and kinks in salivary gland ducts. J Oral Maxillofac Surg. 2001;59(5):484–92. https://doi.org/10.1053/joms.2001.22667.
34. Brown AL, Shepherd D, Buckenham TM. Per oral balloon sialoplasty: results in the treatment of salivary duct stenosis. Cardiovasc Intervent Radiol. 1997;20(5):337–42. https://doi.org/10.1007/s002709900164.
35. Borner U, Anschuetz L, Caversaccio M, et al. A retrospective analysis of multiple affected salivary gland diseases: diagnostic and therapeutic benefits of interventional sialendoscopy [published online ahead of print, 2022 Mar 24]. Ear Nose Throat J. 2022;1455613221081911. https://doi.org/10.1177/01455613221081911 18(5):763-767.
36. Stimson CW, Leban SG. Transplantation of the submandibular duct associated with resection for carcinoma. Oral Surg Oral Med Oral Pathol. 1983;56(2):136–40. https://doi.org/10.1016/0030-4220(83)90277-3.
37. Ord RA, Lee VE. Submandibular duct repositioning after excision of floor of mouth cancer. J Oral Maxillofac Surg. 1996;54(9):1075–9. https://doi.org/10.1016/s0278-2391(96)90163-9.
38. Liu DG, Jiang L, Xie XY, Zhang ZY, Zhang L, Yu GY. Sialoendoscopy-assisted sialolithectomy for submandibular hilar calculi. J Oral Maxillofac Surg. 2013;71(2):295–301. https://doi.org/10.1016/j.joms.2012.02.016.
39. Koch M, Iro H. Salivary duct stenosis: diagnosis and treatment. Stenosi duttali salivari: diagnosie terapia. Acta Otorhinolaryngol Ital. 2017;37(2):132–41. https://doi.org/10.14639/0392-100X-1603.
40. Mandel L. Plunging ranula following placement of mandibular implants: case report. J Oral Maxillofac Surg. 2008;66(8):1743–7. https://doi.org/10.1016/j.joms.2006.08.003.

Chapter 16
Iatrogenic Neurologic Complications

Louis Mandel

Abstract The nerve supply to the major salivary glands exists in an overcrowded anatomic area. The head and neck area is replete with a vast cramped neurologic network. Therefore, operating within the limited anatomic confines of the head and neck, not in the immediate vicinity of the major salivary glands, the surgeon may inadvertently injure a neurologic structure as it travels to a salivary gland. Disruption in normal gland function is the end result. Damage to the chorda tympani nerve during stapes surgery will cause a decrease in submandibular and sublingual gland salivary volume. Furthermore, salivary gland surgical procedures that involve the parotid gland may disrupt a nerve's ability to stimulate the parotid gland (auriculotemporal syndrome) or the paraglandular musculature (facial nerve palsy).

Introduction

Operating within the limited anatomic confines of the head and neck (middle ear, parapharyngeal space, etc.) on pathologic conditions not in the immediate vicinity of the salivary glands, the surgeon may injure neurologic structures that travel to the salivary apparatus and function to maintain normal salivary gland physiology. Similarly, surgical procedures that involve the salivary glands may also cause unpremeditated and unavoidable neurologic disruptions with resulting aberrations that impact upon the function of normal anatomic structures (facial nerve) or alter normal nerve biologic activity (auriculotemporal syndrome).

The aim of this chapter is to review four iatrogenic post-surgical problems that are caused by nerve damage and have come to the attention of the Columbia University Salivary Gland Center. The resulting neurologic abnormalities served as the impetus for the patient's desire to seek care.

© The Author(s), under exclusive license to Springer Nature Switzerland AG 2024

L. Mandel, *Clinical Management of Salivary Gland Disorders*,
https://doi.org/10.1007/978-3-031-50012-1_16

Facial Nerve Palsy

The onset of a facial nerve (FN) palsy can serve as a devastating traumatic psychologic event to a patient. Because the FN supplies motor control to the muscles of facial expression, the patient loses the functioning ability of these muscles to control the eyelid, wrinkle the brow, purse the lips, puff out the cheek, and show teeth (Fig. 16.1). Obvious tell-tale diagnostic signs of FN palsy are facial drooping, and the inability to close the eye due to paralysis of the orbicularis oculi muscle. The facial changes are in direct proportion to the degree of FN injury and are dependent on which FN branch or branches are damaged. Complete FN sectioning during surgery results in an expressionless face limited to the surgically involved side.

Anatomically, the FN exits the cranial cavity via the temporal bone's stylomastoid foramen. After giving off two branches, the posterior auricular nerve and the digastric nerve, it courses through the parotid gland (PG) creating an intimate relationship with the gland. Within the gland, the FN divides into two main trunks which form the parotid plexus. Five branches (frontal, zygomatic, buccal, mandibular, cervical) emerge from the plexus to supply motor function to the facial musculature. The location and distribution of the FN and its branches are such that it artificially separates the PG into a superficial lobe, which is positioned lateral to the nerve, and a deep PG lobe located medial to the FN [1, 2].

A superficial lobectomy of the PG is usually required in the presence of a neoplasm or a parotitis that does not respond to conservative or antibiotic care. Injury to the FN has proven to be the most distressing and common complication that can develop following the parotidectomy (Fig. 16.1). Therefore, FN identification and preservation are crucial requirements during PG surgery. The incidence of FN palsy, usually affecting one or several nerve branches, observed immediately after PG superficial lobectomy, has been reported to vary between 20 and 60% with higher incidences occurring when PG deep lobectomy is performed [3, 4]. Fortunately, postoperative facial palsy can be expected to improve within 24 months with few permanent palsies evolving [4].

Neoplasms, usually a benign pleomorphic adenoma located in the superficial lobe, function as a frequent motive for PG surgery. Additionally, some patients with

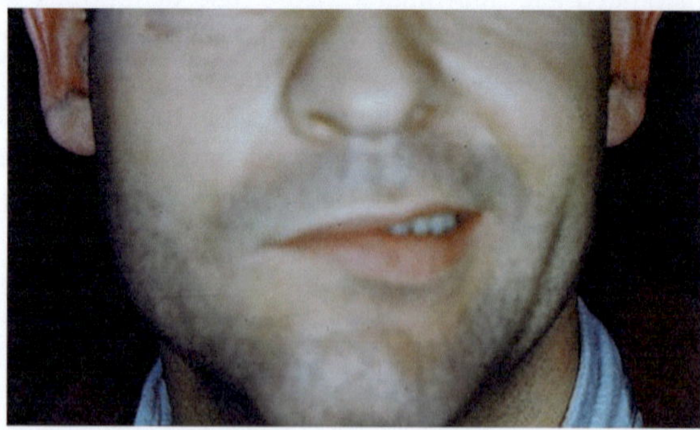

Fig. 16.1 Facial nerve palsy after right parotidectomy for benign pleomorphic adenoma

chronic parotitis may require PG surgery because they develop intractable PG symptoms resulting from repeated inflammatory episodes [5]. Superficial PG lobectomy has been the surgical procedure of choice, but with it came many incidents of FN palsy. Partial superficial parotidectomy, a procedure that preserves any unaffected superficial lobe and involves less FN dissection, has been introduced to decrease injury to the FN [4]. Furthermore, electromyographic nerve monitoring has proven to be extremely useful intraoperatively in identifying the FN branches, mapping their course and avoiding their injury during the surgical procedure [1–4].

Some risk factors that increase the possibility of FN palsy following PG surgery have been identified. Because of anatomic problems with surgical accessibility, pathologic entities involving the deep PG lobe lying medial to the FN are significant elements in the occurrence of FN palsy. Large tumor diameter, malignancy, chronic parotitis, and repetitive surgeries because of needed revisions are additional risk factors [1, 4]. The multiple branches of the FN and the inconsistency in their location and number are additional hazards that increase inadvertent iatrogenic nerve injuries.

Auriculotemporal Syndrome

The auriculotemporal (AT) syndrome is a postoperative complication that commonly develops after a parotidectomy. The syndrome, also known as gustatory sweating or Frey syndrome, is characterized by facial sweating and flushing of the cutaneous tissues overlying the parotid gland (PG) (Fig. 16.2). These features of the syndrome are initiated by salivary stimulation. Most frequently, the syndrome results from damage to the AT nerve during surgery in the parotid area. Occasionally, the AT syndrome can develop following facial trauma, condylar surgery, radical neck dissection, or cervicofacial infection [6]. It is estimated to occur in 4% of the parotidectomy patients during the immediate postoperative period, attains an incidence of 62% by the time 18 months have passed [7], and can even reach 100% if objectively investigated years later [8]. The AT syndrome occurs equally in both sexes and can occur at any age. Discomfort can be present, but it is not a dominant feature. Spontaneous resolution of the socially embarrassing symptomatology is a possibility [9].

Although the syndrome had been recognized for many years, it was not until 1923 that Lucja Frey, a Polish neurologist, defined the generally accepted aberrant regeneration theory of the AT nerve as the pathophysiologic cause of the syndrome [6]. The syndrome arises from the fact that the AT nerve provides both parasympathetic innervation to the PG and sympathetic innervation to sweat glands and subcutaneous blood vessels. Normally, parasympathetic efferents reach the PG by traveling with the AT nerve which is an offshoot of the mandibular branch of cranial nerve V. The AT nerve parasympathetic fibers normally synapse in the otic ganglion and then continue as postganglionic secretomotor fibers to the PG. Concurrently, sympathetic fibers from the spinal cord at level T1–T2 move to the superior cervical ganglion where they synapse with postganglionic fibers. These postganglionic sympathetic fibers eventually pass through the otic ganglion and join the AT nerve [10].

Fig. 16.2 (**a**)
Auriculotemporal syndrome.
Patient A. Facial flush and
sweating are present. (**b**)
Auriculotemporal syndrome.
Patient A. Paper tissue
adheres to moisture caused
by sweating

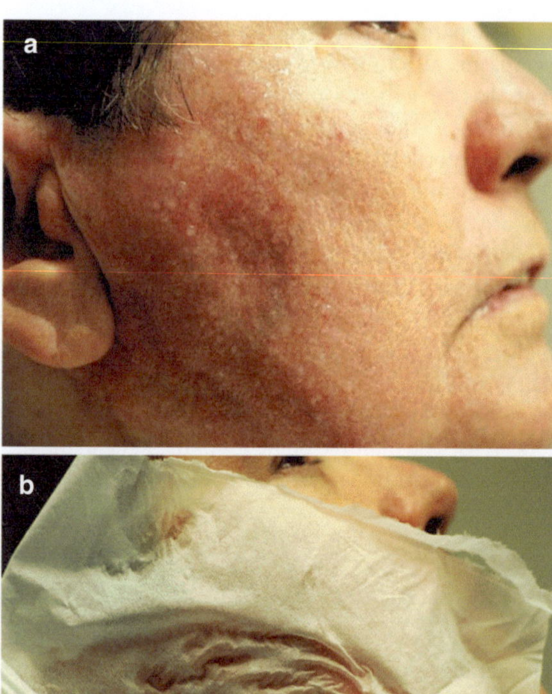

Parotidectomy can damage the AT nerve and its parasympathetic fibers with a consequent interruption of the AT nerve's functional activity. With the passage of time, AT nerve parasympathetic secretomotor fiber regeneration occurs. However, these fibers can no longer navigate their normal course to innervate a now absent PG. The parasympathetic fibers take an alternate path, grow into the vacant sheath of the severed AT nerve's sympathetic fibers, and reach the facial cutaneous sweat glands and blood vessels, normally supplied by the sympathetic fibers that run with the AT nerve. Normally, eating, particularly sour or spicy foods, serves to stimulate PG salivation via the AT nerve. Activation of the AT nerve now causes sweating from the sweat glands and flushing from vascular dilations in the cutaneous pre-auricular area. Symptom severity can range from non-annoying to severe embarrassment, with patients often abstaining from eating in public.

Diagnosis of AT syndrome is readily achieved by incorporating the history of PG surgery with the subsequent onset of facial sweating and flushing. An objective test, the Minor starch test, is available if confirmation is necessary. The test requires iodine to be painted on the involved cutaneous tissue just anterior to the ear and allowed to dry. Starch powder is then dusted on the iodinized area and a sialogogue (lemon candy) is given to the patient. Sweating will now occur from PG stimulation and serve as the fluid medium that mixes the iodine with the starch. A blue-black chemical discoloration of the powdered area functions as a positive result.

Only 10–15% of patients with AT syndrome have symptoms severe enough, usually sweating, to request treatment [9]. A variety of treatments has been advocated for the syndrome [9]. Antiperspirants (aluminum hexahydrate), topical anticholinergics (glycopyrrolate), and tympanic neurectomy have been suggested. Surgeons have tried to prevent the problem by surgically incorporating a tissue barrier between the postganglionic parasympathetic nerve endings and the overlying cutaneous tissue. A partial superficial lobectomy of the PG may also serve to lessen the occurrence of an AT syndrome [9]. A safe and effective therapeutic approach to the syndrome can be obtained with intradermal injections of botulinum toxin A (BT) [8]. The BT prevents the release of acetylcholine at the nerve terminals, thus blocking neurotransmission of the signals to the sweat glands and blood vessels. Unfortunately, repeat BT injections are required as the effects of the toxin wear off, usually 4–6 months afterward. Most patients opt for no treatment because the symptomatology does not significantly impact the quality of their life.

Middle Ear Surgery

The middle ear is that division of the ear that lies between the tympanic membrane (eardrum) and the oval window. The tympanic membrane separates the outer ear from the middle ear, while the oval window is a membrane that serves to separate the middle ear from the inner ear. The bony wall circumscribing the middle ear is the temporal bone's mastoid process which is honeycombed by air cells that are susceptible to secondary infection, often originating from an otitis media. Key structures that inhabit the very limited confines of the middle ear include the ossicles (malleus, incus, stapes) and the chorda tympani nerve (CTN). The ossicles function to transmit sound vibrations from the eardrum to the inner ear, while the CTN has as one of its responsibilities the transport of taste sensation from the anterior two-thirds of the tongue. The CTN has another important and significant role. It also functions to supply secretomotor fibers to the submandibular and sublingual salivary glands (SMSG/SLSG).

Surgery involving the very cramped anatomic quarters assigned to the middle ear is common and consists of procedures such as tympanoplasty, mastoidectomy, and ossiculoplasty. Tympanoplasty involves repair of both a hole in the eardrum and any existing ossicular damage. Mastoidectomy becomes necessary when infection of the mastoid air cells develops and requires removal of the diseased bone. Ossiculoplasty is concerned with any ossicular repair.

A common ossicular problem that demands surgical intervention is otosclerosis. Otosclerosis is a disease of the middle ear characterized by a progressive loss of hearing due to fixation of the stapes. Otosclerosis has been reported to occur in 10% of the population with 60% of these patients having family members who have the problem [11]. A female predilection of 2:1 has also been noted, with the condition occurring bilaterally in 80% of the cases [11]. The sound conducting mechanism, mediated by the ossicles, is impaired when abnormal bone deposition involves the footplate of the stapes and fixes the stapes to the edges of the oval window. This problem of excessive bone deposition occurs despite the fact that there is no inflammatory involvement of the stapes or middle ear mucosa. Excessive bone deposition may have its etiological origins from a genetic background [11].

The surgical procedure to remedy the loss of stapes mobility was first developed by Shea in 1956 [12]. The technique involves surgical removal of the malfunctioning stapes and its replacement by a prosthesis. The prosthesis is a freely moving rod, fixed to the incus, that will act as a stapes substitute and transmit sound vibrations to the oval window. Anatomically, an intimate relationship exists between the ossicular bones, particularly the stapes [13], and the CTN (Fig. 16.3). Unfortunately, because of the very close anatomic position of the CTN to the stapes and the limited physical confines of the middle ear, surgical accessibility to the stapes requires the retraction/stretching or even sectioning of the CTN. The consequent trauma to the nerve can lead to dysgeusia and hyposalivation.

Anatomically, the fibers of the CTN originate from the inferior salivary nucleus in the pons and then join the facial nerve. Moving through the facial nerve canal, the

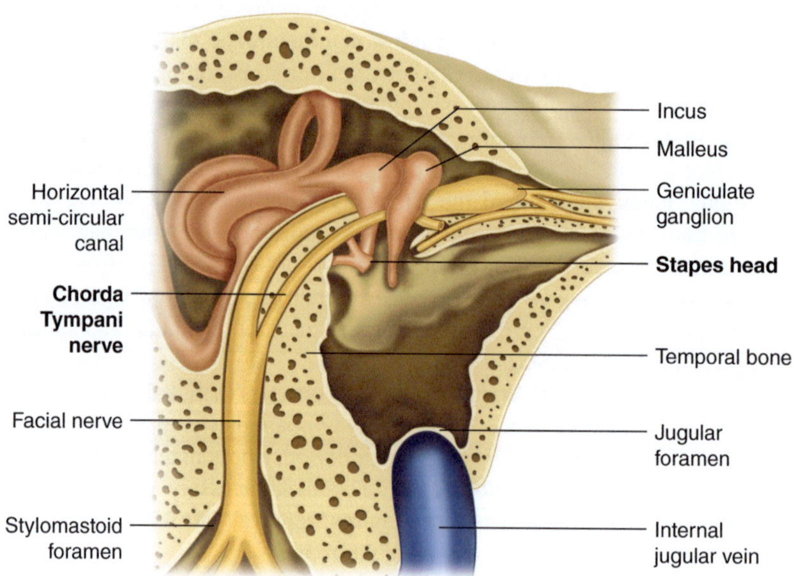

Fig. 16.3 Sketch demonstrates close relationship of stapes to chorda tympani nerve (Louis Mandel. Hyposalivation after undergoing stapedectomy. J Am Dent Assoc. 2012 Jan;143(1):39-42. https://doi.org/10.14219/jada.archive.2012.0016.)

CTN reaches a point several millimeters above the stylomastoid foramen, at which time it separates from the facial nerve and enters the posterior wall of the middle ear whereupon it establishes a close anatomic liaison with the stapes. The CTN now courses anteriorly deep to the neck of the malleus, exits the middle ear, and enters the infratemporal fossa where it joins the lingual nerve traveling to the tongue. In addition to receiving fibers from the anterior two-thirds of the tongue that act as afferents for taste, CTN preganglionic efferent secretomotor fibers are dispatched to the submandibular ganglion. Here after synapsing, a relay of postganglionic secretory fibers proceed to activate the salivary production of the SMSG/SLSG complex.

Injury to the CTN during middle ear surgery has resulted in several postoperative complaints. Dysgeusia is not uncommon, occurring postoperatively in 57% of the patients [14]. Usually, the dysgeusia is transient and recovery can be anticipated within 12 months [15]. Tinnitus and dizziness may also develop. Of great interest is that hyposalivation can be placed into the mix of postoperative complications. Bull [16] reported that 37 of 126 stapedectomy patients developed postoperative hyposalivation. One year later, it was still present in 31 patients. Another side effect of the loss of CTN stimulation involves the contralateral SMSG. A resulting compensatory hypertrophy along with a moderate increase in salivary production has been observed in the contralateral SMSG [17]. Surprisingly, the ipsilateral SMSG, deprived of its stimulation, does not atrophy.

The SMSG/SLSG complex produces approximately 68% of the saliva during periods of rest [18]. Patients who have had stapedectomy with CTN injury will complain that their mouth is dry at rest (nothing in the mouth), but when they eat, sufficient moisture is present. The explanation rests in the fact that with the stimulation that occurs during mastication, the parotid gland increases its salivary production, and this normal consistent physiologic action compensates for the SMSG/SLSG hypofunction. The SMSG/SLSG hyposalivation is most oppressive when there is bilateral CTN damage, a significant possibility considering that otosclerosis is frequently bilateral [19] in its presentation. Because the CTN's secretomotor fibers to the salivary glands are more sensitive and suffer more damage from trauma than the taste afferents, hyposalivation tends to persist for longer periods than dysgeusia, which is usually transient. Bull [16] reported that 101 of 126 cases developed taste alterations in the immediate postoperative period, but only 32 still experienced this problem 1 year later. A metallic taste, bitter taste, or loss of taste acuity may result from the CTN damage. This dysgeusia may be ameliorated by any contralateral uninvolved CTN and will be buttressed by the normally functioning glossopharyngeal and vagus nerves, which convey taste from the posterior third of the tongue and pharynx, respectively.

Treatment of patients who have issues with hyposalivation is best directed at the use of sialogogues. Pilocarpine or cevimeline are medications that can be prescribed. These patients and those who do not have a severe secretory problem may also be encouraged to use sugarless sour candy or chewing gum, oral lubricants, or mouthwashes and to sip water.

First Bite Syndrome

First bite syndrome (FBS) is a painful orofacial condition characterized by unilateral severe paroxysmal spurts of pain in the parotid area whenever food is first placed in the mouth. The bursts of pain tend to moderate with subsequent masticatory bites. When gustatory stimulation stops, the pain gradually disappears. Unfortunately, the pain cycle returns during the next meal when food is introduced into the mouth. Patients often avoid eating due to the severity of the discomfort. The unilateral pain focuses around the parotid gland (PG) and radiates to the ear and upper neck. Sialogogic foods such as citrus intensify the pain. Some diminution of the severity and frequency of the pain occurs across a time span of several months, while total spontaneous resolution may develop within 12–18 months [20].

Although the clinical features of the syndrome were first recognized by Haubrich in 1986 [21], it remained for Netterville and his colleagues [22] to more thoroughly describe FBS symptomatology and simultaneously develop a working hypothesis regarding its pathophysiology. Surgery that involves the parapharyngeal space (PPS), infratemporal fossa (ITF), or deep lobe of the PG (Figs. 16.4 and 16.5) is considered the usual initiating cause of the ipsilateral PG pain cycles, which become manifest several days to several months post-surgically. Surgery in these areas often fails anatomically to avoid involvement of the sympathetic chain's superior cervical ganglion (SCG) and/or the postganglionic fibers of the SCG. Anatomically, the SCG is approximately 3 cm in length and lies posterior to the carotid sheath at the level of the second and third cervical vertebrae. Postganglionic fibers from the SCG run along with the external carotid artery (ECA) as a plexus to supply sympathetic innervation to the myoepithelial cells that peripherally circumscribe the ducts of the PG. Damage to the nerve plexus around the ECA or injury to the SCG or both will lead to a loss of innervation to these sympathetic receptors on the myoepithelial cells. The myoepithelial cells will now develop a denervation hypersensitivity. These myoepithelial cells also possess parasympathetic receptors, but no interruption occurs in the innervation of these myoepithelial cells by the postganglionic parasympathetic fibers originating from the otic ganglion. With salivary stimulation by food, etc., these parasympathetics release acetylcholine which then crosses over to activate the hypersensitive denervated myoepithelial sympathetic receptors. The resulting heightened response of the sympathetic receptors on the myoepithelial cells is thought to cause duct spasms and the acute pain associated with FBS [22].

Linkov et al. [23] reported a 9.6% incidence of FBS in 499 patients who had undergone deep lobe parotid gland surgery or other surgeries involving the PPS and/ or ITF. The most common cause for FBS is surgery in the PPS usually mandated by the presence of a PG deep lobe pleomorphic adenoma (Fig. 16.4) with schwannoma (Fig. 16.5) following as the second most frequent pathologic cause [24]. Cases of FBS have also been reported following carotid endarterectomy, mandibular condyle surgery, styloid surgery, and cervical lymph node surgery [25]. Surgical procedures in the PPS can evade SCG trauma but often require ligation of the ECA and will in

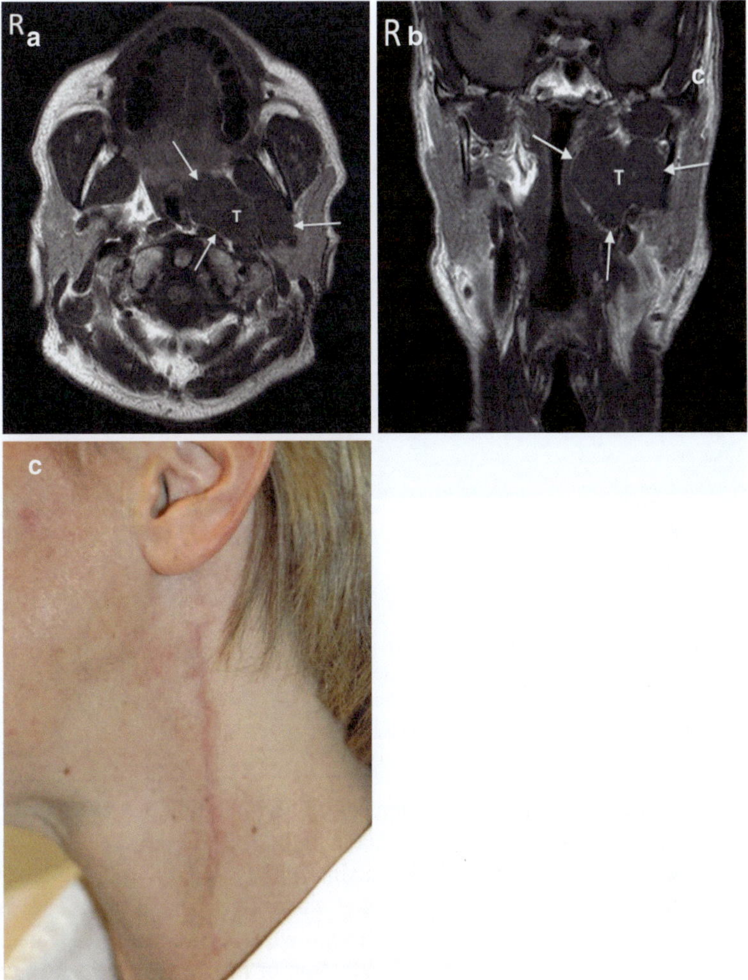

Fig. 16.4 (**a**) First bite syndrome. Patient C. MRI, axial view. Pleomorphic adenoma (T) encroaching on nasopharynx (arrows) (Houle A. J Oral Maxillofac Surg 2014;72:1475). (**b**) First bite syndrome. Patient C. MRI, coronal view. Pleomorphic adenoma (T) impinging on the nasopharynx (arrows) (Houle A. J Oral Maxillofac Surg 2014;72:1475). (**c**) First bite syndrome. Patient C. Surgical scar 5 weeks post-surgery (Houle A. J Oral Maxillofac Surg 2014;72:1475)

the process interrupt the sympathetic plexus accompanying the ECA as it travels to the PG. In some but not all such cases, symptoms of FBS can be expected.

It should be noted that if the SCG is involved, not only will FBS develop, but Horner's syndrome (HS) will also become an issue (Fig. 16.5b). Postganglionic fibers from the SCG also run as a nerve plexus with the internal carotid artery (ICA) to the eye and orbit. Therefore, if there is injury to the SCG or even the ICA, HS will

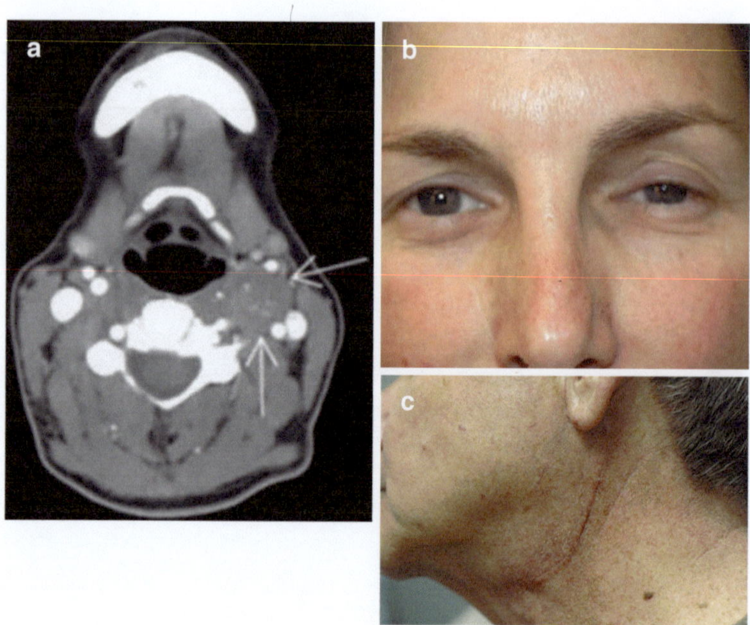

Fig. 16.5 (a) First bite syndrome. Patient B. CT scan. Benign mass, schwannoma (arrows) (Mandel L. JADA 2008;139:1480). (b) First bite syndrome. Patient B. Left eyelid ptosis and left miosis characteristics of Horner syndrome (Mandel L. JADA 2008;139:1480). (c) First bite syndrome. Patient B. Healing surgical site (Mandel L. JADA 2008;139:1480)

be thrown into the symptom mix in patients with FBS and will be recognized by the presence of eyelid ptosis, miosis, and facial anhidrosis [26].

The pain associated with FBS may be misinterpreted as temporomandibular joint (TMJ) pain but can readily be differentiated when TMJ palpation or TMJ movements fail to elicit the pathognomonic pain seen with FBS. Glossopharyngeal neuralgia can be recognized when intraoral palpation of the subtonsillar space creates pain. An intraoral and/or extraoral palpation of the styloid apparatus that elicits pain indicates the presence of Eagle's syndrome and can eliminate a FBS diagnosis.

Successful treatment of FBS has not been achieved. Anti-epileptic medications (carbamazepine, gabapentin), antidepressants (amitriptyline), and analgesics have produced only a limited improvement in symptoms. Radiotherapy has been avoided because of its associated morbidity. Tympanic neurectomy has failed to relieve FBS symptomatology. Botulinum toxin A (BT) injections have been advocated and offer relief following injection into the painful zone of the PG [26]. Because BT represents a relatively new approach to FBS treatment, a protocol has not been firmly established. In addition to these pro-active approaches to the care of FBS, observation is always an option. Resolution of the pain's frequency and intensity can occur with time [20, 25].

References

1. Sajisevi M. Indications for facial nerve monitoring during parotidectomy. Otolaryngol Clin North Am. 2021;54(3):489–96. https://doi.org/10.1016/j.otc.2021.02.001.
2. El Sayed AY, Winters R. Parotidectomy. In: StatPearls. Treasure Island: StatPearls Publishing; 2021.
3. Nouraei SA, Ismail Y, Ferguson MS, et al. Analysis of complications following surgical treatment of benign parotid disease. ANZ J Surg. 2008;78(3):134–8. https://doi.org/10.1111/j.1445-2197.2007.04388.x.
4. Kawata R, Kinoshita I, Omura S, et al. Risk factors of postoperative facial palsy for benign parotid tumors: outcome of 1,018 patients. Laryngoscope. 2021;131(12):E2857–64. https://doi.org/10.1002/lary.29623.
5. Goomany A, Sood S. Superficial parotidectomy for chronic parotid sialadenitis: a case series and review of the literature. J Laryngol Otol. 2021;135(10):883–6. https://doi.org/10.1017/S0022215121002115.
6. O'Neill JP, Condron C, Curran A, Walsh A. Lucja Frey—historical relevance and syndrome review. Surgeon. 2008;6(3):178–81. https://doi.org/10.1016/s1479-666x(08)80115-1.
7. Motz KM, Kim YJ. Auriculotemporal syndrome (Frey syndrome). Otolaryngol Clin North Am. 2016;49(2):501–9. https://doi.org/10.1016/j.otc.2015.10.010.
8. Marchese MR, Bussu F, Settimi S, Scarano E, Almadori G, Galli J. Not only gustatory sweating and flushing: signs and symptoms associated to the Frey syndrome and the role of botulinum toxin A therapy. Head Neck. 2021;43(3):949–55. https://doi.org/10.1002/hed.26561.
9. Sood S, Quraishi MS, Bradley PJ. Frey's syndrome and parotid surgery. Clin Otolaryngol Allied Sci. 1998;23(4):291–301. https://doi.org/10.1046/j.1365-2273.1998.00154.x.
10. Farrell ML, Kalnins IK. Frey's syndrome following parotid surgery. Aust N Z J Surg. 1991;61(4):295–301. https://doi.org/10.1111/j.1445-2197.1991.tb00215.x.
11. Adedeji TO, Indorewala S, Indorewala A, Nemade G. Stapedotomy and its effect on hearing—our experience with 54 cases. Afr Health Sci. 2016;16(1):276–81. https://doi.org/10.4314/ahs.v16i1.36.
12. Shea JJ. Symposium: the operation for the mobilization of the stapes in otosclerotic deafness. Laryngoscope. 1956;66:729–84.
13. Miman MC, Sigirci A, Ozturan O, Karatas E, Erdem T. The effects of the chorda tympani damage on submandibular glands: biometric changes. Auris Nasus Larynx. 2003;30(1):21–4. https://doi.org/10.1016/s0385-8146(02)00027-5.
14. Skoloudik L, Krtickova J, Haviger J, Mejzlik J, Chrobok V. Changes of taste perception after stapes surgery: a prospective cohort study. Eur Arch Otorrinolaringol. 2022;279(1):175–9. https://doi.org/10.1007/s00405-021-06665-0.
15. Michael P, Raut V. Chorda tympani injury: operative findings and postoperative symptoms. Otolaryngol Head Neck Surg. 2007;136(6):978–81. https://doi.org/10.1016/j.otohns.2006.12.022.
16. Bull TR. Taste and the chorda tympani. J Laryngol Otol. 1965;79:479–93. https://doi.org/10.1017/s0022215100063969.
17. Yagmur C, Miman MC, Karatas E, Akarcay M, Erdem T, Ozturan O. Effects of the chorda tympani damage on submandibular glands: scintigraphic changes. J Laryngol Otol. 2004;118(2):102–5. https://doi.org/10.1258/002221504772784531.
18. Dawes C. Salivary flow patterns and the health of hard and soft oral tissues. J Am Dent Assoc. 2008;139 Suppl:18S–24S. https://doi.org/10.14219/jada.archive.2008.0351.
19. Mandel L. Hyposalivation after undergoing stapedectomy. J Am Dent Assoc. 2012;143(1):39–42. https://doi.org/10.14219/jada.archive.2012.0016.

20. Charles-Harris H, Rodriguez B. First bite syndrome: presentation of a patient status-post right carotid endarterectomy. Vasc Endovascular Surg. 2021;55(1):64–8. https://doi.org/10.1177/1538574420954589.
21. Haubrich WS. The first-bite syndrome. Henry Ford Hosp Med J. 1986;34(4):275–8.
22. Netterville JL, Jackson CG, Miller FR, Wanamaker JR, Glasscock ME. Vagal paraganglioma: a review of 46 patients treated during a 20-year period. Arch Otolaryngol Head Neck Surg. 1998;124(10):1133–40. https://doi.org/10.1001/archotol.124.10.1133.
23. Linkov G, Morris LG, Shah JP, Kraus DH. First bite syndrome: incidence, risk factors, treatment, and outcomes. Laryngoscope. 2012;122(8):1773–8. https://doi.org/10.1002/lary.23372.
24. Avinçsal MÖ, Hiroshima Y, Shinomiya H, Shinomiya H, Otsuki N, Nibu KI. First bite syndrome—an 11-year experience. Auris Nasus Larynx. 2017;44(3):302–5. https://doi.org/10.1016/j.anl.2016.07.012.
25. Xu V, Gill KS, Goldfarb J, et al. First bite syndrome after parotidectomy: a case series and review of literature. Ear Nose Throat J. 2022;101:663–7.
26. Mandel L, Syrop SB. First-bite syndrome after parapharyngeal surgery for cervical schwannoma. J Am Dent Assoc. 2008;139(11):1480–3. https://doi.org/10.14219/jada.archive.2008.0073.

Chapter 17
Sublingual Salivary Gland Abnormalities

Louis Mandel

Abstract The sublingual salivary gland (SLSG), because of its superficial location in the floor of the mouth, is susceptible to trauma initiated by an intraorally introduced foreign object or during the performance of adjacent surgery. Trauma to one of the many ducts possessed by this gland may result in salivary leakage. The escaping saliva accumulates and results in the cyst-like ranula. The ranula anatomically manifests itself in different oro-cervical areas. This varied anatomic location of the ranula mandates different surgical therapeutic approaches. In this chapter attention is also called to the anatomic abnormalities that the SLSG occasionally displays.

Sublingual Salivary Gland Overview

Overview

The sublingual salivary gland (SLSG), developing in the eighth week of fetal life [1], is a mixed gland consisting mostly of mucous acini (Fig. 17.1) and some elements of seromucous acini (Fig. 17.2). The gland has no distinct capsule and lies on the oral surface of the mylohyoid muscle (MM) in a bed of connective tissue. The generally accepted anatomic concept that the SLSG consists of one unit has recently been clarified [2–4]. Anatomic dissections have indicated that the SLSG consists of anterior and posterior segments. Small minor ducts, 8–20 ducts of Rivinus, originate from the posterior segment of the SLSG and open directly above their position onto the mucosa of the elevated sublingual fold. The ducts of Rivinus arising from the anterior section of the SLSG may unite to form a single major duct, the duct of Bartholin (BD) [4]. The BD either empties into the Wharton duct (WD) (Fig. 17.3), the SMSG's major duct, or runs along the side of WD and opens independently on

© The Author(s), under exclusive license to Springer Nature Switzerland AG 2024

L. Mandel, *Clinical Management of Salivary Gland Disorders*, https://doi.org/10.1007/978-3-031-50012-1_17

Fig. 17.1 Sublingual salivary gland. Mucous acini

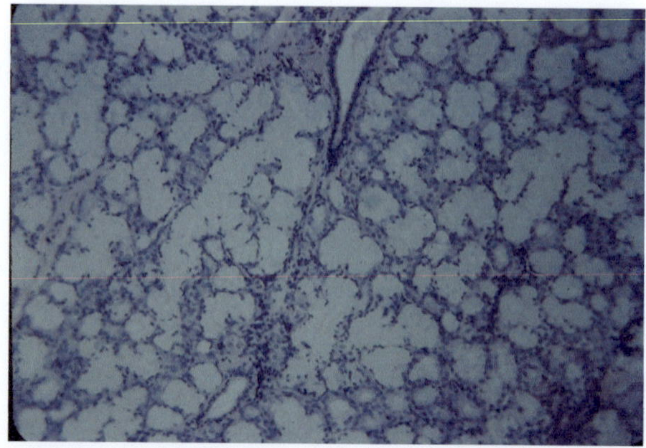

Fig. 17.2 Sublingual salivary gland. Microscopic high-power view of serous demilunes

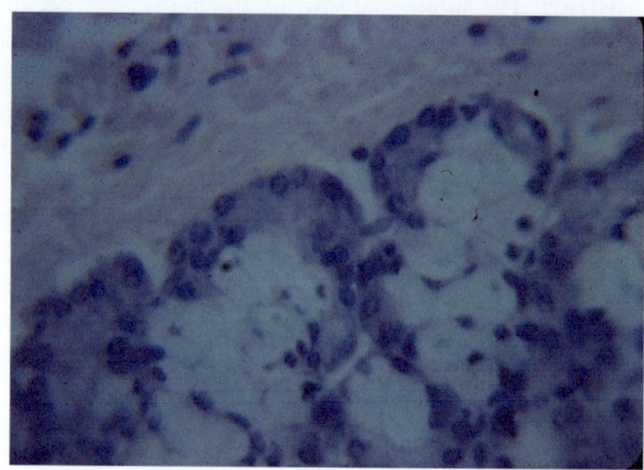

Fig. 17.3 Left submandibular sialogram demonstrates incidental finding of duct of Bartholin (arrows) emptying into anterior portion of the submandibular duct

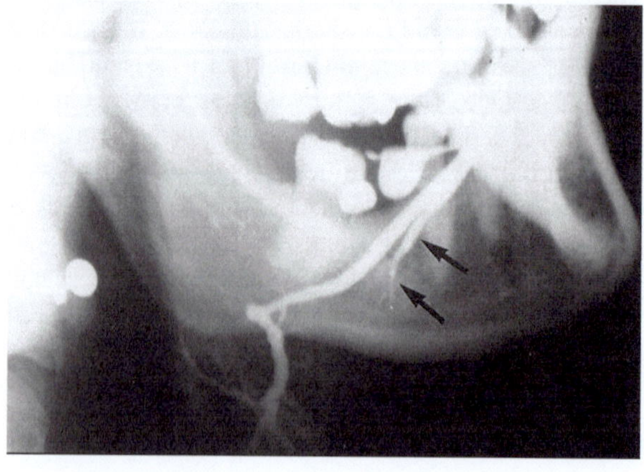

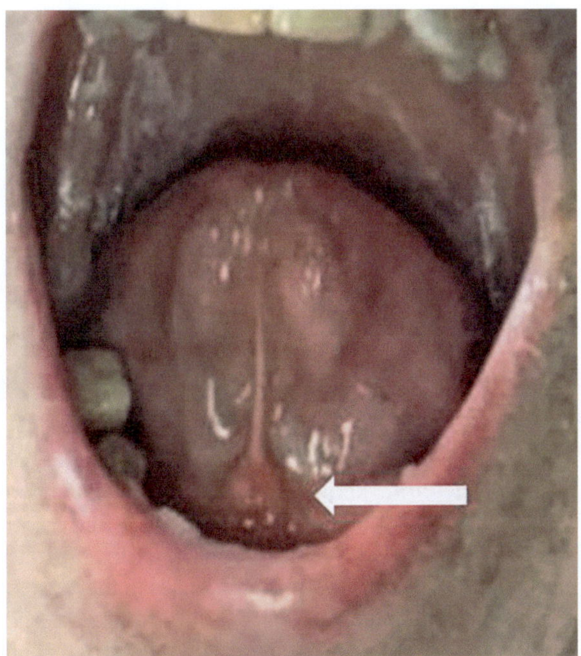

Fig. 17.4 Sublingual caruncle (arrow)

the sublingual papilla (caruncle) (Fig. 17.4) adjacent to the orifice of WD. It has been reported that, when present, 40% of the BDs open into WD, a factor that must be considered when treating a ranula, while the remainder open on the sublingual caruncle [3].

Anteriorly, the SLSG approaches its fellow from the opposite side in the midline area adjacent to the lingual frenum, while posteriorly it advances toward the orally situated deep lobe of the SMSG. Laterally, it is limited by the sublingual fossa on the lingual surface of the mandible. Medially, the SLSG is bordered by the geniohyoid-genioglossus muscle complex, WD, and the lingual nerve. Superiorly, the mucosa of the mouth is projected upward by the physical bulk of the SLSG to form the sublingual fold. Inferiorly, the SLSG is limited by the MM.

Ranula

Ranula in Latin means little frog (rana for frog and ula for the diminutive). Its resemblance to a frog is based on the similarity of the ranula's appearance to the orally filled vocal sac of the frog (Fig. 17.5) and not to its likeness to the frog's belly. As the frog fills its oral vocal sac, ventrally positioned in the mouth floor, with air in preparation for allowing escaping air to make the croaking sound, the sac becomes distended and balloon-like. The filled air sac is then projected upward and outward such that it resembles a ranula.

Fig. 17.5 Distended vocal sac of a frog

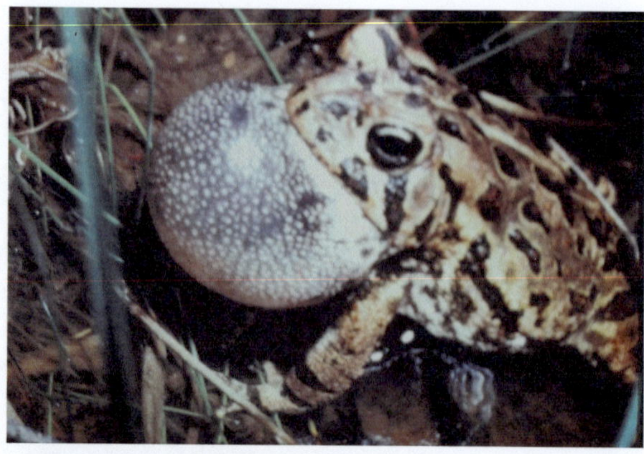

The mylohyoid muscle (MM) plays a very significant role in the development of a ranula. Therefore, knowledge of its anatomy is imperative. Although the MM acts as a floor for the sublingual salivary gland (SLSG), glandular projections through the muscle exist. Cadaver dissections have demonstrated MM defects in 27–45% of the studied specimens [5, 6]. Dehiscences in the muscle layer exist with one or more hiatuses present in the anterior two-thirds of the MM [7, 8]. Units of the SLSG often herniate through these muscle breaks [5] and are responsible for the development of some plunging ranulas (PR) or even the recurrence of a PR.

The ranula is generally thought to result from a traumatic laceration [7, 9] of one of the ducts of Rivinus. However, obstruction of a duct may also play a role in ranula development [10, 11]. Harrison [7] reviewed 19 ranula studies in the literature, all of which concluded that trauma to a duct of Rivinus with resulting salivary leakage was the inciting cause for ranula formation. Following trauma with rupture to one of the SLSG ducts, the extravasation of secretions will accumulate and clinically manifest itself in one of three clinical displays, intraoral, extraoral, or mixed ranulae (Figs. 17.6, 17.7, 17.8, and 17.9) [9]. The more common intraoral ranula (IOR) fluid collection is limited to the oral cavity by the underlying MM. No extraoral signs are evident. The mean age is 21 years [11] and there is a slight female preponderance [9]. The cyst-like fluctuant IOR has a round ovoid shape and gradually increases in size, usually reaching diameters of 2–3 cm [9]. The swelling is subjectively painless and tends to have a bluish tinge caused by the Tyndall effect, a physical phenomenon of light scattering created by the colloidal contents of the ranula. Palpation indicates that the IOR is compressible, fluctuant, and painless. There are no signs of inflammation of the surrounding oral mucosal tissues. The IOR is usually unilateral in its presentation, but it can be seen bilaterally if the fluid content dissects its way across the midline.

The extraoral PR makes its presence known via a cervical area swelling, typically in the submandibular triangle. The PR reaches this anatomic location in one of two ways. The extravasated secretions from an intraoral SLSG lobe can track posteriorly along the oral aspect of the MM. The limiting MM floor ends posteriorly in the third molar area at which point the escaping fluid can drop down cervically into the submandibular triangle. The main occupant of this triangle is the SMSG. Consequently,

Fig. 17.6 (**a**) Intraoral ranula (arrow).
(**b**) Intraoral ranula.
(**c**) Intraoral ranula

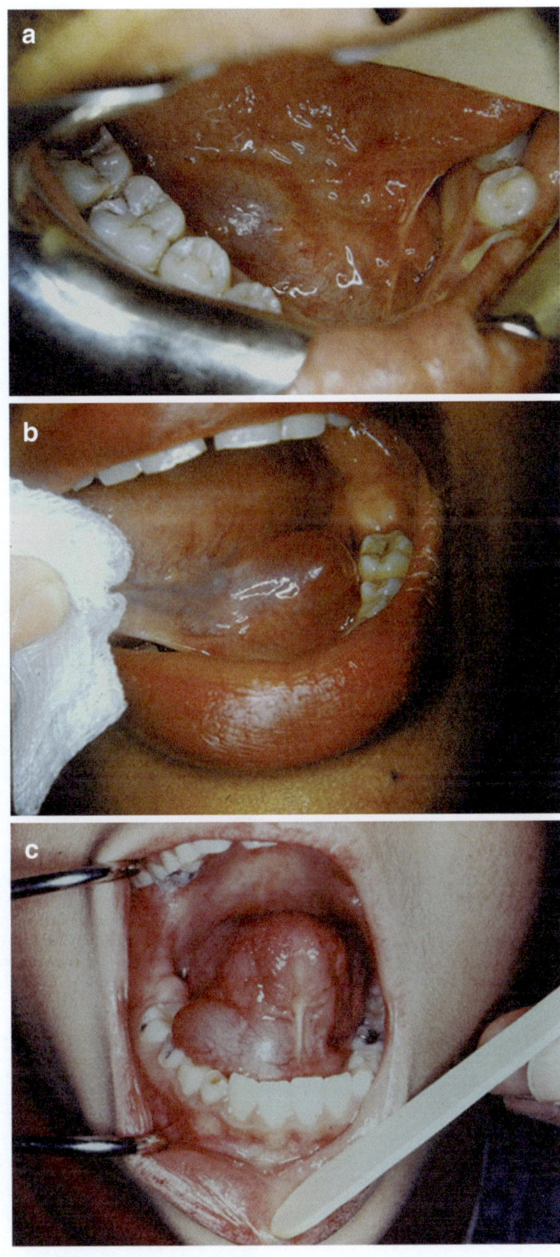

the collecting secretions will mimic a SMSG problem. Another pathway for the development of the extraoral PR is for the escaping SLSG secretions to take a direct route through an existing MM dehiscence. If such a pathway is chosen, secretions can accumulate in the submandibular triangle. However, the fluid buildup may be more anteriorly placed and even involve the submental triangle. This anatomic

Fig. 17.7 (**a**) Plunging ranula. Patient A. Extraoral submandibular swelling. (**b**) Plunging ranula. Patient A. Intraoral swelling. (**c**) Plunging ranula. Patient A. Limiting pseudocystic ranula wall. (**d**) Plunging ranula. Patient A. Ranula cavity after unroofing. (**e**) Plunging ranula. Patient A. Ranula cavity packed with iodoform gauze

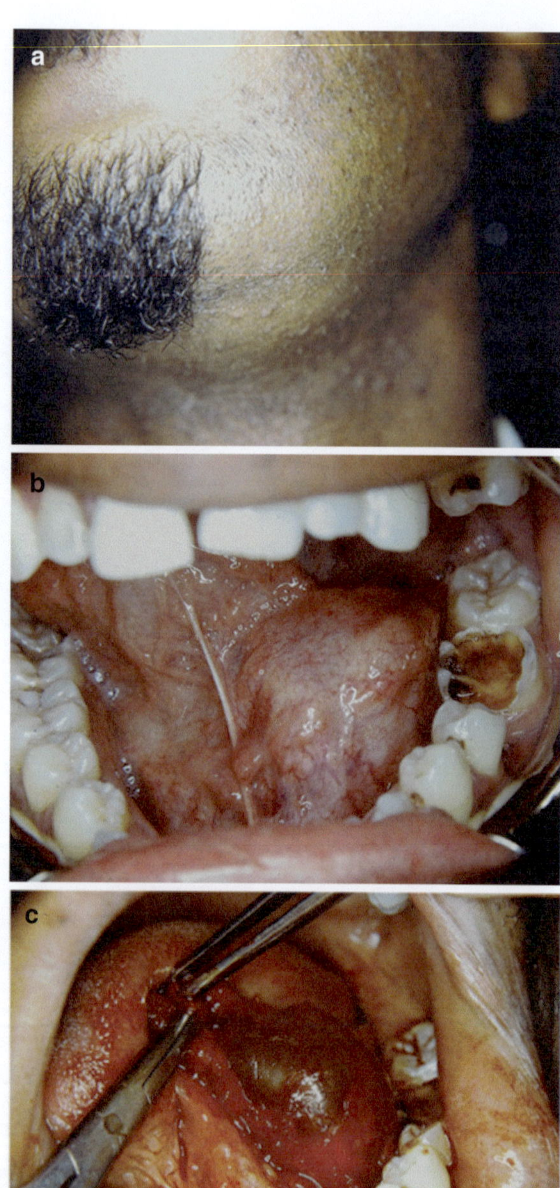

Fig. 17.7 continued

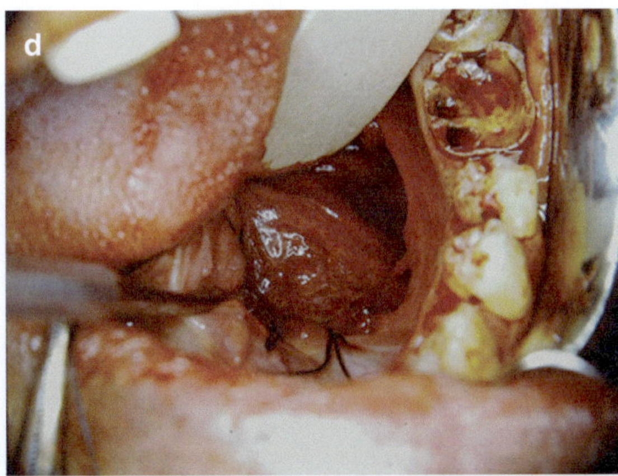

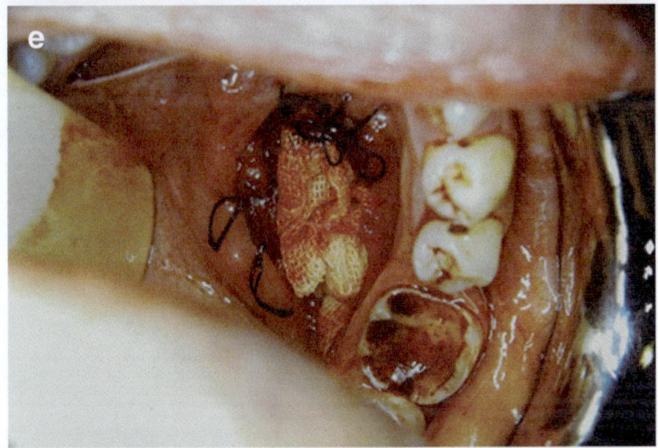

Fig. 17.8 (**a**) Plunging ranula. Patient B. Right submandibular swelling. (**b**) Plunging ranula. Patient B. CT scan, axial view of ranula (R) involving both intraoral and extraoral tissues. (**c**) Plunging ranula. Patient B. CT scan, coronal view of ranula (R)

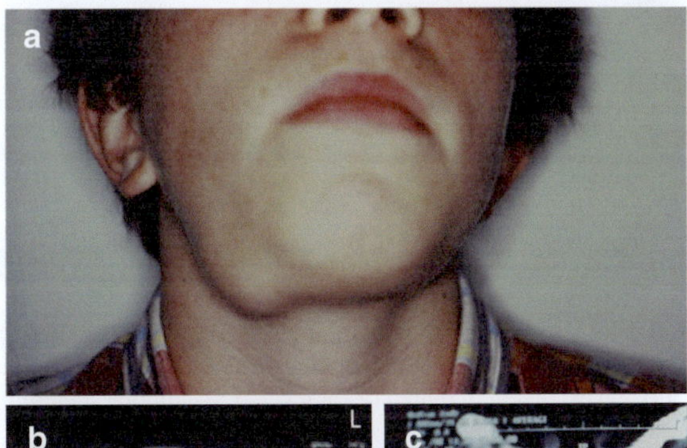

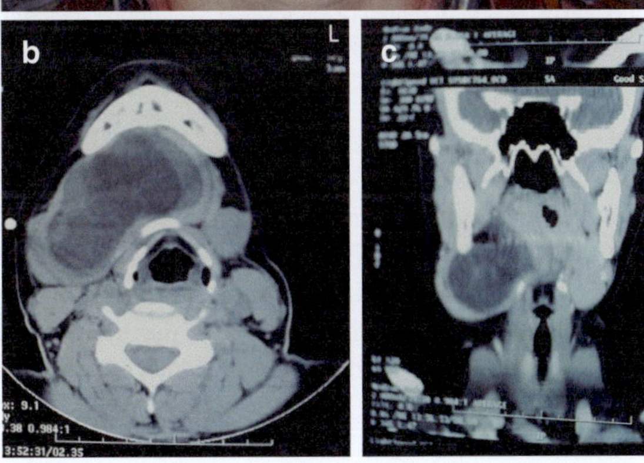

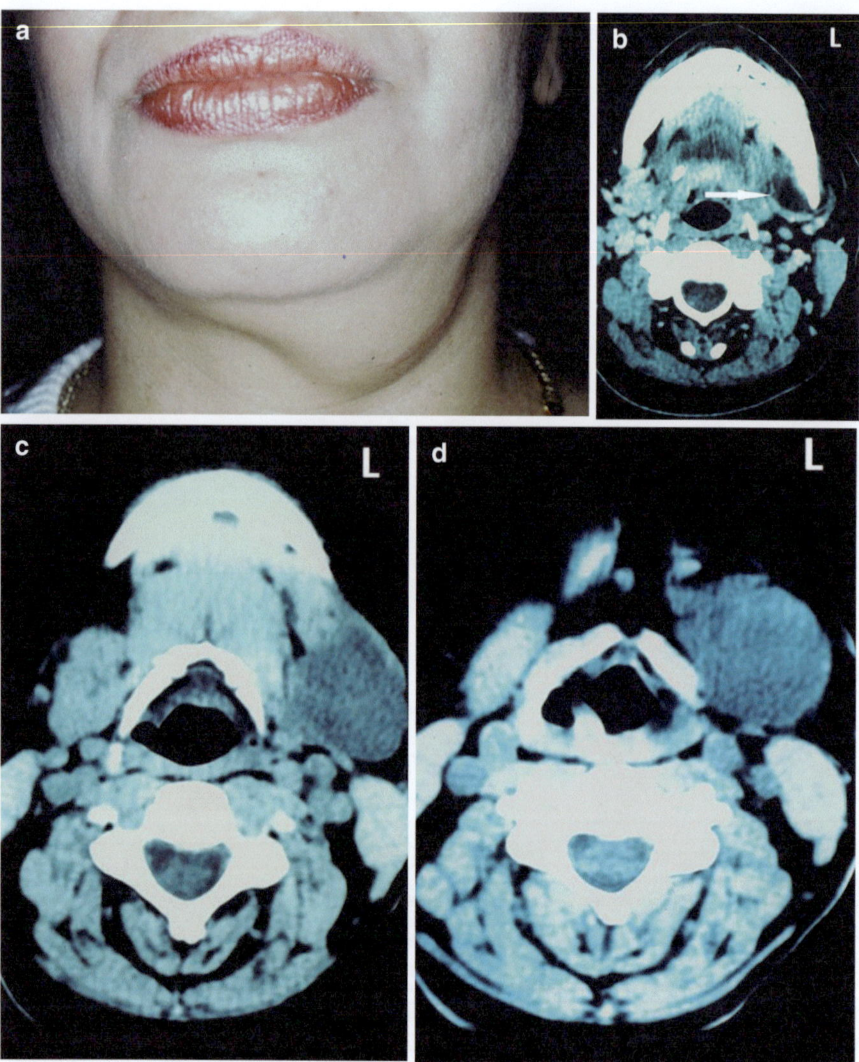

Fig. 17.9 (**a**) Plunging ranula. Patient C. Extraoral swelling. (**b**) Plunging ranula. Patient C. CT scan. Limited intraoral manifestation of ranula (arrow). (**c**) Plunging ranula. Patient C. CT scan. Cervical extension of ranula (R) at level of mandibular mentum. (**d**) Plunging ranula. Patient C. CT scan. Extension of ranula (R) inferior to mandible

submental area location of the PR results from the hiatuses of the MM being mostly present in the anterior portion of the muscle. Another mechanism for the presence of an extraoral PR in the submental/submandibular triangle is a consequence of a herniation of a SLSG unit through a MM dehiscence. Leakage from such a protruding SLSG lobe will directly involve the soft tissues inferior to the MM. If such inferiorly placed glandular tissue is involved in the fluid leakage, an extraoral swelling can develop without any evidence of an intraoral component.

The third clinical variety of ranula is the mixed type. The mixed ranula category probably develops from a long-standing IOR. With persistent leakage, the secretory accumulations eventually find a pathway through a MM dehiscence or posteriorly around the posterior margin of the MM to the cervical area. As such, the ranula will clinically demonstrate both oral and extraoral swellings.

Imaging is not indicated for the evaluation of the IOR. However, the CT scan has a significant role in the diagnosis of the PR because it will demonstrate a cervically oriented well-circumscribed, homogeneous, relatively lucent thin-walled cystic mass. Those IORs that begin their journey to the submandibular triangle by tracking posteriorly along the oral surface of the MM will frequently leave behind a radiolucent trail that can be imaged by a CT scan. This oral lucency, the fluid tail of the ranula, is often considered a pathognomonic feature of a PR and facilitates diagnosis. The imaged fluid tail will help the clinician in the differential diagnosis of similar appearing lucent submandibular lesions. The possible presence of a thyroglossal cyst, branchial cleft cyst, dermoid, or even a lymphatic malformation must always be considered. Besides aiding in differentiation, the scan will also alert the practitioner to what extent adjacent vital structures are compromised.

Histologically, the pseudocystic ranula does not have an epithelial wall. It is lined by granulation tissue and a condensed fibrous connective tissue that represent the body's reaction to the irritation caused by the extravasated secretions. A scattering of chronic inflammation cells will also be evident. Reflecting its origin from a salivary gland, the secretory content of the ranula will have significant levels of amylase.

Some controversy exists regarding a standardized therapeutic surgical approach for the IOR. Certainly, removing the entire SLSG with its leaking component via an intraoral excision will result in the lowest incidence of recurrent disease [11]. However, complications from damage to the Wharton duct (WD), the lingual nerve, and bleeding from small sublingual vessels are not uncommon [12]. A more conservative approach involves the unroofing of the IOR, evacuating its contents and aggressively inserting a gauze packing into the cavity (Fig. 17.7). The pressure of the pack against the adjoining soft tissue acts to simultaneously curb the leak and incite an inflammatory response. In most cases the inflammation is severe enough to stimulate sufficient fibrosis to seal the leak [13]. Although the packing is subjectively uncomfortable, it should be maintained for 7–10 days [13, 14]. With this procedure, recurrences are minimal and have been reported to be in the 10–12% range [15]. Failure demands removal of the guilty SLSG lobe, identified after collapsing the IOR via an incision. Otherwise, the fallback position must be the intraoral excision of the entire SLSG. Total or partial SLSG removal has been advocated by many as the most advantageous surgical approach [16, 17]. No matter what surgical procedure is used for any ranula, the pseudocyst wall will inevitably be surgically perforated, and the fluid contents will escape. The remaining fluid content within the residual pseudocyst requires no intervention by the surgeon because it will be absorbed by the body's normal physiologic activity.

The treatment of the PR differs in that it requires an intrusive approach that mandates the intraoral excision of the entire SLSG [17]. Such surgery will result in a high rate of success. Recurrences may develop and are due to several causes. Incomplete SLSG removal can lead to a recurrence when an orally placed leaking SLSG unit may inadvertently be left behind during surgery. Additionally, secretory leakage may have originated from a segment of the SLSG that has herniated through a MM hiatus. Hidden away from the operator's visual field, the segment can unintentionally be retained following surgery and serve to cause a recurrence. Furthermore, a failure to recognize the existence and anatomic behavior of the Bartholin duct (BD) can lead to a recurrence. On many occasions, the BD empties into WD. Therefore, if the opening of BD into WD is not sealed, secretions from the SMSG, as they pass along WD, will leak out through the residual and open BD junction to create a recurrence [8, 17]. The key to avoiding such a problem is to always tie off an existing BD when performing a SLSG excision [8].

As an alternative to surgery, sclerosing agents (OK-432 or bleomycin) have been advocated as successful treatments for the PR [18]. The carbon dioxide laser has also been utilized for treatment of the PR [18].

Sublingual Salivary Gland Enlargement: Effect on Sublingual Fold

The sublingual salivary gland (SLSG) lies in the floor of the mouth on the mylohyoid muscle, while the mucosa of the mouth floor acts to cover the gland superiorly. The sublingual fold (SLF) is an upward projection of the oral mucosa caused by the underlying physical bulk of the SLSG. Anteriorly, the SLF is most visible in the area of the lingual frenum. It then moves posterolaterally (in a diagonal direction) following the anatomic course of the SLSG as this gland approaches the deep lobe of the submandibular salivary gland in the mandibular molar region.

It is not uncommon for patients to be seen with a significant swelling of the SLF such that its mass tends to overlap into posteriorly existing edentulous mandibular pre-molar/molar areas (Figs. 17.10, 17.11, and 17.12). The projections are caused by enlargements of the underlying SLSG. The enlargements usually are observed equally in both genders in the sixth to seventh decades of life in patients who have no related local or systemic pathologies [19, 20]. Because the SLF swelling is asymptomatic, the patient is often unaware of its existence and duration. Recognition of its presence is usually made during a dental visit. The enlarged SLF may be unilateral or bilateral in its presentation and extend the entire length of the fold, or it may be limited and project into a constricted edentulous area and may even mimic a neoplasm (Fig. 17.12) [21]. No inflammatory changes of the surrounding mucosa are evident. Palpation indicates that the involved tissues are soft, compressible, and painless. The key common denominator that seems to unite patients with this problem is the fact that the tissue proliferations develop in relation to mandibular areas that are edentulous. The elderly are most susceptible to the SLF size alteration because dental loss is a factor in aging. Reduction in alveolar height, associated with dental loss and aging, encourages a SLF expansion into the void created by both the absence of teeth and alveolar bone resorption.

Fig. 17.10 Enlarged sublingual folds (bilateral) (Mandel L, et al. NY State Dent J 2004;70:24)

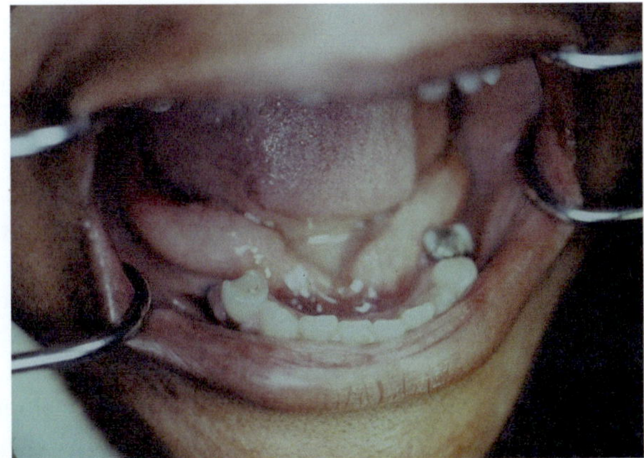

Fig. 17.11 Enlarged sublingual fold overlapping into edentulous mandibular molar area (Mandel L, et al. NY State Dent J 2004;70:24)

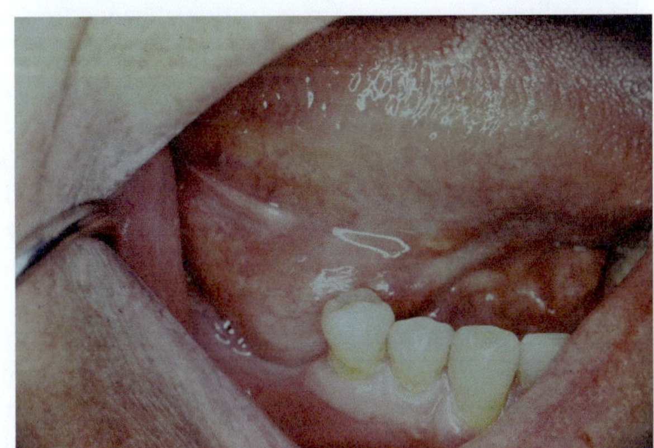

Fig. 17.12 Enlarged sublingual fold (unilateral) (Mandel L, et al. NY State Dent J 2004;70:24)

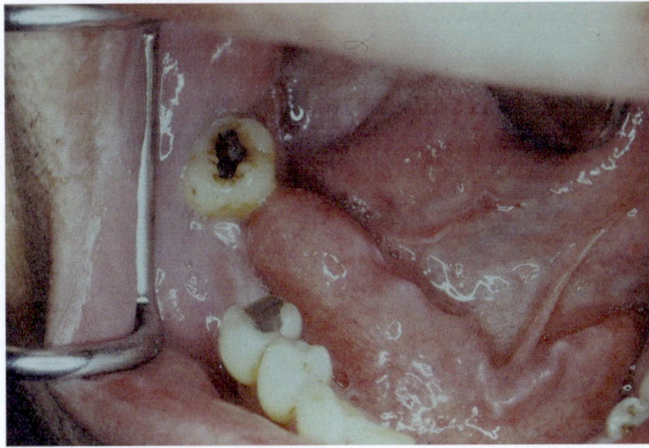

Because many edentulous patients do not exhibit SLF enlargements, it can be assumed that other factors are involved in its development. No etiologic cause has been determined for the SLSG enlargement. Although the common element seen in patients is an existing edentulous void, most mandibular edentulous areas will not demonstrate this unique SLSG/SLF abnormality. It has been suggested that a high insertion of the mylohyoid muscle paired with free tongue movements related to dental loss may be components in a functional adaptation of the mouth floor that may lead to the SLF/SLSG enlargement [22].

The practitioner should be aware that lymphomas do have a tendency to invade salivary gland tissues. Occasionally, enlargement of the SLF/SLSG complex will be seen in which there may be no association with an edentulous area, and the involved tissues are firm and erythematous. These signs are ominous and demand investigation as to the presence of a neoplasm, particularly a lymphoma (Fig. 17.13).

Histologically, the surface mucosa over the enlarged SLF/SLSG exhibits no abnormalities. Microscopic examination obtained from a surgical biopsy of the proliferated mouth floor tissue reveals that the SLSG has a normal cellular pattern [21] and demonstrates no increase in the size of individual glandular cells [20]. Specimens of the involved SLSG have been thoroughly examined histologically in an attempt to find some pathologic aberration. Acinar atrophy and hypoplasia, duct-like structures, and increased deposition of fat and fibrotic tissue have been observed. However, these findings are not pathologic. Rather, they represent the normal aging process [20] of the SLSG that is seen in older age groups, and as stated, the enlargements are usually seen in the elderly.

SLF/SLSG enlargement should not be mistaken for a neoplasm or ranula. It requires no treatment other than reassurance. Recognition avoids concern, misdiagnosis, and unnecessary surgery. Surgical intervention may be necessary if the enlargement interferes with denture construction or denture stability.

Fig. 17.13 Bilaterally enlarged erythematous sublingual folds. Swellings in this case caused by a malignant lymphoma

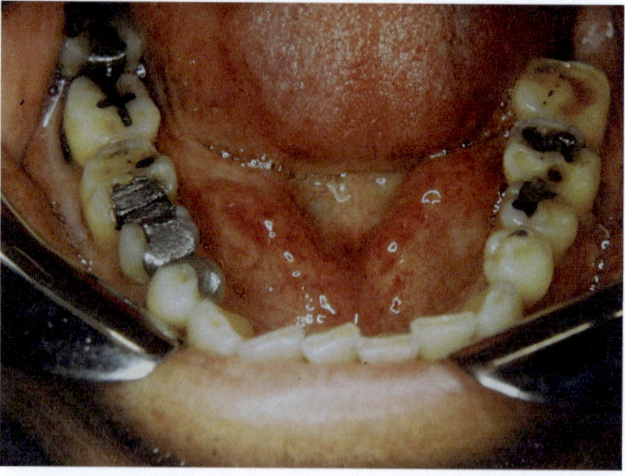

Sublingual Salivary Gland Enlargement: Aplasia Submandibular Salivary Gland

Enlargement of the sublingual salivary gland (SLSG) can result from a compensatory hypertrophy caused by aplasia of other major salivary glands. Salivary gland aplasia is an infrequent congenital disorder with the parotid gland (PG) being more frequently affected than the submandibular salivary gland (SMSG) [23]. Compensatory SLSG hypertrophies have randomly been reported as an aspect of gland aplasia, but only in relation to SMSG aplasia. If both SMSGs are missing, bilateral compensatory hypertrophies of both SLSGs develop [23–26]. Unilateral SMSG absence can lead to ipsilateral SLSG hypertrophy [23–26]. The explanation for this unique SMSG/SLSG relationship may be a result of the fact that both salivary glands share a common secretory nerve innervation via the chorda tympani nerve (CTN). The CTN's preganglionic efferent secretomotor fibers enter the submandibular ganglion. Here, they synapse with postganglionic secretory fibers that proceed to activate the SMSG/SLSG complex. It is possible that those efferent fibers, originally intended to stimulate the now missing SMSG, can move to the SLSG. Consequently, they can have an augmented stimulatory effect on the existing SLSG and serve as the root of the compensatory hypertrophy.

Herniation Sublingual Salivary Gland

In the floor of the mouth, the sublingual salivary gland (SLSG) rests on the mylohyoid muscle (MM). Dehiscences in the MM have been observed in 27–45% of dissections performed on cadavers [5]. The dehiscences can be multiple, are asymptomatic, and usually involve the lateral aspect of the anterior two-thirds of the MM [5, 7]. The defects measure between 5 and 20 mm in size [27–29] with shapes that vary from narrow fissures to broad oval openings [5]. Therefore, it should be no surprise that a lobe of the SLSG accompanied by fatty tissue can prolapse through these anatomic gaps. At the level of the muscular defect, these herniations can have either a wide or constricted base [5]. They are recognized as relatively rare permanent visible extraoral submental asymptomatic nodular swellings (Fig. 17.14). Swallowing or increasing intraoral pressure by blowing up the cheek exacerbates the herniation and causes a conspicuous prominence of the extraoral swelling [29].

Although the persistent extraoral bulge is asymptomatic and nonpathologic, patients seek medical attention because of the cosmetic issue or concern about neoplastic possibilities. No treatment is required except offering the patient reassurance and an explanation of the cause of the problem.

Fig. 17.14 (**a**) Sublingual salivary gland herniation (lateral view). Patient D. (**b**) Sublingual salivary gland herniation (frontal view). Patient D. Submental swelling

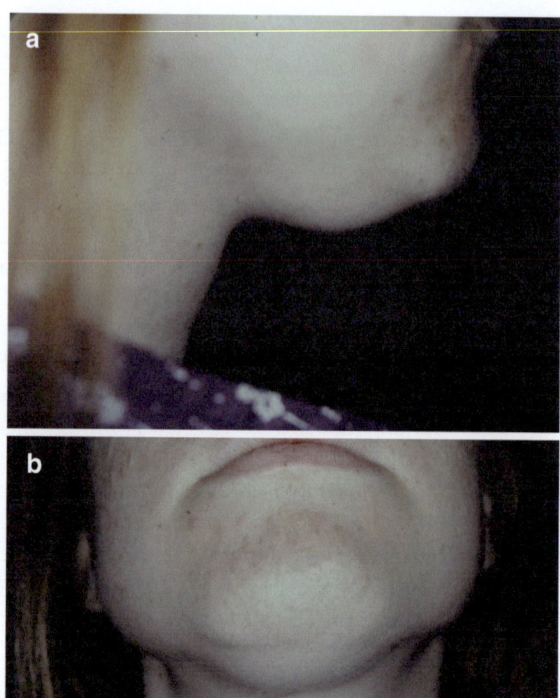

References

1. Grewal JS, Bordoni B, Shah J, Ryan J. Anatomy, head and neck, sublingual gland. In: StatPearls. Treasure Island: StatPearls Publishing; 2022.
2. Batsakis JG. Pathology consultation: sublingual gland. Ann Otol Rhinol Laryngol. 1991;100(6):521–2.
3. Zhang L, Xu H, Cai ZG, et al. Clinical and anatomic study on the ducts of the submandibular and sublingual glands. J Oral Maxillofac Surg. 2010;68(3):606–10. https://doi.org/10.1016/j.joms.2009.03.068.
4. Ab Rahim NAC, Liew YT, Ghauth S, Narayanan P, Abu BZ. A single institution cadaveric study on anatomical variation of the sublingual gland duct. Indian J Otolaryngol Head Neck Surg. 2023;75:347–51. https://doi.org/10.1007/s12070-022-03261-4.
5. Nathan H, Luchansky E. Sublingual gland herniation through the mylohyoid muscle. Oral Surg Oral Med Oral Pathol. 1985;59(1):21–3. https://doi.org/10.1016/0030-4220(85)90109-4.
6. Engel JD, Harn SD, Cohen DM. Mylohyoid herniation: gross and histologic evaluation with clinical correlation. Oral Surg Oral Med Oral Pathol. 1987;63(1):55–9. https://doi.org/10.1016/0030-4220(87)90340-9.
7. Harrison JD. Modern management and pathophysiology of ranula: literature review. Head Neck. 2010;32(10):1310–20. https://doi.org/10.1002/hed.21326.

8. Chen CJ, Guo P, Chen XY. Recurrent sublingual ranula or saliva leakage from the submandibular gland? Anatomical consideration of the ductal system of the sublingual gland. J Oral Maxillofac Surg. 2015;73(4):675.e1–7. https://doi.org/10.1016/j.joms.2014.10.012.

9. Zhao YF, Jia Y, Chen XM, Zhang WF. Clinical review of 580 ranulas. Oral Surg Oral Med Oral Pathol Oral Radiol Endod. 2004;98(3):281–7. https://doi.org/10.1016/S1079210404000800.

10. Yang Y, Hong K. Surgical results of the intraoral approach for plunging ranula. Acta Otolaryngol. 2014;134(2):201–5. https://doi.org/10.3109/00016489.2013.831481.

11. Lee DH, Yoon TM, Lee JK, Lim SC. Treatment outcomes of the intraoral approach for a simple ranula. Oral Surg Oral Med Oral Pathol Oral Radiol. 2015;119(4):e223–5. https://doi.org/10.1016/j.oooo.2015.01.007.

12. Zhao YF, Jia J, Jia Y. Complications associated with surgical management of ranulas. J Oral Maxillofac Surg. 2005;63(1):51–4. https://doi.org/10.1016/j.joms.2004.02.018.

13. Baurmash HD. Mucoceles and ranulas. J Oral Maxillofac Surg. 2003;61(3):369–78. https://doi.org/10.1053/joms.2003.50074.

14. McGurk M. Management of the ranula. J Oral Maxillofac Surg. 2007;65(1):115–6. https://doi.org/10.1016/j.joms.2006.05.033.

15. Baurmash HD. Treating oral ranula: another case against blanket removal of the sublingual gland. Br J Oral Maxillofac Surg. 2001;39(3):217–20. https://doi.org/10.1054/bjom.2000.0606.

16. McGurk M, Eyeson J, Thomas B, Harrison JD. Conservative treatment of oral ranula by excision with minimal excision of the sublingual gland: histological support for a traumatic etiology. J Oral Maxillofac Surg. 2008;66(10):2050–7. https://doi.org/10.1016/j.joms.2008.01.019.

17. Than JK, Rosenberg TL, Anand G, Sitton M. The importance of sublingual gland removal in treatment of ranulas: a large retrospective study. Am J Otolaryngol. 2020;41(3):102418. https://doi.org/10.1016/j.amjoto.2020.102418.

18. Olojede ACO, Ogundana OM, Emeka CI, et al. Plunging ranula: surgical management of case series and the literature review. Clin Case Rep. 2017;6(1):109–14. Published 2017 Nov 29. https://doi.org/10.1002/ccr3.1272.

19. Domaneschi C, Maurício AR, Modolo F, Migliari DA. Idiopathic hyperplasia of the sublingual glands in totally or partially edentulous individuals. Oral Surg Oral Med Oral Pathol Oral Radiol Endod. 2007;103(3):374–7. https://doi.org/10.1016/j.tripleo.2006.04.012.

20. Sá JC, Tolentino Ede S, Azevedo-Alanis LR, Iwaki Filho L, Lara VS, Damante JH. Morphology and morphometry of the human sublingual glands in mouth floor enlargements of edentulous patients. J Appl Oral Sci. 2013;21(6):540–6. https://doi.org/10.1590/1679-775720130342.

21. Campos LA. Hyperplasia of the sublingual glands in adult patients. Oral Surg Oral Med Oral Pathol Oral Radiol Endod. 1996;81(5):584–5. https://doi.org/10.1016/s1079-2104(96)80052-7.

22. Iwaki Filho L, Damante JH, Consolaro A, Bonachela WC, Damante CA. Mouth floor enlargements related to the sublingual glands in edentulous or partially edentulous patients: a microscopic study. J Appl Oral Sci. 2006;14(4):264–9. https://doi.org/10.1590/s1678-77572006000400010.

23. Yilmaz M, Karaman E, Isildak H, Enver O, Kilic F. Symptomatic unilateral submandibular gland aplasia associated with ipsilateral sublingual gland hypertrophy. Dysphagia. 2010;25(1):70–2. https://doi.org/10.1007/s00455-009-9238-8.

24. Herrera-Calvo G, García-Montesinos-Perea B, Saiz-Bustillo R, Gallo-Terán J, Lastra-García-Barón P. Unilateral submandibular gland aplasia with ipsilateral sublingual gland hypertrophy presenting as a neck mass. Med Oral Patol Oral Cir Bucal. 2011;16(4):e537–40. Published 2011 Jul 1. https://doi.org/10.4317/medoral.16.e537.

25. Chung J, Lee YW. Functional compensation of a hypertrophied sublingual gland and the absence of the ipsilateral submandibular gland. Br J Oral Maxillofac Surg. 2019;57(8):813–6. https://doi.org/10.1016/j.bjoms.2019.06.019.

26. Tatsis D, Mantevas A, Kilmpasani M, Karafoulidou I, Venetis G. Unilateral submandibular gland aplasia with ipsilateral sublingual ranula—a case report. Ann Maxillofac Surg. 2020;10(2):543–6. https://doi.org/10.4103/ams.ams_63_20.

27. Sher ZA, Tan G. Unilateral sublingual salivary gland hypertrophy with herniation through a boutonniére defect and contralateral sublingual gland hypoplasia. BJR Case Rep. 2016;2(3):20150382. Published 2016 Jul 28. https://doi.org/10.1259/bjrcr.20150382.
28. Taji SS, Savage N, Holcombe T, Khan F, Seow WK. Congenital aplasia of the major salivary glands: literature review and case report. Pediatr Dent. 2011;33(2):113–8.
29. Yerli H. Dynamic sonography and CT findings of unilateral submandibular gland agenesis associated with herniated hypertrophic sublingual gland. J Clin Ultrasound. 2014;42(3):176–9. https://doi.org/10.1002/jcu.22072.

Chapter 18
Minor Salivary Glands

Louis Mandel

Abstract The minor salivary glands are an integral part of the salivary gland complex. Their dispersion throughout the oral cavity makes them subject to a variety of pathologic insults. It is not unusual for a minor salivary gland to reflect pathologic changes in association with a disease process that involves the major salivary glands. The presence of these pathologic changes in a minor salivary gland has been recognized and utilized as key or adjunctive aids in attaining a definitive diagnosis of a systemic disease process. The role of the labial salivary gland biopsy in attaining the diagnosis of some systemic diseases is highlighted. It is the availability and accessibility of the labial salivary gland that makes it the prime subject for histologic examination via a biopsy. In addition, the clinician should be aware that there are several pathologic processes that primarily target the minor glands (mucocele, necrotizing sialometaplasia).

Introduction

The minor salivary glands (MSGs) develop in the third month of fetal life, and with the exception of the anterior hard palate, gingiva, and dorsum of the tongue, they can be found scattered throughout the oral cavity. Approximately 800–1000 MSGs [1], lacking true capsules, exist as individual nodules, with each MSG nodule measuring 1.0–2.0 mm in diameter. The MSGs are located submucosally and fixed in position by the surrounding submucosal connective tissue [2]. Their secretions, amounting to approximately 10% of the total salivary secretions, are delivered directly into the oral cavity by short ducts that open onto the surface mucosa immediately above the glandular nodule.

Each MSG usually consists mostly of mucous cells with some serous demilunes. However, some are composed completely of serous cells (von Ebner), and on occasion a mixed pattern of mucous and serous cells (Blandin-Nuhn) may be observed.

L. Mandel, *Clinical Management of Salivary Gland Disorders,*
https://doi.org/10.1007/978-3-031-50012-1_18

The MSG secretions play a critical role in the protection, by secreting high concentrations of immunoglobulin A [3], and lubrication of the oral mucosa. These glands are also the mainstay of secretions during sleep and are involved in the development of the dental biofilm. Their saliva, consisting essentially of water, ions, and proteins [4], is secreted by groupings of mucous and groupings of serous cells circularly arranged around a central lumen. Tapered mucous cells, in clusters of 8–12 cells, congregate to form individual spherical acini. The broad base of each mucous cell rests peripherally on a basement membrane. The narrowed opposite end of the cell abuts the lumen into which the cellular secretions are deposited. The nuclei of the mucous cells are displaced to the cell's base and are flattened by the accumulation of intracellular mucigen [5]. The centrally located acinar lumen normally contains secreted viscous mucin.

Pyramid-shaped serous cells, with dark round nuclei centrally positioned in the cytoplasm, also are deployed in acinar groupings of 8–12 cells. Serous cells contain a multitude of highly refractive apically located zymogen granules that are the precursors of amylase. The serous cell produces an aqueous amylase containing secretion that is delivered into the acinar lumen. The lumen of the serous acini tends to be smaller in diameter than that seen in mucous acini, probably reflecting the ease of transporting an aqueous rather than a viscous secretion.

MSGs display a ductal system similar to the major glands, but with shorter tracts [6, 7] because of their very superficial anatomic location. Intercalated ducts serve as the initial duct secretory transport route from the acinar lumen to the oral cavity. The intercalated ducts may harbor pluripotential cells that produce replacement cells [7]. The intralobular (striated) duct, a continuation of the smaller intercalated duct, functions to regulate secretions and electrolytes. The terminal collecting ducts serve to reabsorb ions from the saliva as the saliva makes its way to the oral cavity and exits on mucosal pores. The movement of MSG secretions to the oral cavity is facilitated by contractile myoepithelial cells. The myoepithelial cell is characterized by spider-like tentacles resting on the periphery of the acinar's basement membrane [8]. Upon contraction, they function to move cellular secretions through the duct system to the oral cavity.

Although the MSGs are dispersed in the oral cavity, their deployments in distinct locations where they serve unique functions have led to their identification with eponyms that honor their discoverer: Weber, von Ebner, and Blandin-Nuhn. Weber's mucous glands are found in close relation to the moats surrounding lingual tonsillar nodules. Here, their secretions function to flush and cleanse the tonsillar crypts. In juxtaposition to the taste buds located on circumvallate and foliate papillae, von Ebner's serous glands produce secretions that carry food's chemical tastants to the taste buds. On the anterior ventral surface of the tongue, an array of mixed serous and mucous glands, the glands of Blandin-Nuhn (BN), are located on either side of the midline. Their seromucous secretions, co-mingled with the secretions of all MSGs, participate in the maintenance of oral health. Because of BN's location and proximity to the incisal edges of the mandibular anterior teeth, these ventrally positioned tongue glands are often subjected to trauma and mucocele formation.

As with all tissues, the MSGs are subject to pathologic insult. There are several primary disease processes that home in on these minor glands. It is these primary conditions that this chapter will highlight. In addition, the role of the MSG biopsy in the diagnosis of existing systemic diseases that have pathologic manifestations in the MSG will be briefly reviewed.

Labial Mucocele

Numerous minor salivary glands (MSGs) scattered throughout the oral cavity are located superficially just beneath the overlying oral mucosa. Their location, particularly in the lower lip, makes the ducts of these mucous glands susceptible to trauma with resulting duct lacerations. Extravasation of secretions from a ruptured duct into the surrounding connective tissue will lead to the development of an extravasation mucocele (ME) (Fig. 18.1a). Alternatively, duct obstruction from scar tissue, foreign body, or even a sialolith can cause mucus retention and the much rarer mucus retention cyst (MR). Both the ME and MR will cause classic soft localized fluid filled swellings, the oral mucocele, that predominantly involve the lower and upper lips, respectively.

The oral mucocele is not an uncommon lesion, with a reported prevalence of 2.5 per 1000 individuals and is seen equally in both sexes [9]. The ME occurs most frequently in the 15- to 24-year age group, while the rarer MR variety tends to affect older patients [9]. Although the ME mostly affects the lower lip, it can also involve the buccal mucosa, retromolar area, upper lip, and mouth floor. The increased incidence in lower lip ME occurrence is a reflection of the lower lip's susceptibility to trauma during mastication, as well as its obvious exposure to external offending irritating factors.

Mucoceles have a sudden onset and are self-limiting. They are superficially placed, painless, fairly well-circumscribed fluid-filled soft lesions with a bluish tinge. The commonly observed blue discoloration is due to the Tyndall effect, a light scattering phenomenon caused by colloidal suspensions such as the mucus in the mucocele [10]. Clinically, the mucocele usually measures from a few millimeters to 1.5 cm in diameter [9], but most approximately 1 cm. Interference with mastication and speech can develop and obviously is dependent upon size and location of the mucocele. Mucoceles often have a clinical history of rupturing spontaneously, collapsing, and then recurring. The duration of the mucocele can vary from a few days to several years [9].

The ME undergoes three developmental phases [11]. Initially, mucus secretions exit from a leaking duct and infiltrate diffusely into the surrounding connective tissues. Subsequently, a second phase develops with the formation of a limiting granulation tissue barrier (Fig. 18.1e). With the passage of time, the third phase manifests itself with the body's attempt to localize and even absorb the extravasated mucus. A pseudo-encapsulation by a fibrous tissue wall will evolve as the body's defensive mechanisms strive to isolate the fluid extravasation (Fig. 18.2).

Clinically, the appearance of the uncommon MR mimics the ME. However, the MR tends to be seen in the upper lip and even in the palate and cheek of older individuals [9]. Histologically, the MR mucocele is considered a true cyst because it is lined by a well-developed epithelial wall derived from the duct epithelium. It is the absence of this cystic epithelial wall in the ME that differentiates the ME from the MR.

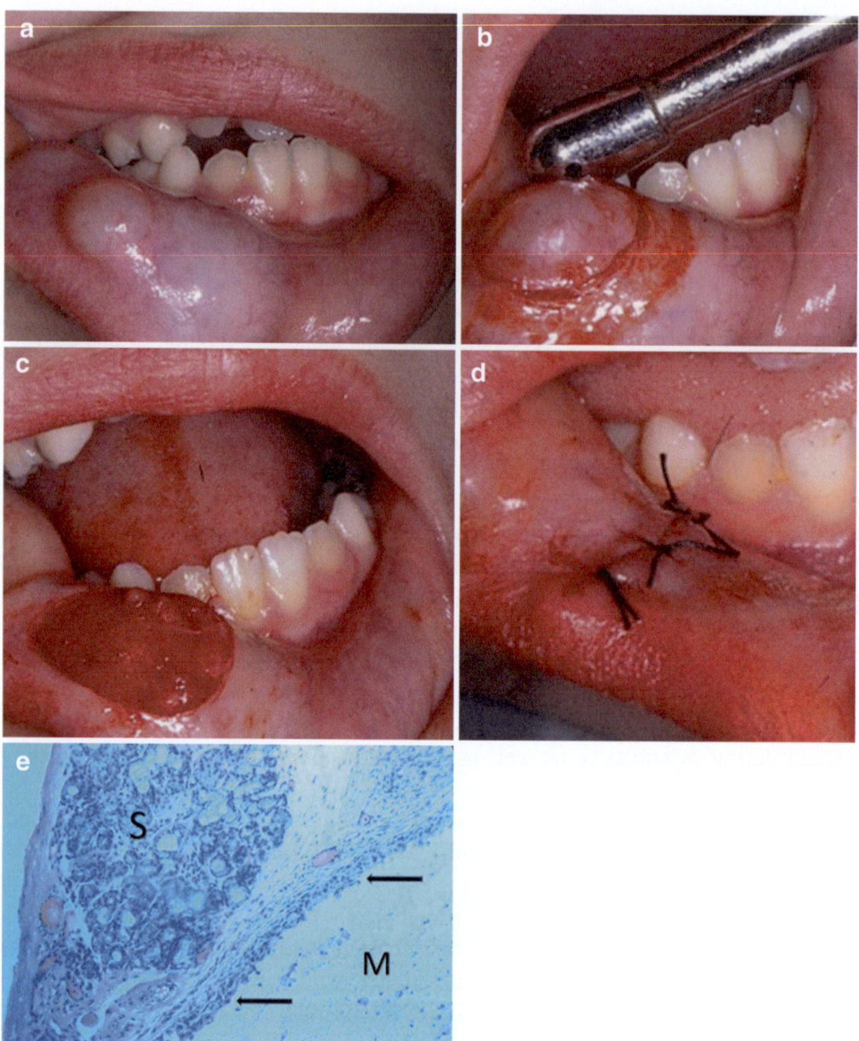

Fig. 18.1 (**a**) Labial mucocele. Patient A (Zeng Q, et al. NYS Dent J 2019;85:42). (**b**) Labial mucocele. Patient A. Circumscribing incision (Zeng Q, et al. NYS Dent J 2019;85:42). (**c**) Labial mucocele. Patient A. Exposure of orbicularis oris muscle after mucocele excision (Zeng Q, et al. NYS Dent J 2019;85:42). (**d**) Labial mucocele. Patient A. Sutures placed to close surgical wound (Zeng Q, et al. NYS Dent J 2019;85:42). (**e**) Labial mucocele. Microscopic view. Minor salivary gland (S) Mucocele cavity (M). Granulation tissue wall (arrows)

Several therapeutic regimens have been proposed for mucocele treatment, but surgical intervention remains the treatment most often employed [12]. Removal of the common labially located mucocele is best accomplished by surgically circumscribing the lesion via a mucosal incision that extends down to the underlying orbicularis oris muscle. Dissection of the circumscribed ME is then performed using the orbicularis oris muscle layer as an anatomic cleavage plane (Fig. 18.1). Care must be taken to avoid the labial filaments of the mental nerve. These nerve fibers lie on the surface of the orbicularis oris muscle just beneath and/or alongside the mucocele. Surgical trauma to a nerve filament will lead to paresthesia/anesthesia of that segment of the lower lip to which the filament supplies sensory fibers. Another complication that can arise is damage to an adjacent MSG duct which then can cause another mucocele.

Attempts to bluntly dissect the ME in toto are usually met with failure (Fig. 18.3). It must be remembered that the ME has only a granulation tissue wall rather than the well-defined epithelial wall seen in cysts (Fig. 18.1e). The occasional success that is achieved with blunt dissection tends to originate from a ME that has been present for a prolonged period (Fig. 18.2). The passage of time has given the body's defense mechanisms the opportunity to form a well-defined fibrous capsular wall around the ME. It is this fibrous walling-off process that facilitates successful in toto dissection.

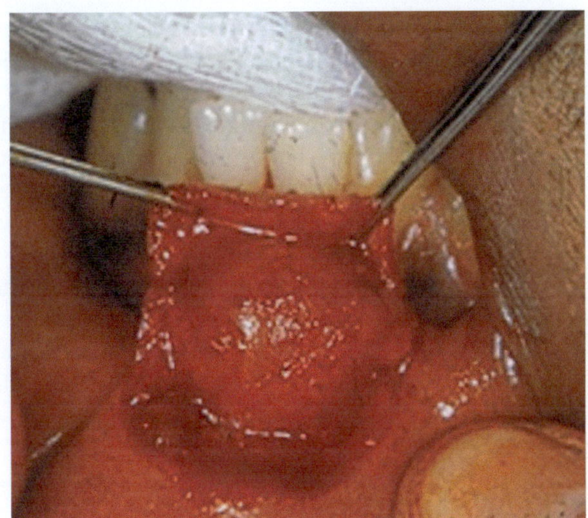

Fig. 18.2 Labial mucocele. Patient B. Successful blunt dissection of 7 months old mucocele (Zeng Q, et al. NYS Dent J 2019;85:42)

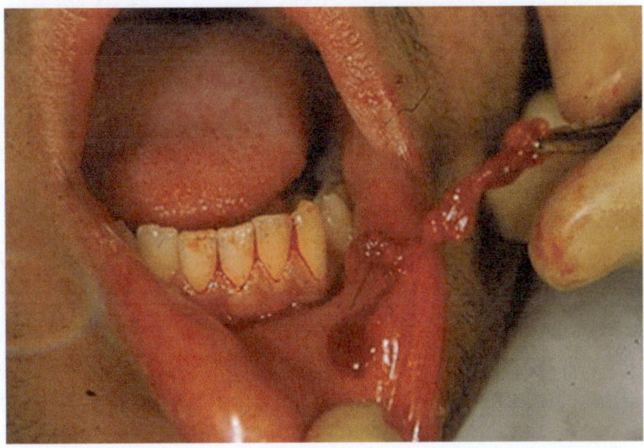

Fig. 18.3 Labial mucocele. Patient C. Collapsed mucocele after attempted blunt dissection (Zeng Q, et al. NYS Dent J 2019;85:42)

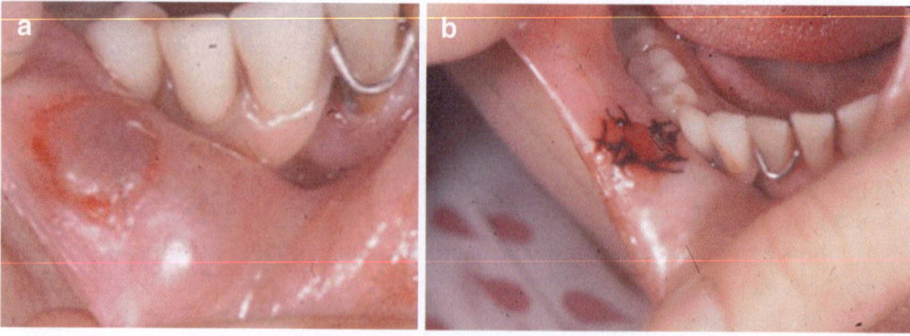

Fig. 18.4 (**a**) Labial mucocele. Patient D. Marsupialization. Unroofing of mucocele (Zeng Q, et al. NYS Dent J 2019;85:42). (**b**) Labial mucocele. Patient D. Suturing of marsupialized mucocele (Zeng Q, et al. NYS Dent J 2019;85:42)

Surgical marsupialization represents another surgical approach used in the treatment of the ME (Fig. 18.4) [13]. The technique is simple because it involves only the removal of the roofing mucosa and allows the surgically exposed ME granulation tissue floor to epithelialize. Because the removal of the ME's causative MSG is not achieved, recurrence rates for marsupialization are high. Nevertheless, the technique, with its relatively high recurrence rate, is recommended for those large mucoceles whose surgical excision will be traumatic and disfiguring. If a failure occurs with marsupialization, success can be attained with a second attempt utilizing a standard surgical excision.

The use of sclerosing agents (OK-432 [14], sodium tetradecyl sulfate [15], polidocanol [16]), has been reported to represent a successful nonsurgical therapy for the treatment of a mucocele. Cryotherapy and lasers have also been advocated for the care of the mucocele [9, 13].

Superficial Mucocele

The superficial mucocele (SM), first described by Eveson [17], is a variant of the classic oral mucocele and has an unknown etiology. Clinically, the SMs are seen as small discrete painless tense translucent, solitary, or multiple vesicle-like nodules (Fig. 18.5) that spontaneously appear, rupture, heal within a few days, and then recur unpredictably at varying time intervals. The ruptured vesicles expose erosive bases that cause a mild discomfort which is relieved by the rapid healing that ensues. These small mucin-filled vesicles, measuring 1–4 mm in diameter, tend to occur in crops. They usually involve a non-inflamed normal-appearing mucosa of the soft palate and occasionally the retromolar pad or buccal mucosa, locations where trauma is an unlikely etiological factor. The SM most commonly occurs in single locations but can be present simultaneously in the multiple oral cavity sites that harbor minor salivary glands. Women 30 years and older [18–20] are most likely to develop the

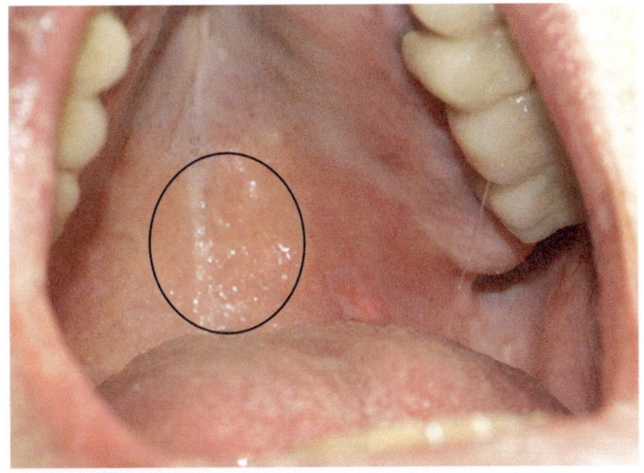

Fig. 18.5 Superficial mucoceles posterior palate (circled)

condition, which clinically has often been misdiagnosed as pemphigoid or bullous lichen planus [21]. However, the bullae in these two entities are large, flaccid, and opaque rather than the small, tense, and translucent vesicles seen in the SM [22].

Microscopically, the SM forms just below the surface epithelium where it cleaves a space for itself at the interface between the overlying mucosal epithelial surface and the underlying connective tissue (Fig. 18.6). There is no evidence of a continued active extension of this subepithelial separation at the lesion's periphery. The SM is mostly surrounded by mucosal epithelium that is represented by a thinned epithelial layer visible along its roof. A connective tissue barrier serves as the limiting floor of the SM. This confining connective tissue wall is usually infiltrated by a chronic inflammatory response reminiscent of that seen in lichen planus (LP). The well-defined cavity of the SM contains a pool of amorphous mucin and a scattering of lymphocytes. Ducts of adjacent minor salivary glands are often seen in the immediate vicinity of the SM.

Diagnosis of the SM can readily be attained from recognition of its clinical signs and symptoms. Therefore, surgical biopsy for diagnostic purposes is unnecessary. Although the etiology of the SM is in doubt, a clinical association with oral LP has been observed in SM patients [23]. Furthermore, SMs have also been reported to be present in many graft-versus-host disease patients with many of these patients exhibiting lichenoid signs (Fig. 7.21) [23, 24]. These observed relationships of LP and lichenoid lesions to the SM lend credence to the theory that mucosal epithelial changes and/or the subepithelial inflammatory infiltrates associated with LP and lichenoid changes may initiate the salivary duct obstruction and rupture that leads to mucus extravasation and SM formation [23, 25].

With no defined etiology established, effective treatment has been hindered. Because SMs are recurrent and can cause discomfort, surgical excision, laser vaporization, and cryotherapy [18] are therapeutic procedures that have been recommended. However, because they are self-limiting and relatively asymptomatic, monitoring, tinctured with reassurance, is always a viable option.

Fig. 18.6 Superficial
mucocele beneath oral
mucosa (E).
Microscopic view

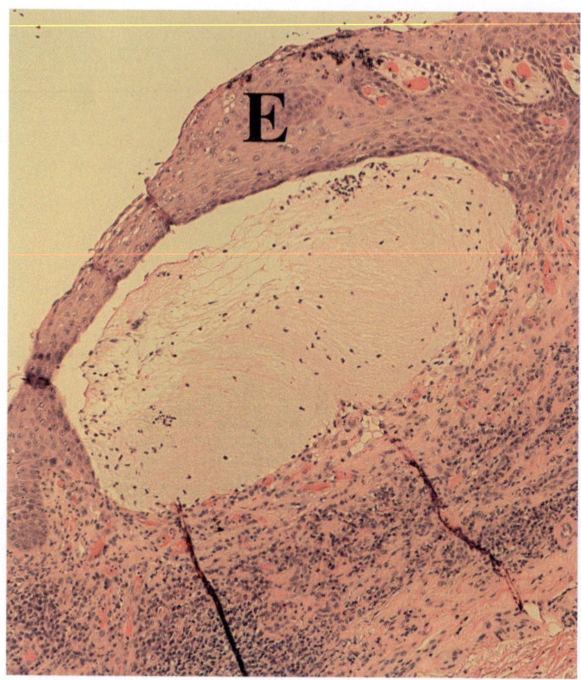

Mucocele of Glands of Blandin-Nuhn

The glands of Blandin-Nuhn (BN) are mixed mucous and serous glands that are anatomically located bilaterally in the anterior ventral aspect of the tongue. These glands are situated just beneath an overlying thin mucosa and are considered part of the minor salivary gland complex. They extend laterally and posteriorly in a longitudinal fashion. Combined bilaterally, they mimic a horseshoe configuration. The open end of the horseshoe faces posteriorly toward the tongue root. The longitudinal section of the horseshoe measures approximately 12–25 mm anteroposteriorly and has a width of approximately 8 mm [26]. Each lateral segment of the horseshoe has 5–7 small ducts exiting from individual lobes with their orifices medial to the plica fimbriata and lateral to the lingual frenum.

It is not unusual for mucoceles to originate from the BN (Fig. 18.7). Young females seem to be more susceptible to its development, with most lesions occurring in the first two decades of life [27]. However, older males have also been victimized. Epidemiological studies indicate that the incidence of BN mucoceles ranges from 2 to 8% of all mucoceles [28]; thus, it should not be considered a rarity.

The mucoceles of BN occur in a tongue area that is subject to trauma. The constant motion of the tongue during mastication, speech, or from a thrusting habit exposes its ventral surface to dental trauma from the mandibular incisors. Duct laceration with extravasation of secretions, as is seen in the more frequently observed labial mucocele, is the end result. As with the relatively common labial mucocele,

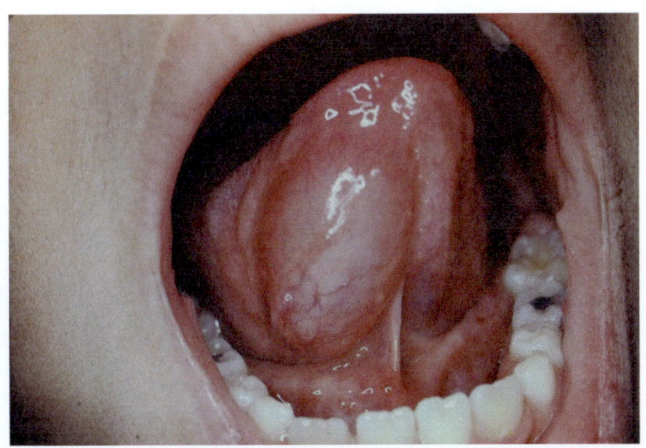

Fig. 18.7 Mucocele of gland of Blandin-Nuhn

the fluid leakage excites an inflammatory response with the formation of a granulation tissue wall [29].

Most mucoceles of BN are observed as longitudinal swellings, lateral and parallel to the ventral tongue's midline. Despite the small size of the gland, the long axis of the mucocele that forms can be quite extensive. Nevertheless, many will involve the midline and tend to be polypoid in shape [30]. Clinically, they replicate the signs and symptomatology of the labial mucocele. Asymptomatic fluid-containing soft and fairly well-circumscribed painless blue tinted lesions are tell-tale diagnostic signs. Because of their location and continued exposure to trauma during tongue movements, they are inclined to rupture, only to heal and recur.

Because BN mucoceles represent extravasation phenomena, they do not have an epithelial lining. Rather than a well-defined epithelial wall, a granulation tissue wall surrounding escaped fluid makes the removal via blunt in toto dissection a demanding and practically impossible challenge. Cryotherapy, lasers, sclerosing agents, and intralesional injections of cortisone have been therapeutically advocated. Nevertheless, a circumscribed surgical excision, facilitated by its superficial location, has proven to be the option of choice. Removal of the BN mucocele en bloc, down to the underlying muscle base, is required. Care must be taken to avoid the lingual vein and filaments of the lingual nerve.

Sialolithiasis

Sialolithiasis, calcific deposits within the ductal system of a salivary gland, has usually been reported as a clinical entity that affects a major salivary gland. Various statistical incidences have been noted indicating that approximately 80–90% of the sialoliths involve the submandibular salivary gland, 6–19% the parotid gland, and most of the remainder occurring in the sublingual salivary or minor salivary glands (MSG), with only 2% reported to occur in a MSG [31]. When considering MSG sialoliths, the upper lip is most often implicated with decreasing occurrences of

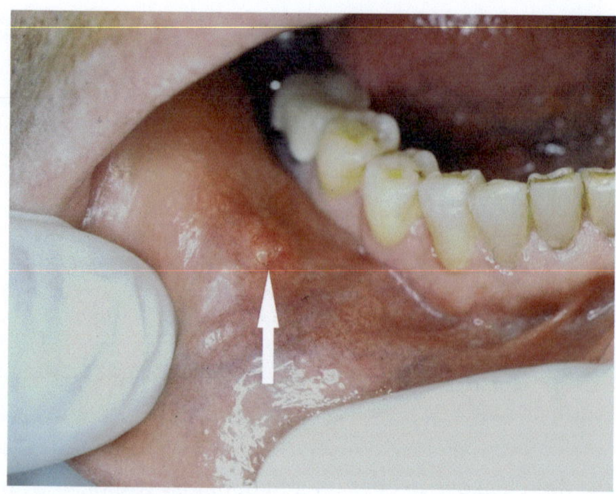

Fig. 18.8 Sialolithiasis has caused nodular swelling in lower lip (arrow)

MSG sialoliths in the buccal mucosa and lower lip (Fig. 18.8). The incidence of MSG sialolithiasis is higher in males, with the sialolithiasis most frequently occurring in the sixth decade of life [31].

A precise etiology for sialolith formation in the MSG has not been determined. However, it is believed that initially an irritant, such as invading bacteria, foreign body, or trauma, causes duct inflammation with intraluminal shedding of cellular debris, which results in a nidus that narrows and blocks the lumen. Salivary flow is impeded, and the resulting stasis then allows for the precipitation of salts that function to form the sialolith [32].

Clinically, the MSG containing a sialolith is noted to be a firm movable nodule that elevates a usually normal-appearing overlying mucosa. Pain becomes an issue only when secondary infection develops. A suppurative discharge will then become visible at the ostium of the MSG. Most MSG sialoliths are small, measuring 1–2 mm, but can approach 5 mm in size [32]. At times, multiple sialoliths are present in the MSG and occasionally the sialolith is spontaneously delivered into the oral cavity [33].

Diagnosis of a MSG sialolith is challenging because of a lack of specific clinical symptoms. Imaging can be unreliable because the sialolith is small and often radiographically undetectable due to its poor calcification. A soft tissue radiograph, using a low radiation dose, may be a diagnostic help (Fig. 4.20b). Demonstration of the calcific body aids in clinically differentiating the nodular lesion from a neoplasm or mucocele. Final and definitive diagnosis awaits a microscopic examination that reveals the sialolith with its associated glandular changes.

Histologically, a calcific body will be seen located in a dilated duct (Fig. 4.21). The ductal epithelium surrounding the sialolith often demonstrates a squamous metaplasia [34]. Chronic inflammation and acinar atrophy, reflecting the presence of a MSG sialadenitis, can also be observed. If infection has developed secondary to sialolith obstruction, manifestations of an acute inflammatory process with suppuration will be evident.

Because the culpable MSG nodule is localized and movable, a simple circumscribing surgical excision, using the underlying musculature as a dissecting plane, is the therapeutic approach of choice.

Stomatitis Nicotina

Smoking is a worldwide health problem that is responsible for high levels of mortality and morbidity. Although tobacco use contributes to many systemic pathologic conditions, it also has a local harmful effect that can be observed in the oral cavity and includes the minor salivary glands (MSG). Prolonged use of any tobacco smoking product, whether it be pipe smoking, cigars, or cigarettes, will lead to oral mucosal and palatal gland changes. The most common form of tobacco use is the cigarette. Patients who smoke at least 15 cigarettes each day for many years are the ones most likely to develop the signs of stomatitis nicotina (SN) of the palate from the effects of the heat associated with smoking [35]. Direct contact of high-temperature smoke, not the exposure to the chemical irritants in smoke, leads to the pathologic changes associated with SN.

SN, a not uncommon pathologic condition involving the hard palate, is more often observed in pipe and cigar users rather than cigarette smokers because the pipe and cigar generate more heat to affect the palate. During smoke inhalation, the temperature in the oral cavity reaches 190 °C [36]. This interior oral heat induces an inflammatory reaction that leads to both hyperkeratinization of the palatal mucosal epithelium and palatal gland inflammation. Similar changes have been noted in individuals who frequently drink extremely hot beverages. Confirmation of the deleterious effect of smoking can be derived from the fact that when the hard palate in smokers is partially covered by a removable prosthesis, there will be signs of SN on the exposed areas of the palate, but none beneath the protective prosthetic appliance. Further confirmation of heat's role can be derived from the fact that oral heat is intensified in individuals who reverse smoke. More severe epithelial changes, with progression to epithelial dysplasia or carcinoma, tend to occur in these reverse smokers [37].

Clinically, SN is an asymptomatic visible lesion that starts as an erythematous area. With long-term heat exposure, the mucosa eventually takes on a gray/white discoloration reflecting the development of hyperkeratosis (Fig. 18.9a). Acanthosis may also be present [35], but dysplasia is not usually observed in SN. In later stages, numerous slightly elevated papules, representing hyperplasia of the underlying palatal mucous glands, develop in response to the chronic thermal irritation (Fig. 18.9a). Few papular changes are noted in the soft palate or anterior third of the hard palate because these areas have decreased numbers of MSG. Each elevated papule commonly has a central depressed visible red dot representing the underlying palatal gland's inflamed duct orifice. Chronic inflammation from heat also causes a squamous metaplasia of the gland's duct wall and a subepithelial inflammatory infiltrate (Fig. 18.9b, c). Melanin deposition, a protective reaction to heat exposure, often is seen in the basal epithelial layer and the lamina propria [38].

Fig. 18.9 (**a**) Stomatitis nicotina. Patient E. Palatal hyperkeratinization, elevated nodules of palatal glands, and red inflamed duct orifices are clinically visible. (**b**) Stomatitis nicotina. Patient E. Palatal mucous gland (**a**) and metaplasia of duct epithelium (**b**). Low-power microscopic view. (**c**) Stomatitis nicotina. Patient E. Periductal chronic inflammatory cell infiltration (arrows). High power microscopic view

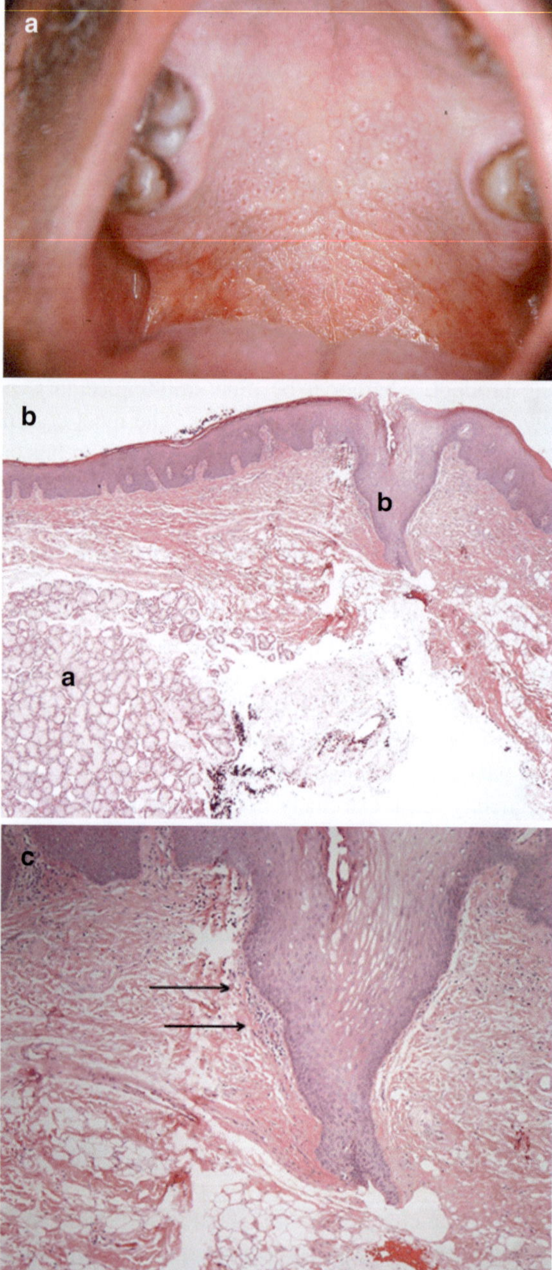

The diagnosis of SN is based upon the clinical history, location, appearance, and absence of subjective symptoms. Because the condition is readily recognizable and reversible with the cessation of smoking, biopsies are not indicated to demonstrate the microscopic features of SN for diagnostic substantiation. If remission of the clinical picture of SN does not materialize after 1–2 months of smoking cessation, the presence or absence of more serious tissue alterations must be determined via further investigation.

Once the patient stops smoking, any existing hyperkeratosis and acanthosis that are present regress and are replaced by a normal epithelial histology. The papules which represent hyperplastic palatal glands will also recede as these glands recover from the thermal effects of smoking. As can be anticipated, the inflamed red orifices of the ducts of the palatine mucous glands will also visually disappear with the loss of the thermal irritant's inflammatory effect.

Upon reaching a confident clinical diagnosis of SN, the patient must be impressed with the need to stop smoking. In addition, a follow-up visit is mandatory in order to ascertain the return to normality of the palatal tissues. If no significant improvement has occurred, a tissue specimen should be obtained via a surgical biopsy. Never forget, epithelial dysplasia or even a malignancy is always a lurking threat and demands appropriate aggressive therapeutic measures.

Necrotizing Sialometaplasia

Necrotizing sialometaplasia (NS) is a localized benign ulcerative lesion that can occur in any area harboring salivary gland tissue. Although it can develop in a major salivary gland, larynx, tongue, retromolar trigone, or buccal mucosa, NS most commonly involves the minor salivary glands (MSG) in the posterior hard palate (Fig. 18.10). There seems to be a gender predilection regarding NS that favors males, with the average age for occurrence being 49 years [39]. NS is a relatively

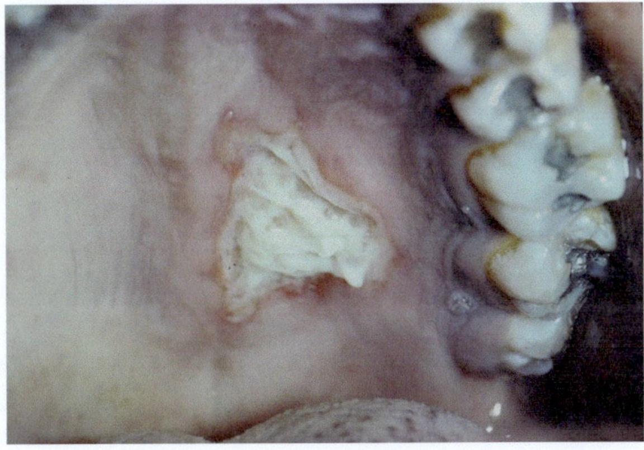

Fig. 18.10 Necrotizing sialometaplasia. Clinical view of hard palate ulcer

uncommon lesion whose significance rests in the fact that it may be misdiagnosed as a manifestation of a mucoepidermoid or a squamous cell carcinoma.

The blood supply to the MSGs of the hard palate is mainly provided through the greater palatine artery. Events that compromise this vessel's vascular nourishment to the palatine mucous glands have been accepted as the causative factor in the onset of NS. Systemic and local factors can affect vascularity and lead to ischemia, infarction, and ulcer formation. Causative systemic conditions that alter vascularity encompass atherosclerosis, diabetes, sickle cell anemia, Buerger's disease, and autoimmune problems that include vasculitis [39]. The blood supply can also be compromised by local factors such as local injections that contain a vasoconstrictor, trauma from a prosthesis, cocaine use, alcohol, and thermal irritations from the use of tobacco [40, 41]. Although an association of NS with bulimia has been recognized, a cause has not been clearly defined [40, 42].

A prodromal sign of numbness, probably caused by the initial ischemia of the involved area, is often experienced. Initially, the NS begins visually as an erythematous swelling which rapidly ulcerates. Clinically, a large ulcer 1.0–3.0 cm in diameter develops. Despite the ulcer's size and the possibility of palatal bone exposure, subjective pain can be mild. Sharp erythematous non-indurated margins surround the ulcer. The ulcer is self-limiting in extent, and spontaneous healing by secondary intention takes place within 6–12 weeks. The palatal NS is usually unilateral in its presentation, but occasionally it can manifest itself bilaterally.

The linchpin for a confident NS diagnosis is obtaining multiple serial sections of a biopsied specimen. An accurate histologic diagnosis can then be based on microscopically observing the maintenance of the general globular configuration of the preexisting salivary gland lobules (Fig. 18.11). Squamous epithelial metaplasia of the ducts, acinar atrophy, and varying amounts of a nonspecific chronic inflammation are also present [43].

Because the ulcer rapidly granulates and epithelializes spontaneously, only palliative care is indicated. Analgesics can be prescribed if pain is an issue. Good oral hygiene must be maintained. The key element in the management of NS is to side-step a misdiagnosis in view of the ulcer's clinical similarity to a malignancy.

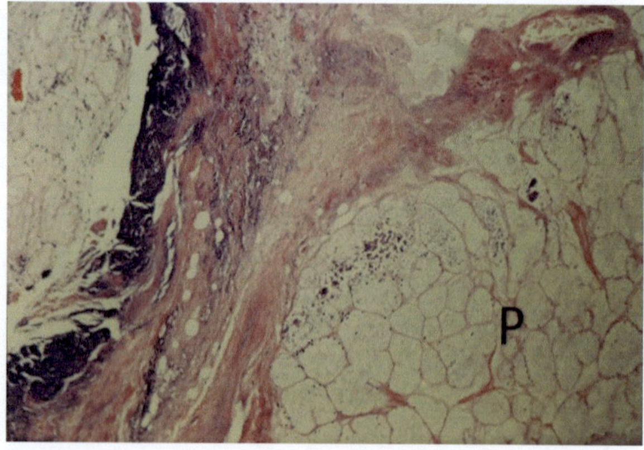

Fig. 18.11 Necrotizing sialometaplasia. Microscopic view. Globular configuration of pre-existing palatal gland (P) is maintained

Cheilitis Glandularis

Cheilitis glandularis (CG) is a poorly understood rare inflammatory condition that usually involves the surface mucosa of the lower lip vermilion and the underlying labial salivary glands (LSG). Palpation of the lip will reveal multiple submucosal nodules that represent inflamed and enlarged LSG. Occasionally, the upper lip, palate, or buccal mucosa is implicated. Varying degrees of macrocheilia with red dilated ostia of the LSG are present (Fig. 18.12). A viscous mucoid secretion can be expressed from these dilated ostia. The signs and symptoms probably result from a primary surface mucosal change that extends submucosally to cause a secondary LSG involvement. Although the etiology has not been specifically delineated, CG probably represents a chronic salivary gland reaction to a surface irritant. The irritating factor may be exposure to the sun, but wind, smoking, alcohol, and mechanical irritations may also have roles in CG development [44]. The susceptibility of fair-skinned individuals, particularly albinos, suggests that sunlight is a significant factor in the pathogenesis of CG [45].

Enlargement, eversion, and hardening of the lower lip in an adult male in the fifth to seventh decades of life [46] are the usual presenting signs. Clinically, three types of CG have been identified and may represent a progression of one type into the next [44, 47]. The simple type is recognized when palpation reveals lip induration and swollen LSG nodules. A thick mucopurulent secretion, exiting from dilated red depressed LSG ostia, can be obtained upon exerting mild pressure on the lip. The superficial suppurative variety (Baelz's disease), the second type of CG, is probably a result of pathologic extension from the simple type. Swelling and lip induration associated with a suppurative discharge from the LSGs' ostia are also evident but are more pronounced than what is present in the simple variety. Continued progression of the pathologic process is thought to lead to the deep suppurative third category of CG. This deep-seated inflammation probably represents a process that started in the lip's surface epithelium and progressed to the underlying LSGs. Significant scar formation and a copious mucopurulent discharge from the LSG's ostia are pathognomonic signs. The clinician should be aware that the deep suppurative CG has been considered to be premalignant, and the development of a

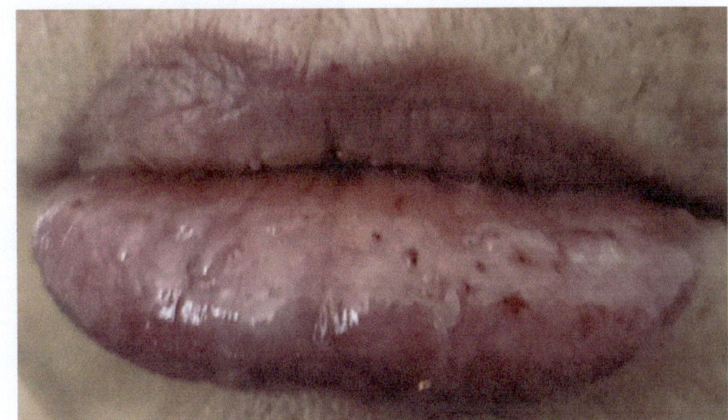

Fig. 18.12 Cheilitis glandularis (Stoopler ET, et al. JADA 2022;153:480)

squamous cell carcinoma (SCC) is a possibility [48, 49]. It is also possible that the SCC is an incidental occurrence reacting independently to chronic actinic trauma [46]. Superimposition of a significant bacterial infection can also become an issue, particularly in long-standing CG lesions [49].

Histologically, CG is characterized by the presence of a chronic LSG sialadenitis with evidence of duct ectasia and metaplasia. Mucin or a mucopurulent accumulation in the ducts can be observed. An inflammatory infiltrate and a significant fibrosis are present [46].

Conservative treatment involves the removal of all irritants, antibiotics when indicated, topical and/or intralesional steroids, and lip balms. Because of its persistent nature and malignant threat, surgical vermilionectomy has been advocated for the suppurative varieties of CG. The removal of the damaged vermilion should be accompanied by excision of all underlying swollen abnormal LSG nodules [45, 48, 49]. The excised lip mucosa can be replaced with skin grafts.

Labial Salivary Gland Biopsy

Numerous surgically accessible minor salivary glands are present in the lower lip (Figs. 18.13 and 18.14). Gentle pressure against the lower lip with the tongue readily results in feeling the presence of scattered nodules that represent the superficially positioned labial salivary glands (LSG). Each LSG, measuring 1–2 mm, is enclosed in a thin layer of connective tissue and rests on the orbicularis oris muscle. Few are located in the lip's midline with most being positioned laterally. Filaments of the mental nerve, the sensory supply of the lower lip, course just beneath and beside the individual LSG nodule, while the vascular supply (inferior labial artery) to the lip runs deep to the LSG.

As a component of the salivary gland apparatus, the LSG is subject pathologically to a variety of systemic diseases that affect the major salivary glands. Because

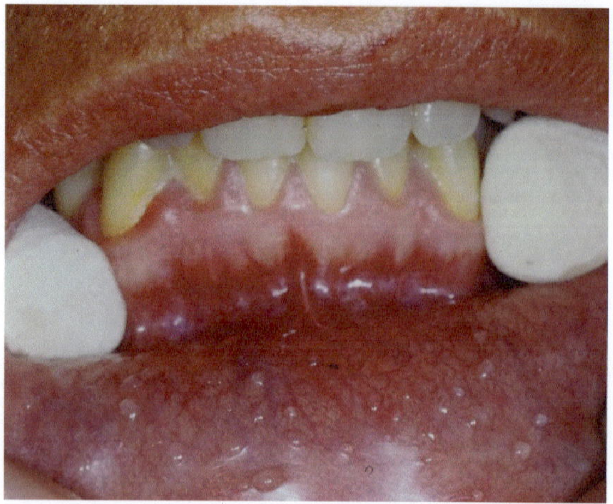

Fig. 18.13 Droplets of saliva exiting from normal labial salivary glands

Fig. 18.14 Histologic view of normal labial salivary gland

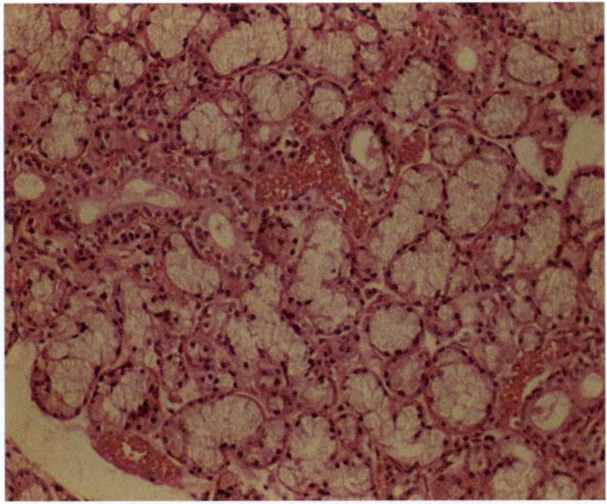

the LSG is readily accessible, biopsies are indicated to aid in the diagnosis of the associated systemic disease. The following list of systemic diseases represents conditions for which a histologic examination of a LSG specimen can serve, albeit to a limited extent, as an aid in diagnosing the causative systemic pathologic entity.

Indications

Sjögren syndrome (SS). The surgical removal of several LSG and their microscopic examination are considered crucial components in the diagnosis of Sjögren syndrome (SS) [50], an autoimmune disease. Histologically, a diagnosis of SS is made when one or more foci of mononuclear cells (mostly lymphocytes) are identified in the glandular parenchyma. A focus is defined as 50 or more mononuclear cells in a 4 mm^2 of gland tissue. One focus is consistent with a diagnosis of SS, while more than one focus is considered the gold standard for diagnosis (Fig. 18.15).

The development of non-Hodgkin's lymphoma (NHL), characterized by a B cell hyperactivity, is a known negative event associated with SS. Recent studies have underlined the diagnostic ability of the LSG biopsy in the development of an NHL originating from SS [51–53].

Sarcoidosis is a chronic systemic granulomatous disease that involves multiple organ systems, including the salivary gland complex, and is characterized by the presence of non-caseating granulomas. Diagnosis is based upon radiologic identification of distinctive lung infiltrates, mediastinal lymphadenopathy, and elevated levels of angiotensin-converting enzyme. However, a final diagnosis awaits histologic evidence obtained from a surgical biopsy of an involved structure. An LSG biopsy may have a low diagnostic yield. Nevertheless, it can demonstrate the pathognomonic non-caseating granulomas (Figs. 8.3c and 8.4c) in patients with sarcoidosis [54, 55], particularly in those patients with sarcoid uveitis.

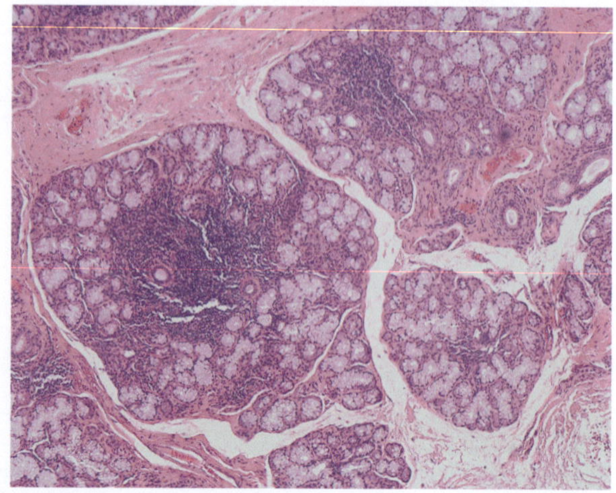

Fig. 18.15 Sjögren syndrome. Labial salivary gland. Several foci are evident (Courtesy of Dr. Khanh Trinh)

IgG4-related systemic disease. The LSG biopsy has proven to be a useful procedure in the diagnosis of IgG4-related systemic disease (IgG4-RD) [56], particularly if chronic sclerosing sialadenitis involving the submandibular salivary gland is a presenting condition. The salivary and lacrimal glands are involved in up to 50% of the IgG4-RD patients [57]. Other target organs (pancreas, lung, liver, biliary duct, gastrointestinal tract) can be difficult to access for a biopsy. The LSG's location makes it a convenient available structure that can aid in diagnosing IgG4-RD. A diffuse plasmacytic infiltrate, with more than half of these cells staining positive for anti-IgG4, will be noted. A storiform fibrosis and obliterative phlebitis may be present histologically. Unfortunately, the LSG biopsy is not suitable as a single diagnostic procedure because of its low sensitivity in IgG4-RD patients without major salivary gland (SG) lesions. However, the LSG biopsy, combined with clinical findings, including serum IgG4 and multiple organ involvement, may contribute toward a diagnosis of IgG4-RD even without SG lesions involving the major glands [58].

Amyloidosis. Extracellular deposition of fibrillary proteins (amyloidosis) in multiple organs impairs function. Diagnosis of systemic amyloidosis demands identification of amyloid deposits in the tissue of one of the involved organs. Because it is a safe procedure that avoids vital structures and because of its accessibility, biopsy of the LSG has been advocated for diagnosis of systemic amyloidosis [59, 60]. A high positive sensitivity rate of 88% for an LSG biopsy has been reported by Jamet et al. [61].

Chronic graft-versus-host disease (cGVHD). Patients who have had an allogenic hematopoietic stem cell transplantation can develop cGVHD. The disease may involve the oral mucosa, salivary glands, skin, liver, gastrointestinal tract, and lymphoid system. The LSG often is involved, but the histologic features seen with cGVHD are not pathognomonic. Regardless, LSG biopsy has been used as an adjunctive aid in diagnosing the early symptomatology of the salivary gland

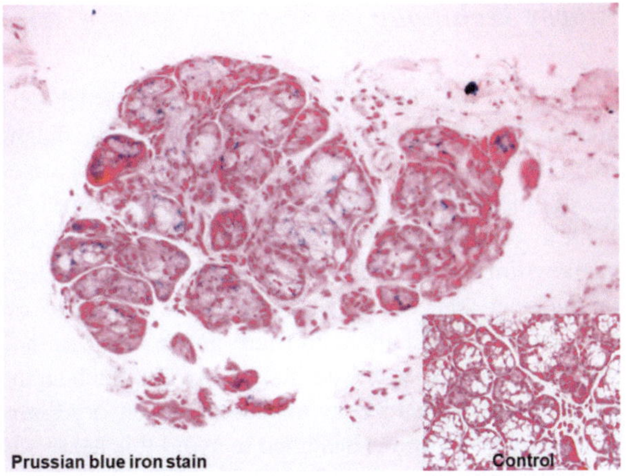

Fig. 18.16 Neonatal hemochromatosis. Iron depositions revealed by Prussian blue stain (Courtesy of Dr. K.C. Chan)

involvement that develops in cGVHD. Interstitial fibrosis in the LSG has been observed in 92.7% of the cGVHD patients, while a lichenoid histology may be seen in the surface epithelium and the underlying connective tissues [62].

Diffuse infiltrative lymphocytosis syndrome (DILS). Patients with HIV may present themselves with DILS, a subset of HIV. As part of the pathology associated with DILS, an exuberant lymphoproliferation can develop in the major and minor salivary glands. One or more lymphocytic foci, similar to that seen in SS, are usually observed in the LSG but differ from SS in that the lymphocytic infiltrate is dominated by CD8 lymphocytes rather than the CD4 cell majority seen in SS [63]. Acinar atrophy, ductal ectasia, moderate fibrosis, and the lymphocytic infiltration which is mainly periductal are also observed.

Neonatal hemochromatosis (NH) is a fatal neonatal iron storage disease in which iron deposits in multi-organs lead to organ failure [64]. Iron deposition occurs within hepatic and extrahepatic sites. The microscopic examination of a LSG biopsy can be useful as a diagnostic aid in NH diagnosis. The diagnosis of NH is facilitated when a Prussian blue stain demonstrates hemosiderin in the epithelial cells of the LSG (Fig. 18.16) [65].

Cystic fibrosis. A diagnosis of cystic fibrosis (CF) is usually made from clinical symptoms, a sweat chloride test, and genetic testing. However, for patients with limited phenotypes, the LSG biopsy can be of adjunctive value in diagnosis [1]. Mucin accumulation and eosinophilic acinar plugs are reported to be present in the LSGs of CF patients [1, 66, 67].

Chronic hepatitis C patients have an inflammatory infiltrate into their LSGs that is dominated by CD3 and CD20 lymphocytes. A focal pattern of inflammatory cells was present in 43% of LSG biopsies, while a diffuse pattern of inflammatory cell distribution was noted in the remaining 57% of LSG biopsies [68]. Some histologic similarities with SS exist, but a difference rests in the fact that the infiltration is pericapillary rather than the periductal infiltration seen in SS [68].

Biopsy Technique

By virtue of their ready accessibility, the LSGs lend themselves to surgical removal and microscopic study. Surgical harvesting for diagnostic purposes may be indicated because pathologic extension of systemic diseases into the LSG is not unusual. Local infiltration anesthesia with a vasoconstrictor is used to isolate the biopsy site. With a surgical assistant stabilizing, extending, and everting the lower lip, a very shallow linear 1.5- to 2.0-cm incision is made through the normal surface mucosa on the inner aspect of the lip between the lip midline and the commissure. The incision should run a diagonal postero-anterior course in the area midway between the mucobuccal fold and the dermal lip margin. Such an incision is created to run parallel to the path taken by the mental nerve sensory filaments that are on their way to innervate the lip and is designed to avoid this nerve's transection.

If effective lip stretching and eversion are implemented following the surgical incision, nodules of protruding LSGs, enveloped in a thin connective tissue covering, will immediately become evident. Blunt dissection will release an intact LSG from its surrounding tissues. Sensory filaments of the mental nerve may be visible and with care can be avoided (Fig. 7.14). The individual glandular nodules are easily separated from the underlying orbicularis oris muscle upon which they are based. Each LSG should be removed in toto in order to prevent subsequent mucocele formation from retained residual glandular remnants. Because the extent of pathologic change can vary in each gland nodule, four glands should be harvested for microscopic examination. Two or three sutures, engaging the margins of the thin incised overlying mucous membrane, can be placed and will result in a primary tension-free closure. Postoperatively, some minimal pain and swelling, occasional cutaneous ecchymosis, and hopefully only an infrequent localized numbness from a traumatized mental nerve filament may develop.

References

1. Shen D, Ono K, Do Q, et al. Clinical anatomy of the inferior labial gland: a narrative review. Gland Surg. 2021;10(7):2284–92. https://doi.org/10.21037/gs-21-143.
2. Hand AR, Pathmanathan D, Field RB. Morphological features of the minor salivary glands. Arch Oral Biol. 1999;44(Suppl 1):S3–S10. https://doi.org/10.1016/s0003-9969(99)90002-x.
3. Aframian DJ, Keshet N, Nadler C, Zadik Y, Vered M. Minor salivary glands: clinical, histological and immunohistochemical features of common and less common pathologies. Acta Histochem. 2019;121(8):151451. https://doi.org/10.1016/j.acthis.2019.151451.
4. Dawes C, Wood CM. The composition of human lip mucous gland secretions. Arch Oral Biol. 1973;18(3):343–50. https://doi.org/10.1016/0003-9969(73)90157-x.
5. Tandler B, Riva A. Salivary glands. In: Mjör IA, Fejerskov O, editors. Human oral embryology and histology. Copenhagen: Munksgaard International Publishers; 1986. p. 243–84.
6. Tandler B, Denning CR, Mandel ID, Kutscher AH. Ultrastructure of human labial salivary glands. 3. Myoepithelium and ducts. J Morphol. 1970;130(2):227–45. https://doi.org/10.1002/jmor.1051300208.

7. de Paula F, Teshima THN, Hsieh R, Souza MM, Nico MMS, Lourenco SV. Overview of human salivary glands: highlights of morphology and developing processes. Anat Rec (Hoboken). 2017;300(7):1180–8. https://doi.org/10.1002/ar.23569.

8. Redman RS. Myoepithelium of salivary glands. Microsc Res Tech. 1994;27(1):25–45. https://doi.org/10.1002/jemt.1070270103.

9. More CB, Bhavsar K, Varma S, Tailor M. Oral mucocele: a clinical and histopathological study. J Oral Maxillofac Pathol. 2014;18(Suppl 1):S72–7.

10. Kauzman A, Rei N, Avon SL. The blue nevus: a rare lesion of the oral cavity. Gen Dent. 2014;62(5):e22–6.

11. Chaitanya P, Praveen D, Reddy M. Mucocele on lower lip: a case series. Indian Dermatol Online J. 2017;8(3):205–7.

12. Zeng QC, Mandel L. Surgical management of the labial mucocele. NYState Dent J. 2019;85:42–4.

13. Nallasivam KU, Sudha BR. Oral mucocele: review of literature and a case report. J Pharm Bioallied Sci. 2015;7(Suppl 2):S731–3.

14. Ohta N, Fukase S, Suzuki Y, Aoyagi M. Treatment of salivary mucocele of the lower lip by OK-432. Auris Nasus Larynx. 2011;38(2):240–3. https://doi.org/10.1016/j.anl.2010.07.003.

15. Shetty VM, Rao R, Pai BS. Sclerotherapy in mucocele: a novel therapeutic approach. J Cutan Med Surg. 2018;22(6):652–3. https://doi.org/10.1177/1203475418775376.

16. Liu JL, Zhang AQ, Jiang LC, et al. The efficacy of polidocanol sclerotherapy in mucocele of the minor salivary gland. J Oral Pathol Med. 2018;47(9):895–9. https://doi.org/10.1111/jop.12764.

17. Eveson JW. Superficial mucoceles: pitfall in clinical and microscopic diagnosis. Oral Surg Oral Med Oral Pathol. 1988;66(3):318–22.

18. Jinbu Y, Tsukinoki K, Kusama M, Watanabe Y. Recurrent multiple superficial mucocele on the palate: histopathology and laser vaporization. Oral Surg Oral Med Oral Pathol Oral Radiol Endod. 2003;95(2):193–7.

19. Inoue A, Ikeda S, Mizuno Y, Ogawa H. Superficial mucoceles of the soft palate. Dermatology. 2005;210(4):360–2.

20. Venugopal DC, Warrier SA, E S, T H, Ramesh P. Superficial mucocele: a rare presentation. Cureus. 2021;13(9):e18038. Published 2021 Sep 17.

21. Bermejo A, Aguirre JM, López P, Saez MR. Superficial mucocele: report of 4 cases. Oral Surg Oral Med Oral Pathol Oral Radiol Endod. 1999;88(4):469–72.

22. Xu GZ, Yang C, Yu CQ, He D, Zhang S. Multiple superficial mucoceles on lower lip, soft palate, retromolar region, and floor of mouth. J Oral Maxillofac Surg. 2010;68(10):2601–3.

23. Lv K, Liu J, Ye W, Wang G, Yao H. Multiple superficial mucoceles concomitant with oral lichen planus: a case series. Oral Surg Oral Med Oral Pathol Oral Radiol. 2019;127(4):e95–e101. https://doi.org/10.1016/j.oooo.2018.08.017.

24. Treister NS, Stevenson K, Kim H, Woo SB, Soiffer R, Cutler C. Oral chronic graft-versus-host disease scoring using the NIH consensus criteria. Biol Blood Marrow Transplant. 2010;16(1):108–14.

25. Campana F, Sibaud V, Chauvel A, Boiron JM, Taieb A, Fricain JC. Recurrent superficial mucoceles associated with lichenoid disorders. J Oral Maxillofac Surg. 2006;64(12):1830–3.

26. Graillon N, Mage C, Le Roux MK, Scemama U, Chossegros C, Foletti JM. Mucoceles of the anterior ventral surface of the tongue and the glands of Blandin-Nuhn: 5 cases. J Stomatol Oral Maxillofac Surg. 2019;120(6):509–12.

27. Jinbu Y, Kusama M, Itoh H, Matsumoto K, Wang J, Noguchi T. Mucocele of the glands of Blandin-Nuhn: clinical and histopathologic analysis of 26 cases. Oral Surg Oral Med Oral Pathol Oral Radiol Endod. 2003;95(4):467–70.

28. Eversole LR. Oral sialocysts. Arch Otolaryngol Head Neck Surg. 1987;113(1):51–6.

29. Andiran N, Sarikayalar F, Unal OF, Baydar DE, Ozaydin E. Mucocele of the anterior lingual salivary glands: from extravasation to an alarming mass with a benign course. Int J Pediatr Otorhinolaryngol. 2001;61(2):143–7.

30. Joshi SR, Pendyala GS, Choudhari S, Kalburge J. Mucocele of the glands of Blandin-Nuhn in children: a clinical, histopathologic, and retrospective study. N Am J Med Sci. 2012;4(9):379–83.
31. Ben Lagha N, Alantar A, Samson J, Chapireau D, Maman L. Lithiasis of minor salivary glands: current data. Oral Surg Oral Med Oral Pathol Oral Radiol Endod. 2005;100(3):345–8.
32. Abe A, Kurita K, Hayashi H, Minagawa M. A case of minor salivary gland sialolithiasis of the upper lip. Oral Maxillofac Surg. 2019;23(1):91–4.
33. Anneroth G, Hansen LS. Minor salivary gland calculi. A clinical and histopathological study of 49 cases. Int J Oral Surg. 1983;12(2):80–9.
34. Favia G, Capodiferro S, Turco M, Cortelazzi R. Lithiasis of minor salivary glands of the upper lip. Clinico-pathological report of a case with unusual presentation. Minerva Stomatol. 2004;53(4):179–83.
35. Taybos G. Oral changes associated with tobacco use. Am J Med Sci. 2003;326(4):179–82.
36. Prabowo D, Widodo H. Nicotine stomatitis in smokers: a case report. J Dentomaxillofac Sci. 2018;3(1):58–60.
37. Bouquot JE, Speight PM, Farthing PM. Epithelial dysplasia of the oral mucosa—diagnostic problems and prognostic features. Curr Diagn Pathol. 2006;12(1):11–21.
38. Bharath TS, Kumar NG, Nagaraja A, Saraswathi TR, Babu GS, Raju PR. Palatal changes of reverse smokers in a rural coastal Andhra population with review of literature. J Oral Maxillofac Pathol. 2015;19(2):182–7.
39. Mandel L, Kaynar A, DeChiara S. Necrotizing sialometaplasia in a patient with sickle-cell anemia. J Oral Maxillofac Surg. 1991;49(7):757–9.
40. Salvado F, Nobre MA, Gomes J, Maia P. Necrotizing sialometaplasia and bulimia: a case report. Medicina (Kaunas). 2020;56(4):188. Published 2020 Apr 19.
41. Shin SA, Na HY, Choe JY, et al. Necrotizing sialometaplasia: a malignant masquerade but questionable precancerous lesion, report of four cases. BMC Oral Health. 2020;20(1):206. Published 2020 Jul 14. https://doi.org/10.1186/s12903-020-01189-1.
42. Imai T, Michizawa M. Necrotizing sialometaplasia in a patient with an eating disorder: palatal ulcer accompanied by dental erosion due to binge-purging. J Oral Maxillofac Surg. 2013;71(5):879–85.
43. Carlson DL. Necrotizing sialometaplasia: a practical approach to the diagnosis. Arch Pathol Lab Med. 2009;133(5):692–8.
44. Stoopler ET, Carrasco L, Stanton DC, Pringle G, Sollecito TP. Cheilitis glandularis: an unusual histopathologic presentation. Oral Surg Oral Med Oral Pathol Oral Radiol Endod. 2003;95(3):312–7.
45. Lourenço SV, Gori LM, Boggio P, Nico MM. Cheilitis glandularis in albinos: a report of two cases and review of histopathological findings after therapeutic vermilionectomy. J Eur Acad Dermatol Venereol. 2007;21(9):1265–7.
46. Stoopler ET, Kulkarni R, Riegel R, Sollecito TP, Alawi F. Chronic lip swelling. J Am Dent Assoc. 2022;153(5):480–3.
47. de Morais Medeiros HC, Del Carmen Martinez Vargas Y, Gonzaga AKG, et al. Co-existence of cheilitis glandularis and actinic cheilitis—an update. Oral Maxillofac Surg. 2021;25(1):113–7.
48. Nico MM, de Melo JN, Lourenço SV. Cheilitis glandularis: a clinicopathological study in 22 patients. J Am Acad Dermatol. 2010;62(2):233–8.
49. Piperi E, Georgaki M, Andreou A, Pettas E, Tziveleka S, Nikitakis NG. Cheilitis glandularis: a clinicopathologic study with emphasis on etiopathogenesis [published online ahead of print, 2022 Feb 3]. Oral Dis. 2022. https://doi.org/10.1111/odi.14144.
50. Shiboski CH, Shiboski SC, Seror R, et al. 2016 American College of Rheumatology/European League Against Rheumatism classification criteria for primary Sjögren's syndrome: a consensus and data-driven methodology involving three international patient cohorts. Ann Rheum Dis. 2017;76(1):9–16.
51. Theander E, Vasaitis L, Baecklund E, et al. Lymphoid organisation in labial salivary gland biopsies is a possible predictor for the development of malignant lymphoma in primary Sjögren's syndrome. Ann Rheum Dis. 2011;70(8):1363–8.

52. Keszler A, Adler LI, Gandolfo MS, et al. MALT lymphoma in labial salivary gland biopsy from Sjögren syndrome: importance of follow-up in early detection. Oral Surg Oral Med Oral Pathol Oral Radiol. 2013;115(3):e28–33.

53. Kapsogeorgou EK, Papageorgiou A, Protogerou AD, Voulgarelis M, Tzioufas AG. Low miR200b-5p levels in minor salivary glands: a novel molecular marker predicting lymphoma development in patients with Sjögren's syndrome. Ann Rheum Dis. 2018;77(8):1200–7.

54. Mandel L, Kaynar A. Sialadenopathy: a clinical herald of sarcoidosis: report of two cases. J Oral Maxillofac Surg. 1994;52(11):1208–10.

55. Bernard C, Kodjikian L, Bancel B, Isaac S, Broussolle C, Seve P. Ocular sarcoidosis: when should labial salivary gland biopsy be performed? Graefes Arch Clin Exp Ophthalmol. 2013;251(3):855–60.

56. Doe K, Nozawa K, Okada T, et al. Usefulness of minor salivary gland biopsy in the diagnosis of IgG4-related disease: a case report. Int J Clin Exp Pathol. 2014;7(5):2673–7. Published 2014 Apr 15.

57. Carubbi F, Alunno A, Gerli R, Giacomelli R. Histopathology of salivary glands. Reumatismo. 2018;70(3):146–54. Published 2018 Oct 3.

58. Moriyama M, Ohta M, Furukawa S, et al. The diagnostic utility of labial salivary gland biopsy in IgG4-related disease. Mod Rheumatol. 2016;26(5):725–9.

59. Sacsaquispe SJ, Antúnez-de Mayolo EA, Vicetti R, Delgado WA. Detection of AA-type amyloid protein in labial salivary glands. Med Oral Patol Oral Cir Bucal. 2011;16(2):e149–52. Published 2011 Mar 1.

60. Lecadet A, Bachmeyer C, Buob D, Cez A, Georgin-Lavialle S. Minor salivary gland biopsy is more effective than normal appearing skin biopsy for amyloid detection in systemic amyloidosis: a prospective monocentric study. Eur J Intern Med. 2018;57:e20–1.

61. Jamet MP, Gnemmi V, Hachulla É, et al. Distinctive patterns of transthyretin amyloid in salivary tissue: a clinicopathologic study of 92 patients with amyloid-containing Minor salivary gland biopsies. Am J Surg Pathol. 2015;39(8):1035–44. https://doi.org/10.1097/PAS.0000000000000430.

62. Santos PS, Coracin FL, Barros JC, Gallottini MH. Histopathologic diagnosis of chronic graft-versus-host disease of the oral mucosa according to the National Institutes of Health consensus. Einstein (Sao Paulo). 2014;12(2):204–10.

63. Rivera H, Nikitakis NG, Castillo S, Siavash H, Papadimitriou JC, Sauk JJ. Histopathological analysis and demonstration of EBV and HIV p-24 antigen but not CMV expression in labial minor salivary glands of HIV patients affected by diffuse infiltrative lymphocytosis syndrome. J Oral Pathol Med. 2003;32(7):431–7.

64. Knisely AS. Neonatal hemochromatosis. Adv Pediatr. 1992;39:383–403.

65. Chan KC, Edelman M, Fantasia JE. Labial salivary gland involvement in neonatal hemochromatosis: a report of 2 cases and review of literature. Oral Surg Oral Med Oral Pathol Oral Radiol Endod. 2008;106(1):e27–30.

66. Doggett RG, Bentinck B, Harrison GM. Structure and ultrastructure of the labial salivary glands in patients with cystic fibrosis. J Clin Pathol. 1971;24(3):270–82.

67. Sweney LR, Hedrick MC, Meskin LH, Warwick WJ. The involvement of the labial mucous salivary gland in patients with cystic fibrosis. II. The heterozygote state. Pediatrics. 1967;40(3):421–4.

68. Caldeira PC, Oliveira e Silva KR, Vidigal PV, de Mattos Camargo Grossmann S, do Carmo MAV. Inflammatory cells in minor salivary glands of patients with chronic hepatitis C: immunophenotype, pattern of distribution, and comparison with liver samples. Hum Immunol. 2014;75(5):422–7.

Chapter 19
False Positives

Louis Mandel

Abstract A great variety of head and neck conditions have the ability to mimic salivary gland pathology. Achievement of an accurate and definitive diagnosis is based on the ability of the investigator to use the available diagnostic armamentarium. Bringing analytic tools such as the patient's history, physical and clinical examinations, imaging, evaluation of saliva, serology and histologic study into play will serve to differentiate a false/positive from a true salivary gland disorder. The false/positives in the head and neck area usually take the form of a tissue swelling or calcification. Because they are in close anatomic relationship with a salivary gland, diagnostic mistakes are common and patients are referred for needless therapy. Surprisingly, this cohort of misdirected and misdiagnosed patients represent the largest patient category seen in the Salivary Gland Center. A review of these false/positives will serve to alert the clinician and sharpen diagnostic skills.

Introduction

Many patients with a great variety of salivary gland (SG) pathophysiologies have been seen in the Columbia University Salivary Gland Center (SGC). An accurate diagnosis for these patients requires an array of techniques, with the individual diagnosis only achieved after integrating the clinical picture with a wide range of investigative procedures. Detailed study of a SG problem includes a thorough history, physical and clinical examinations, evaluation of saliva, serology, imaging, and biopsy. Despite these efforts to reach an accurate SG diagnosis, there is a group of patients whose signs and symptomatology cannot be related to any known SG condition. These patients usually are false-positives and represent a large cluster of extraglandular pathologies. With the goal of alerting the practitioner to these pitfalls, this chapter will classify the false-positives, some of which are unusual, that have been seen in the SGC during the past 33 years. Surprisingly, this cohort of

L. Mandel, *Clinical Management of Salivary Gland Disorders*, https://doi.org/10.1007/978-3-031-50012-1_19

misdirected and misdiagnosed patients has proven to be the largest patient category examined in the SGC. Their significant symptomatology and the major means of differentiating their problem from true SG pathology will be reviewed. Improvement in diagnostic skills will evolve and will act to avoid needless referrals and therapy.

Somatoform Disease

A high percentage of patients referred to the Salivary Gland Center (SGC) with salivary issues have no discernible organic salivary gland (SG) disease and/or objective secretory dysfunction. Their complaint appears to be somatoform in origin, wherein their mental state, often depression, is manifested by a physical complaint with no recognized organic basis [1, 2]. The lifetime prevalence rate of depression is as high as 16% with stress being a significant underlying cause [3]. Many of these patients are caught in a self-perpetuating cycle in which symptoms of common minor problems are magnified to such an extent that they are interpreted as being serious physical disorders. Often, they have complaints concerning salivary quality or quantity and for which no known pathologic origin has been determined. The patients are convinced that something is wrong and that the symptoms are causing a decreased quality of life [4]. They are relentless in their search for a solution and have visited numerous professionals without a resulting satisfactory outcome.

Most somatoform patients seen in the SGC have salivary concerns that involve hyposalivation, hypersalivation, and drooling or salivary quality. Objective salivary volume measurements fail to verify the presence of hyposalivation or hypersalivation. Patients often state that there is an intensification of their salivary problems as the day progresses and they have difficulty with sleeping. Their complaints can also be somewhat odd and even bizarre. These include a fancied oral dryness or excessive salivation. The salivary complaint may be limited to only one area, and there may be a perceived need to constantly expectorate or swallow. Salivary spraying during speech and constant drooling may also play roles in their complaint. In fact, no such events are usually observed during the prolonged examination process. Patients have been seen because they believe their saliva is too thick, gritty, or slimy or that it adheres to specific oral areas. Frothy bubbly saliva also is a frequent patient concern that prompts a professional visit (Fig. 19.1). The explanation for frothiness rests in the fact that a normally clear aqueous saliva exits from the duct orifices and accumulates in the mouth floor. Speech and its related oral muscular activity then cause a whipping action with salivary aeration that results in saliva's foamy appearance. In many somatoform patients, salivary taste alterations, often limited to a defined oral area, also serve as an impetus for a visit. The caveat here is that the clinician should be aware that some medications and systemic diseases will modify taste, and their role, if any, in the patient's complaint must be determined.

Common denominators in somatoform patients include histories of emotional disturbance for which in the past or present psychotherapeutics with anticholinergic side effects have been prescribed. The modest hyposalivation effect of each of these medications and the patient's awareness of their action can function as an instigator

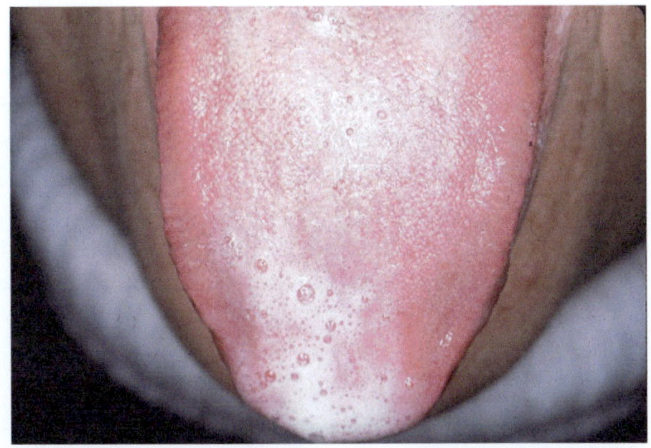

Fig. 19.1 False positives. Frothy saliva results from aeration during speech and tongue movement

or accentuator of the patient's subjective xerostomic complaint. The root of the problem can be exposed by objectively measuring salivary flow. A mild decrease in whole unstimulated saliva may be noted. However, when saliva is stimulated and volume measured in medication-related hyposalivation, normal salivary returns will be obtained because stimulation overrides any anticholinergic effect of the drug on the unstimulated SG. Conversely, true pathology-related hyposalivation (Sjögren syndrome) will produce a reduced whole stimulated saliva flow even when the gland is activated with a stimulant such as sour candy.

Patients may attribute their frequent sleep difficulties and night awakenings to their perceived oral dryness when in reality it is their mental state that keeps them awake. On many occasions, patients bring extremely detailed written (Osler's "la maladie du petit papier") chronologic histories of their symptoms, numerous medical visits, and medications [5]. Their multiple medical consultations with varied specialists have not solved their problem and have prompted the ongoing dogged search for an answer to their perceived trouble. Questioning often reveals that some oral event, often a dental procedure or another form of oral trauma, that focused attention on the mouth was the starting point for their problem. Contributing causes include stressful work and social or family situations whose details can be elicited during a thorough interviewing process.

Concurrently, many patients will display subjective conditions that may have psychogenic aspects. Burning mouth, bruxing, clenching, difficulty with sleep, dysgeusia and atypical pain patterns may be part of their symptom complex for which no pathologic reason can be ascertained. A frequently observed triad of a peculiar unverified salivary complaint, oral burning, and altered taste (often metallic) should alert the diagnostician to a suspicion of a somatoform disorder and the need for a multidisciplinary approach. In these patients, helping them to understand the origin of their perceived symptoms may lead to its alleviation. Often, patients require psychologic consultation but frequently resist the suggestion for such help. It is quite possible that modern medicine does not have the ability to recognize an organic etiology for the problem nor the ability to effectively treat the condition. Undoubtedly, future scientific advances will produce the required answers. With evidence pointing to elevated levels of salivary cortisol in depressed patients [3], a step forward has been taken.

Masseteric Hypertrophy

In the Columbia University Salivary Gland Center, the most common entity mistaken for parotid gland (PG) enlargement is bilateral, occasionally unilateral, masseteric muscle hypertrophy (MH) (Figs. 19.2 and 19.3). It is this muscle's proximity to the PG that causes the confusion and misdiagnoses. Anatomically, the masseter muscle (MM) is a thick quadrate muscle, composed of two layers, arising from the inferior and deep surfaces of the zygomatic arch and inserting for the most part onto

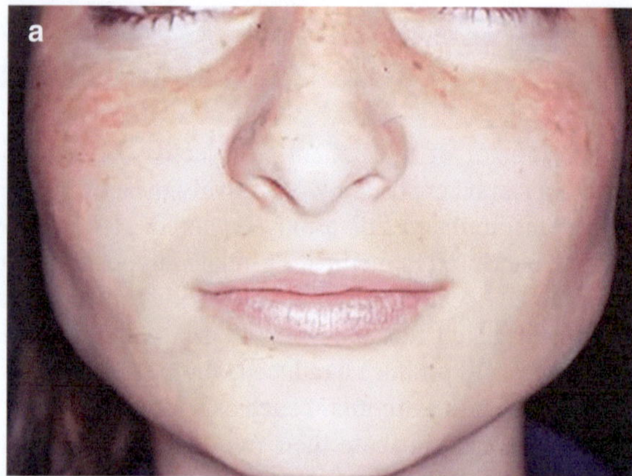

Fig. 19.2 (**a**) Masseteric hypertrophy. Patient A. Bilateral masseter enlargement (gum chewer). (**b**) Masseteric hypertrophy. Patient A. CT scan. Bilateral masseteric (M) enlargement

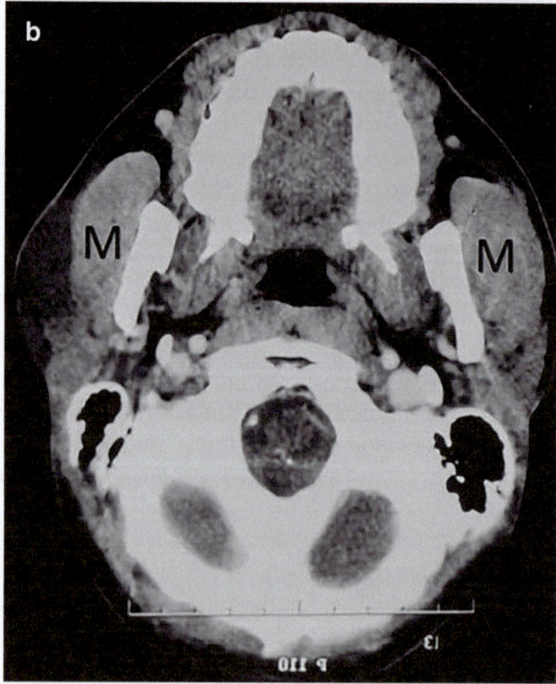

Fig. 19.3 (**a**) Masseteric hypertrophy. Patient B. Bilateral masseteric enlargement (bruxer). (**b**) Masseteric hypertrophy. Patient B clenches and masseter muscle bundles become prominent

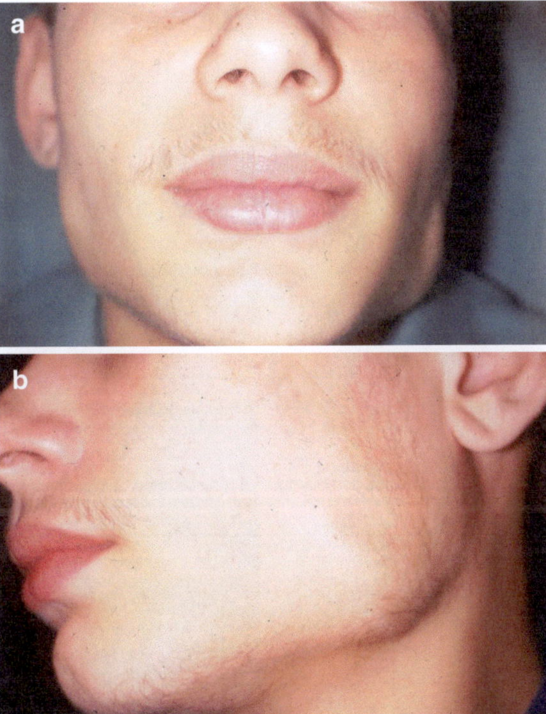

the inferior lateral aspect of the ramus. Most of the muscle's bulk is present along the inferior portion of the mandibular ramus and its gonial area, the region where the facial contour normally tapers. Any increase in bilateral MM mass in the mandibular gonial angle areas causes the face to acquire a characteristic rectangular configuration (Figs. 19.2a and 19.3a). Although there is some overlap with the MM, the PG bulk occupies a higher facial level, mostly pre-auricular, and its enlargement tends to accentuate facial ovality.

MH is considered to result from a work hypertrophy [6], with stress often serving as a common underlying etiologic factor. Other reported risk factors include anxiety disorders, sleep apnea, and increased consumption of alcohol or tobacco [7]. The MH can be caused by bruxism during sleep, a clenching habit during the day, or constant gum chewing. Usually seen in young adults, it is uncommon in the elderly because dental deterioration progresses with aging and causes discomfort with an inability to clench when teeth are brought into active occlusion. Inspection reveals that the facial swelling corresponds to the anatomic outline of the MM. The swelling itself is normal in tone and painless and results from excessive movement-induced hypertrophy of the MM. When the patient activates the muscle by clenching, bulging and rippling of the musculature can be observed extraorally (Fig. 19.3b). What was previously a soft mass now becomes palpably firm and demonstrates a distinct and prominent MM outline with conspicuous visible muscle bundles. Orally, tooth attrition resulting from the bruxing/clenching habit may be present (Fig. 19.4).

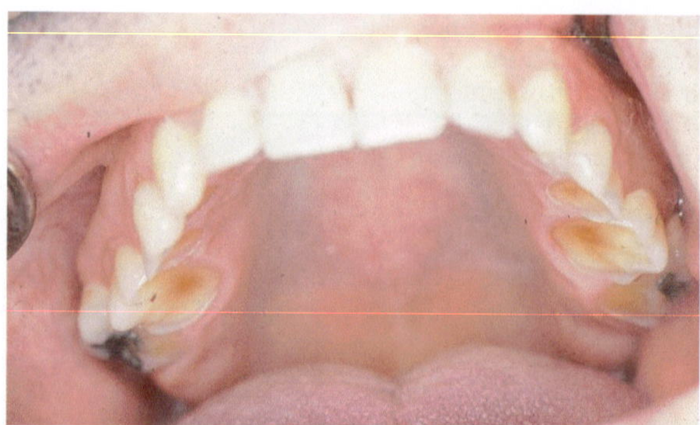

Fig. 19.4 Masseteric hypertrophy. Dental attrition from bruxing/clenching

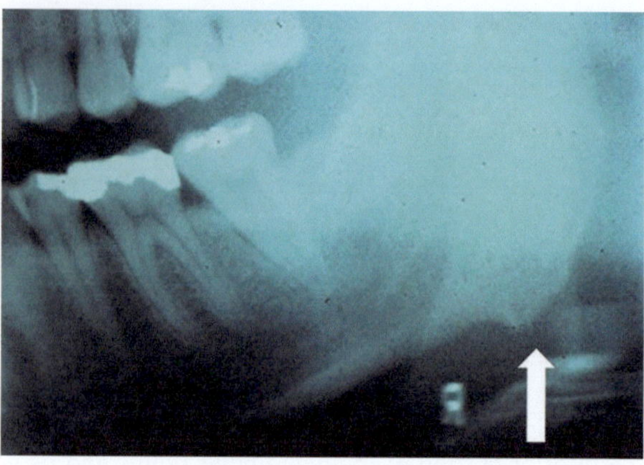

Fig. 19.5 Masseteric hypertrophy. Bone exostosis at gonial angle (arrow)

Patients with MH often state that the swellings are larger upon awakening or at certain specified times during the day. The answer for this behavior pattern is derived from the fact that the patient probably had actively bruxed while sleeping or clenched during a stressful daytime situation. This increased period of MM activity has caused a muscle hyperemia and "pumped up" a large MM to become even larger because of its increased vascular content. With discontinuation of the activation, the hyperemia subsides and the muscle returns to its normal resting enlarged state.

Radiologic findings in MH (CT, panoramic) often show a compensatory bony hyperplasia that is a reaction to the increased muscular force exerted at the MM's mandibular gonial angle insertion. Consequently, a bone spur/exostosis or scalloping can develop at the gonial angle (Fig. 19.5). In addition, an overall ramus enlargement can be discerned as well as a change in the gonial angle's measurements. Panoramic radiographs will clearly show any bony changes incited by the MM. Cephalometric radiographs have demonstrated that in males, the average gonial angle measures 125°, while females have an angle measurement that averages 115°. In MH patients, the angle becomes less obtuse (averaging 106°) because of the additional deposition of bone responding to the increased MM stress exerted by the hypertrophied musculature at its insertion [8].

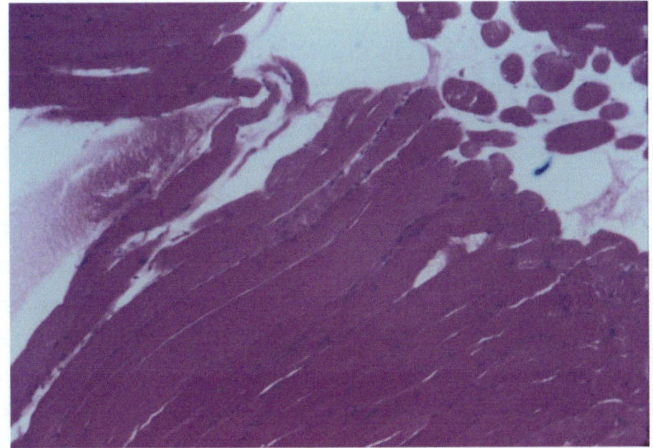

Fig. 19.6 Masseteric hypertrophy. Microscopic view of normal musculature

Imaging (CT, MRI) can be a key factor in the diagnosis of MH. It will show a larger than normal MM (Fig. 19.2b). A normal-sized PG with an absence of glandular pathology will be imaged. Bony changes will also be apparent.

Histologic examination of a biopsy specimen from an involved muscle reveals no abnormal pathology (Fig. 19.6). However, significant increases in muscle fiber length and diameter have been reported [8].

The only entity that can reasonably be confused with MH is PG enlargement. Again, the clinician should be alerted to the fact that MH increases facial rectangularness, while PG swelling tends to cause increased facial ovality. Differential diagnosis is readily achieved by closely observing the facial contour and activating the muscle by asking the patient to clench. A thorough medical history and examination will eliminate systemic conditions that could cause PG enlargement. Furthermore, the normal clear salivary return at the PG duct orifice in a MH patient will rule out PG inflammation. A patient with parotitis will have a cloudy saliva, pain, and a history of recurrent swellings associated with eating.

Therapy for MH is usually unnecessary other than for a cosmetic issue or for any undue stress on the temporomandibular joint that may cause discomfort. Nonsurgical treatment modalities include reassurance, tranquilizers, muscle relaxants, and occasionally psychiatric care. Surgical reduction of the muscle bulk or mandibular bone can be performed [9, 10] via an intraoral or extraoral approach but is rarely indicated. Botulinum toxin injections [11] inactivate the MM and have proven to be effective in bringing about MM atrophy, but repeat injections are necessary until the initiating habit is terminated.

Paraglandular Opacities: Overview

The soft tissues of the head and neck harbor a great variety of calcifications, all of which lend themselves to radiographic visualization. The introduction of the various imaging systems (panoramic, cone beam, CT, MRI, etc.) has ushered in an enhanced ability to observe anatomic features that are or are not in the immediate dentoalveolar field. The clinician has now been afforded the opportunity to visualize both normal and abnormal conditions that are located in areas not previously imaged by standard oral radiography. These readily available investigative imaging tools have exposed the presence of calcifications unrelated to the salivary glands but located in the vicinity of the parotid (PG) or submandibular (SMSG) salivary glands. Consequently, a variety of paraglandular dystrophic and pathologic calcifications are imaged and often present diagnostic dilemmas. Because these opacities are in close anatomic relationship to the salivary glands, the relatively common salivary gland sialolith has been entertained again and again as the provisional diagnosis. Needless misdiagnoses and referrals for treatment of sialolithiasis have been made. Such errors can be avoided with a thorough examination that must include the medical history and physical and clinical examinations. Diagnosing a paraglandular calcification demands the integration of the practitioner's knowledge of anatomy and pathology, combined with the results of the examination. Integration of the gathered accumulated data inevitably leads to an accurate diagnosis. The intent of the following section is to familiarize the clinician with those paraglandular opacities that may imitate the appearance of a sialolith.

Paraglandular Opacities: Carotid Artery Calcification

Cerebrovascular accidents (CVAs) are among the leading causes of death. These CVAs or strokes are classified as either ischemic or hemorrhagic. In both cases, the brain is deprived of the critical supply of the oxygenated blood that is needed to avoid rapid cell death. The majority of the CVAs are ischemic in nature and are due to arterial blockage by blood clots or result from the gradual intravascular buildup of fatty plaque in a vessel's intimal layer which often calcifies. The plaque accumulation with its ability to calcify (atherosclerosis) frequently involves the carotid artery. Eventually, a thickened and elevated calcified plaque protrudes into the vessel's lumen. The hemodynamic force of blood passing through the now narrowed carotid lumen causes the shedding of emboli from the plaque. These emboli can then hematogenously migrate intracranially and plug cranial arteries to create an ischemic stroke.

Carotid artery atherosclerosis can often be detected as an incidental finding on a panoramic film because of its anatomic position and its calcium content. The presence of a carotid calcified plaque was identified in 3–5% of the patients when their panoramic films were viewed [12]. A mean age of 64 years has been reported for these patients [13]. Age is an important factor in the development of these calcifications. Young adults are significantly less likely to have these calcifications than patients over 60 years of age [14]. Carotid atheromas, often located in the region where the carotid artery bifurcates into the internal and external carotid arteries or within the wall of the internal carotid artery, are a common cause of stroke. Carotid artery atherosclerotic

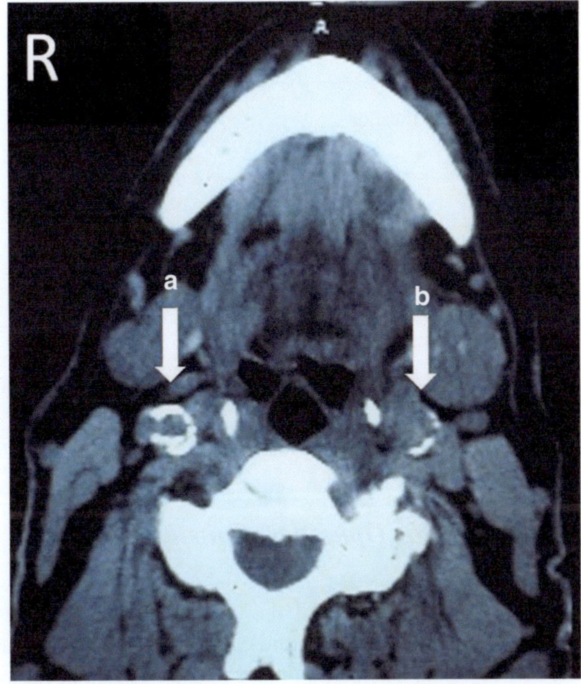

Fig. 19.7 Opacities. Carotid artery calcifications. CT scan. Almost total calcification right carotid artery wall (arrow A) with incomplete calcification left carotid artery wall (arrow B)

disease accounts for about 20% of all ischemic strokes [13]. The calcified carotid atheromas in this critical site can be visualized radiographically as being circular, linear, or irregular in shape (Fig. 19.7). Their presence serves as heralds of future cardiovascular events. When viewing panoramic radiographs, the calcified carotid atheromas are located posterior and inferior to the mandibular angle, at about 45 degrees from the angle of the mandible [15, 16] (Fig. 19.8). They are aligned at a level corresponding to the position of cervical vertebrae 3 and 4, and because they occupy the region of the carotid bifurcation, they are located within 40 mm of the mandibular angle. Here its position in relation to the submandibular salivary gland (SMSG), located in the submandibular triangle, is such that calcified carotid atheromas have been misdiagnosed as SMSG sialoliths or even as calcified cervical lymph nodes.

Besides the panoramic film, the CT scan also has proven to be a reliable means of incidentally identifying carotid calcifications because it is exquisitely sensitive to minute amounts of calcium. Nevertheless, medical centers and offices now utilize ultrasound for definitively diagnosing the presence of carotid artery calcifications. The procedure is cost-effective and widely available.

In order to avoid the possibility of an impending stroke or cardiovascular accident, the identification of a carotid calcification demands a medical referral for a detailed evaluation. If the plaque blocks more than 60% of the artery's luminal diameter, carotid endarterectomy or stenting is usually recommended [17].

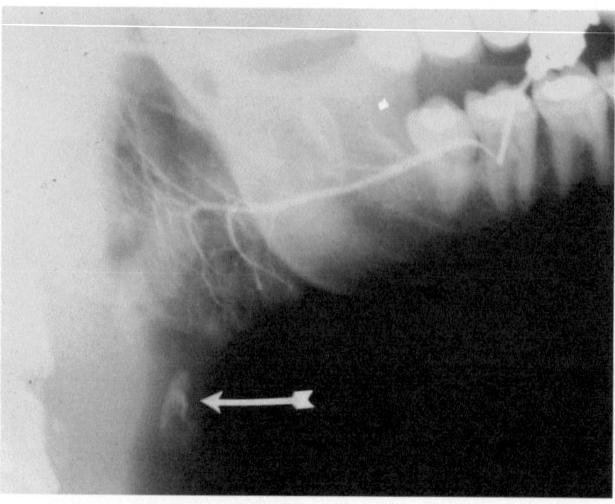

Fig. 19.8 Opacities.
Carotid artery calcification.
Parotid sialogram.
Incidental finding of
carotid artery calcification
(arrow)

Paraglandular Opacities: Tonsillolith

Waldeyer's ring consists of the tonsillar tissue found in the glossopalatine tonsil, nasopharyngeal tonsil (adenoid), lingual tonsil, and tubal tonsillar tissue adjacent to the orifice of the Eustachian tube. These clusters of lymphoid tissue are strategically situated at the entrance to the aerodigestive tract. Here, they serve a useful purpose by intercepting and destroying invading bacteria and viruses with which they come into contact.

The surface of the glossopalatine tonsil is marked by the presence of many crypts. Organic material consisting of dead bacteria, inflammatory debris, and food particles can be trapped at the base of a crypt and act as a nidus for a salt precipitation from saliva that mainly consists of carbonates and phosphates of calcium and magnesium. With salt deposition into the nidus, a calcified tonsillolith forms and tends to grow with additional salt accretions. When the head/neck region is examined by computed tomography, the tonsillolith has been found to be an incidental occurrence in a high percentage (16–40%) [18–20] of the patients, equally in males and females, with a mean age of 39.8 years and an increased presence as the patient ages [19].

The glossopalatine tonsillolith is often an asymptomatic discovery made during a routine panoramic radiographic or CT examination. Tonsilloliths may occur singly or frequently in multiples and may be unilateral or bilateral in their presentation (Fig. 19.9). Their size customarily varies from 1 to 7 mm but can even be larger [20]. Larger tonsilloliths tend to occur alone (Fig. 19.9a) and are often associated with bouts of sore throat, bad odor, and dysphagia. Smaller tonsilloliths are usually asymptomatic and are seen in multiples (Fig. 19.9b, c). The panoramic film will image palatine tonsilloliths as calcific bodies superimposed upon the ramus in the region of the parotid gland and its duct. A consequent misdiagnosis of parotid stones can be avoided because of a demonstrated random distribution and frequent multiplicity of the tonsil calcifications. In contrast, parotid stones are linearly aligned following the course of the parotid duct and are infrequently multiple or bilateral in occurrence. The presence of a normal salivary return, and absence of periods of parotid pain and swelling, can also serve to negate the existence of parotid sialolithiasis.

The panoramic film does not indicate the exact dimensional location of the displayed calcifications. Are they medial or lateral to the ramus or even within the ramus? Their location can be determined via an axial CT image (Fig. 19.9c). Glossopalatine tonsilloliths will be clearly imaged in tonsillar tissue medial to the mandibular ramus and in close relation and lateral to the lucent nasopharyngeal space.

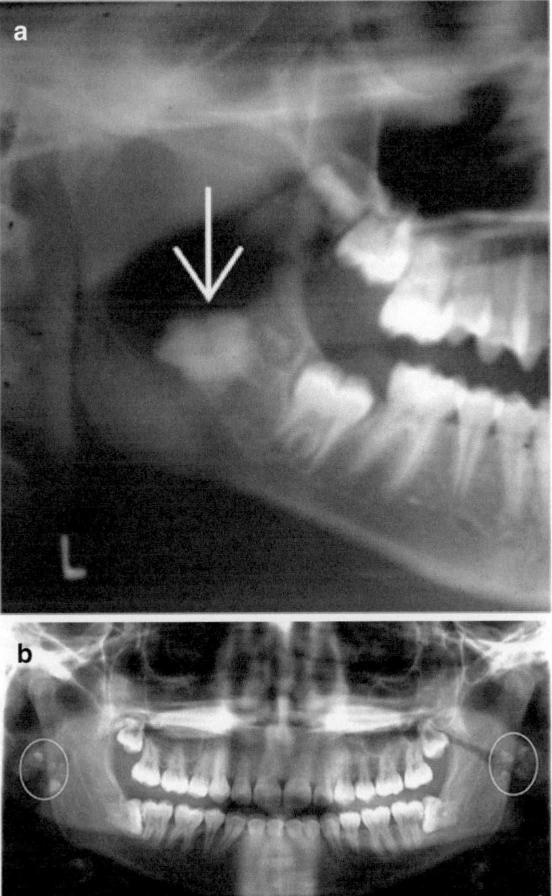

Fig. 19.9 (a) Opacities. Unilateral tonsillolith (palatine) is large and superimposed on ramus (arrow). (b) Opacities. Patient C. Panoramic film. Bilateral multiple palatine tonsilloliths (circled). (c) Opacities. Patient C. CT scan, bony window. Bilateral multiple palatine tonsilloliths (arrows)

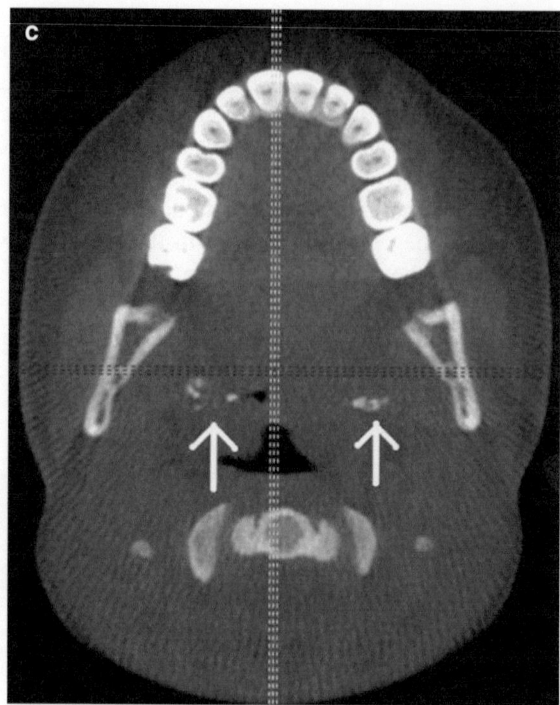

Fig. 19.9 continued

Tonsilloliths may also involve the lingual tonsil (LT) (Fig. 19.10). The LT is located at the base of the tongue posterior to the circumvallate papilla. The LT tonsillar tissue exhibits varying numbers of discrete round nodules that project upward. Each nodule has a central crypt formed by an invagination of the overlying epithelium. As with the glossopalatine tonsil and via the same mechanisms, a tonsillolith can develop at the base of the crypt. When present, a panoramic film will reveal the LT calcification. However, when calcifications are centrally located, such as a LT tonsillolith, their panoramic radiographic image will be subject to the ghost shadow paradox, and the calcifications will be factitiously imaged bilaterally in the parotid gland area (Fig. 19.10a) [21]. Ghost shadows result when an imaged structure is not in the focal trough of the panoramic radiographic unit. A solution to the confusion regarding the exact position of a LT tonsillolith can be achieved with a CT study (Fig. 19.10b).

Tonsilloliths, being mostly asymptomatic, require no treatment. Those that cause symptomatology should be removed via manual compression, curettage, or a simple incision. Tonsillectomy is indicated in the presence of multiple tonsilloliths that are causing subjective symptoms.

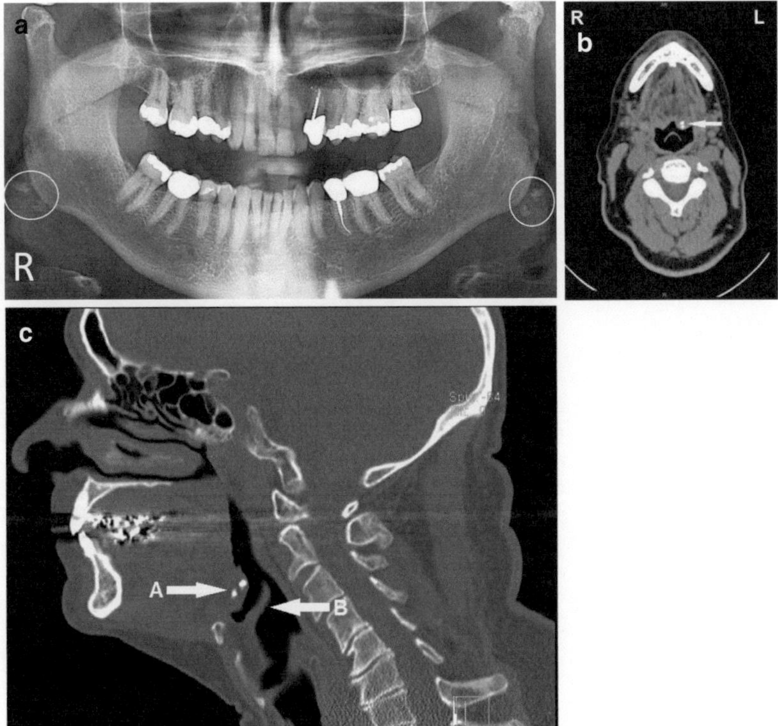

Fig. 19.10 (**a**) Opacities. Patient D. Lingual tonsilloliths (left and circled). Panoramic film with ghost images on right side (circled). (**b**) Opacities. Patient D. CT scan. Lingual tonsilloliths (left, arrow). (**c**) Opacities. Patient D. CT scan, bony window (sagittal view). Lingual tonsilloliths (arrow A) and epiglottis (arrow B)

Paraglandular Opacities: Phlebolith

Phleboliths are calcified thrombi found within a vascular channel. They may originate from a thrombus forming after injury to a vessel wall or result from a stagnant blood flow that tends to clot as it sluggishly moves through a vascular malformation's (VM) tortuous vascular plexus. Injury can result in damage to the vessel's intima, while the healing that follows involves the formation of a protective thrombus. The slow flow of blood that occurs in the convoluted vascular channels present in a VM also favors thrombus formation. Coagulopathy is a recognized complication of almost any form of vascular anomaly. Regardless of the origin of the thrombus, dystrophic calcification of the thrombus, the phlebolith, can develop (Fig. 19.11).

The phlebolith consists of a mixture of calcium carbonate and calcium phosphate salts [22]. It usually has a radiolucent core. A fibrous component attaches itself to the developing phlebolith, and in turn it becomes calcified. Repetition of this

Fig. 19.11 (**a**) Opacities. Phleboliths. Buccal soft tissue (arrows). (**b**) Opacities. Phleboliths. Submandibular area. (**c**) Opacities. Phleboliths. Microscopic view of phlebolith in arteriole

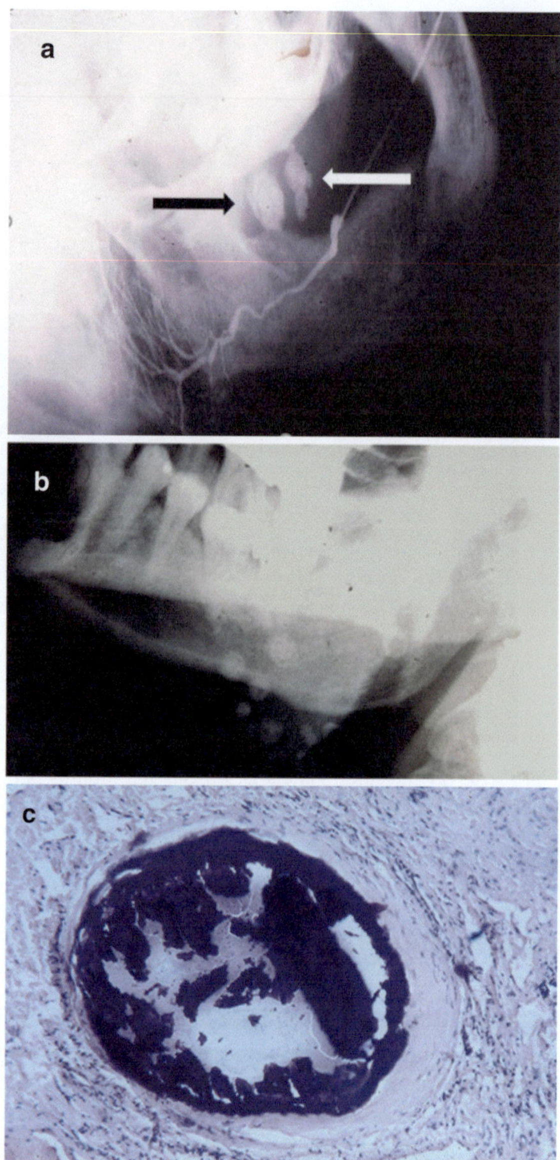

process causes a layering effect such that the phlebolith characteristically has a lamellated or onion-like appearance when viewed radiographically.

Phleboliths are most frequently seen in the pelvic area, with the head and neck region representing the next most common location. They are asymptomatic incidental findings that can be found during routine imaging studies of a parotid (PG) area swelling (Fig. 19.11a) that is actually vascular in origin [23] and usually represents an intramasseteric VM. Occasionally, the VM with contained phleboliths can involve the region of the submandibular salivary gland (SMSG) (Fig. 19.11b) [24].

Because the phleboliths are often located in close proximity to the PG or SMSG, differentiating the phlebolith from a sialolith is imperative. As a rule, the phlebolith's concentric ring appearance distinguishes it from the uniformly opaque sialolith. Phleboliths usually are circular, while sialoliths often are elongated in shape, a result of their molding by the walls of the salivary duct. Multiple phleboliths are frequently present, while sialoliths mostly appear as single calcifications. Furthermore, the absence of salivary gland obstructive symptomatology (pain and swelling) suggests an extraglandular rather than a glandular calcification. Moreover, because phleboliths are often associated with VMs, a persistent swelling mimicking a neoplasm, rather than the periodic swelling that occurs in relation to a sialadenitis, will be seen.

Because phleboliths are associated with vascular entities, the MRI can best substantiate an initial clinical diagnosis [25]. The vascular component will enhance brightly on an MRI film because of its free water content. The CT scan and ultrasound are alternative diagnostic imaging tools that can identify vascularity and calcific bodies. A histologic examination will reveal a calcified body within a vascular lumen (Fig. 19.11c).

The phlebolith requires no treatment, but intervention is indicated for any associated VM. Sclerotherapy, embolization, and radiation have all been suggested, in lieu of surgical removal, as appropriate approaches that avoid the perioperative hemorrhage experienced with the surgical removal of a VM.

Paraglandular Opacities: Cervical Lymph Node Calcification

Cervicofacial lymph nodes (CFLN) have been classified anatomically into five nodal groups: preauricular (parotid), facial, submandibular, submental, and cervical. Calcifications of these lymph nodes can occasionally develop and may be identified during routine dental panoramic radiography, cone beam, or CT examinations. These imaging techniques have proven to be extremely useful in revealing the presence of and aiding in the diagnosis of any existing unusual calcifications.

CFLN calcifications occur in relation to a variety of pathologic processes. The healing process of an inflamed node can result in calcification of the node. It is also not uncommon to see nodal calcifications in relation to granulomatous diseases, particularly tuberculosis and sarcoidosis. In addition, CFLN calcifications can develop in relation to histoplasmosis, blastomycosis, and coccidioidomycosis. Some cases of amyloidosis, rheumatoid arthritis, or scleroderma can also develop CFLN calcifications. Furthermore, malignant nodal disease from thyroid or breast metastases or a lymphoma may affect the CFLN and can result in nodal calcification [26].

CFLN calcifications most often stem from a prior granulomatous infection, especially tuberculosis [27] (Fig. 19.12). CFLN involvement in tuberculosis results from hematogenous or lymphatic bacterial dissemination, usually from the primary respiratory site. Contaminated sputum may also play a role. Tuberculosis causes a caseous necrosis of the diseased lymph nodes. With healing, calcification of the compromised nodes usually occurs. Tuberculous nodal calcification in the head and neck area most frequently implicates the submandibular and/or cervical lymph node

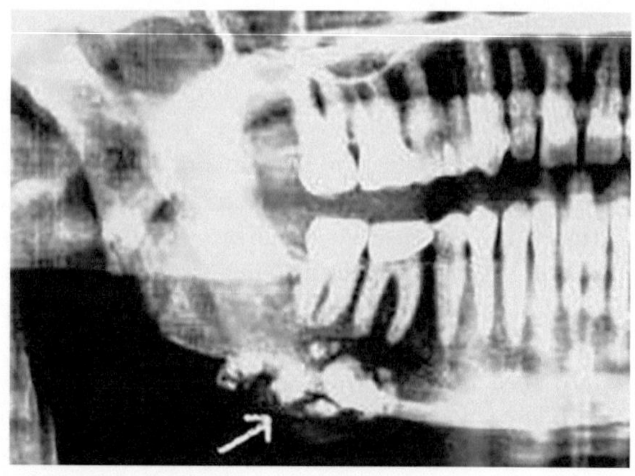

Fig. 19.12 Opacities. Calcified lymph nodes, tuberculosis (arrow)

chains [28] and is referred to as scrofula. Because the calcifications involve a nodal chain, multiple calcified nodes are seen aligned anatomically coinciding with the chain's directional pathway. The calcifications are irregular in outline and tend to have a cauliflower-like configuration.

Diagnostic problems arise when the tuberculous calcified nodes involve the submandibular lymph nodes. Their submandibular location acts to mimic the presence of sialolithiasis (Fig. 19.12). Differentiation is achieved by factoring in the patient's tubercular history and the absence of the signs and symptoms associated with a sialolith induced obstructive sialadenitis. Furthermore, sialoliths usually occur singly, along the anatomic path of the submandibular duct and have defined rather than irregular borders.
Diagnostic recognition of the calcified lymph node and its etiologic origin is the justification for no therapeutic intervention regarding the node. The calcification represents healing secondary to the disease's intrusion into the lymph node. However, investigation as to the primary cause of the nodal calcification is indicated.

Lymphadenopathy: No Calcification

Lymph nodes in the orofacial area (cervicofacial nodes) can anatomically be organized into five groupings: facial, pre-auricular (parotid), submandibular, submental, and cervical. Because many of these nodes are positioned in close proximity to the salivary glands, the presence of a lymphadenopathy has often been misdiagnosed as a salivary gland swelling. An understanding of anatomy, plus a knowledge of the patient's medical history and the many pathological entities that home in on lymph nodes, will serve to differentiate lymphadenopathy from sialadenopathy.

The etiology of lymphadenopathy has proven to be extremely varied. Most frequently, the enlarged cervicofacial lymph nodes seen in the Salivary Gland Center are bacterial in origin and caused by a lymphadenitis (Fig. 19.13). Most infected areas in the oral cavity, particularly the teeth and the side of the face, are drained by afferent lymphatic channels that lead to the submandibular lymph nodes. Pain and swelling of these nodes are the end result. All too frequently, this submandibular

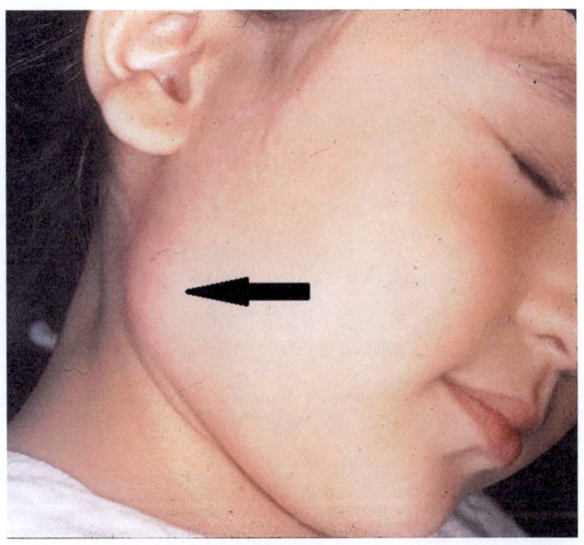

Fig. 19.13 Lymphadenitis (arrow) secondary to middle ear infection

lymphadenitis is misinterpreted as having a salivary gland origin, whereas an infected tooth is the usual cause. In addition, because of its juxtaposition to the salivary glands, cervicofacial lymphadenopathy caused by a variety of systemic conditions has even been misinterpreted as a sialadenopathy. Cat scratch disease and its associated cervicofacial lymphadenitis in a patient who has hugged cats [29] is an example of a bacterial disease process that is often thought to represent swelling of the submandibular salivary gland (Fig. 19.14). Besides bacteria, viral, mycotic, and protozoan organisms can cause a lymphadenitis of the cervicofacial nodes [30].

There are numerous other causes for lymphadenopathy. Granulomatous diseases often involve the lymph nodes that are in salivary gland areas. Tuberculosis can cause a lymphadenitis of the submandibular and cervical nodes, a common extrapulmonary manifestation of this systemic disease, and lead to a misdiagnosis of a submandibular sialadenitis. The intraparotid lymph nodes are also subject to the development of a tuberculous lymphadenitis [31] as well as a variety of systemic lymphoidal pathologies. In addition, sarcoidal granulomas in submandibular lymph nodes have been reported [32].

When considering a persistent lymphadenopathy, malignant neoplasms must be placed at the forefront of the diagnostic mix. Lymph nodes frequently serve as foci for metastatic malignancies. Metastases that invade the submandibular/submental lymph nodes often originate from malignancies of the oral cavity (Figs. 19.15 and 19.16). Metastases from distant anatomic locations can also affect cervicofacial nodes. Furthermore, lymphomas can primarily involve lymph nodes in the cervicofacial area and usually represent Hodgkin's disease. Non-Hodgkin's lymphomas may also develop, and its manifestations tend to be widely disseminated throughout the body. In addition, differential diagnosis should also include the systemic lymphoproliferative diseases that are known to involve the cervicofacial nodes.

Clinical criteria that include a thorough history and physical and clinical examinations of the patient, collated with knowledge of lymphatic pathology, anatomy, and drainage patterns, must be appreciated in attaining a definitive diagnosis. The

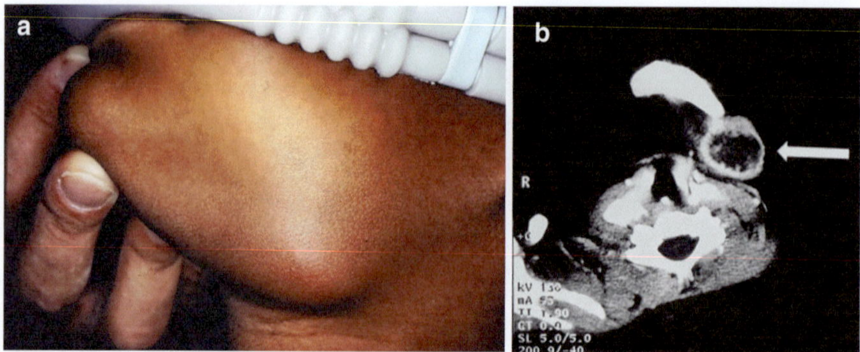

Fig. 19.14 (**a**) Lymphadenitis. Patient E. Cat scratch disease. (**b**) Lymphadenitis. Patient E. CT scan. Cat scratch disease. Abscessed lymph node (arrow)

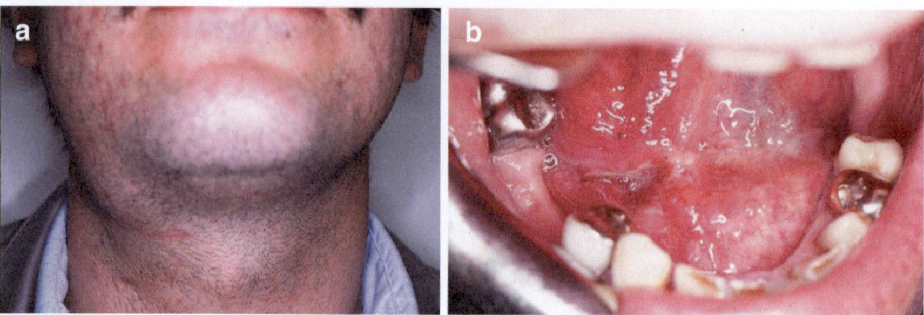

Fig. 19.15 (**a**) Metastatic lymphadenopathy. Patient F. Extraoral view. (**b**) Metastatic lymphadenopathy. Patient F. Intraoral view of mouth floor carcinoma

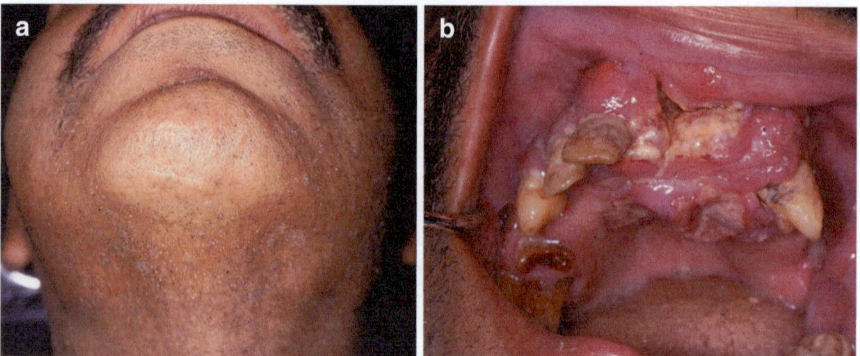

Fig. 19.16 (**a**) Metastatic lymphadenopathy. Patient G. Extraoral view. Bilateral submandibular lymphadenopathy. (**b**) Metastatic lymphadenopathy. Patient G. Intraoral view. Midline maxillary carcinoma

sudden onset of swelling and tenderness in a node that is movable and circumscribed suggests the presence of a lymphadenitis. Neoplastic nodes tend to be persistent, firm, often fixed in position, and usually painless. All nodal swellings demand local and systemic investigations regarding the origin of their abnormality.

A simple method to differentiate a lymphadenopathy from a sialadenitis is to observe whether expressed saliva exiting from the suspected gland's duct is cloudy or clear. Cloudiness indicates the presence of pus associated with a sialadenitis, while clear saliva implies a normal gland and suggests an extraglandular pathologic process. The absence of the glandular pain and swelling associated with eating serves as another diagnostic clue. Imaging (MRI, CT) can demonstrate an enlarged node and may indicate the cause. Biopsy, whether it be a fine-needle aspiration biopsy or a surgical tissue biopsy, is a critical aspect of the diagnostic workup and will also serve to differentiate a reactive node from a neoplastic node.

Paraglandular Pathology: Overview

Anatomically, the salivary glands do not exist in an isolated anatomic neighborhood. They are positioned close to adjacent anatomic structures. The relationship of the glands to these structures can only be appreciated from a familiarity with anatomy.

The bulk of the parotid gland (PG) lies on the lateral posterior aspect of the ramus and posterior aspect of the masseter muscle. A portion (the deep lobe) wraps itself around the posterior border of the mandibular ramus on its way to a relationship with the posterior medial aspect of the ramus. An artificial plane created by the facial nerve and its branches serves to separate the large PG superficial lobe from its smaller deep lobe. The PG's large superficial lobe rests partly on the posterior lateral aspect of the masseter muscle as the muscle inserts onto the lateral surface of the ramus. Therefore, because of this intimate liaison of the PG with the masseter muscle, pathology that involves the muscle or the submasseteric space can be misinterpreted as originating from the PG. Similarly, some extraglandular pathologic conditions that involve the mandibular ramus, the submandibular space (the home of the submandibular salivary gland), or the sublingual space (the home of the sublingual salivary gland) can be misdiagnosed as salivary gland disease.

The Columbia University Salivary Gland Center has had the opportunity to examine many patients with a variety of extraglandular pathologies whose initial diagnosis was misinterpreted as a salivary gland problem because of their intimate relationships with the salivary gland. These are the entities that are being reviewed in this False/Positives section.

Paraglandular Pathology: Ramus Pathology

The body of the mandible is the anatomic home of the mandibular dental apparatus. As such in addition to pathology primarily associated with bone, the mandible is subject to a unique set of pathologic insults by entities that have odontogenic origins. The mandibular ramus can serve as a victim of many of these conditions. Ramus pathology may originate from within the ramus, by extension from the mandibular body or even result secondarily as a metastatic pathologic manifestation from a distant site. Regardless, the anticipated inevitable growth within the ramus of the disease process will eventually cause a bulging or perforation of the lateral cortical plate of the ramus. In so doing, the masseter muscle and the overlying parotid gland (PG) are displaced laterally causing a lateral bulge of the external facial contour that resembles PG swelling. Many patients with ramus abnormalities have been referred to the Salivary Gland Center with a misdiagnosis of PG swelling.

Cysts such as the odontogenic keratocyst or dentigerous cyst are unique to the teeth-harboring jaws. Their relentless and often asymptomatic growth can by extension involve the ramus. The cysts' continued growth will eventually cause expansion of the ramus's lateral cortical plate or even perforate the ramus and displace laterally the overlying soft tissue structures and cause a facial swelling that can imitate a PG swelling. Neoplasms that involve the ramus act in the same way. The ameloblastoma (Fig. 19.17) serves as an example of a neoplastic pathologic growth that can affect the ramus primarily or by extension from the mandibular body [33, 34]. In addition, metastatic malignancies, particularly from the breast, can invade the ramus [35]. Whether the lesion primarily originates in the ramus or whether it finds a secondary home in the ramus as a result of metastasis or extension from the

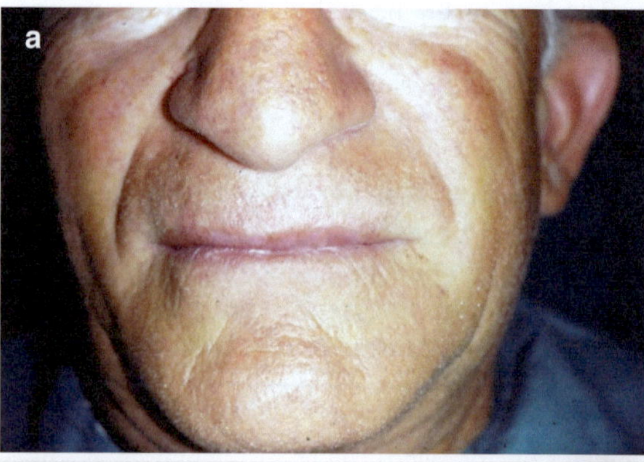

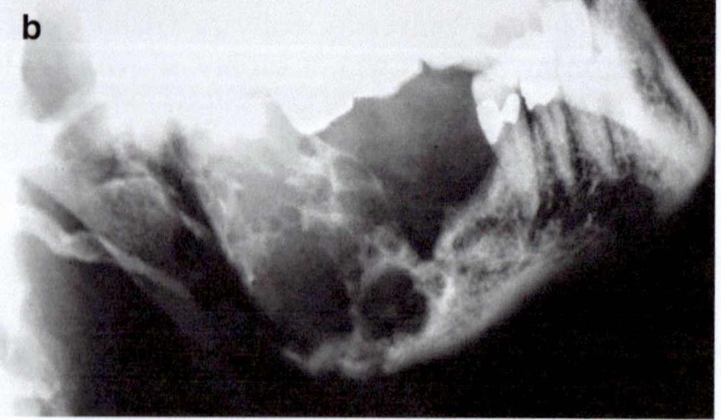

Fig. 19.17 (**a**) Paraglandular. Patient H. Extraoral view ameloblastoma left mandible. (**b**) Paraglandular. Patient H. Ameloblastoma left mandibular ramus

mandibular body, its continued growth will cause the facial asymmetry that often is misinterpreted as a PG problem.

The key to an accurate diagnosis rests in imaging. Radiographs, CT scans, and MRI will indicate that pathologic involvement of the ramus is the cause of the parotid area facial swelling. A detailed normal salivary gland history and the intra-oral visualization of a normal salivary return are measures that can rule out the PG as the cause of the swelling. A definitive diagnosis awaits the obtaining of a surgical specimen followed by its microscopic examination.

Paraglandular Pathology: Masseteric Intramuscular Hemangioma

The intramuscular hemangioma (IMH) is a vascular malformation (VM) that involves skeletal muscle. Despite the name hemangioma, most IMHs probably are VMs and are not true vascular neoplasms as suggested by the term hemangioma. Although more commonly seen in the pelvic area, the head and neck region is where 10–15% of IMHs occur, with 36% of these involving the masseter muscle (MM) [36]. The IMH is considered a congenital and benign VM that results from an error in vessel morphogenesis [37]. Although present but not readily apparent at birth, the VM grows proportionately with the body as the individual matures. Eventually a swelling develops in early adult life and becomes cosmetically visible. Trauma or infection may serve as causative precipitating factors in the IMH's growth.

Because the persistent IMH swelling involves the MM and because the muscle lies in a close anatomic relationship with the parotid gland (PG) and is even to some extent overlapped by the PG, IMH patients have been seen in the Salivary Gland Center with presumptive diagnoses of PG swelling. To further muddy the diagnostic waters, phleboliths, often interpreted as PG sialoliths, are present in many of the IMHs (Fig. 19.18). A phlebolith starts with the formation of a protective thrombus at any point of vascular wall injury. Alternatively, blood slowly flowing through the tortuous channels of an IMH tends to stagnate and thrombose. In either case, a mature phlebolith evolves if dystrophic calcification develops within the thrombus. Phleboliths are uncommon in the oral region, and their presence suggests an IMH. Although phleboliths can occur in the absence of vascular lesions, they are most often associated with vascular abnormalities. The incidence of phlebolith formation in all IMH lesions has variously been reported to be 3–50% [38].

Because it is embedded within muscle tissue, clinically diagnosing the masseteric IMH is difficult. Pulsation and bruits generally are not recognized because of the lesion's depth and sluggish nature of the blood flow. In addition, the depth of the IMH prevents skin discoloration. Palpation usually indicates that the IMH swelling is painless, soft, compressible, and not circumscribed. A gradual increase in size with cosmetic asymmetry develops and eventually serves as the impetus for the patient to seek consultation.

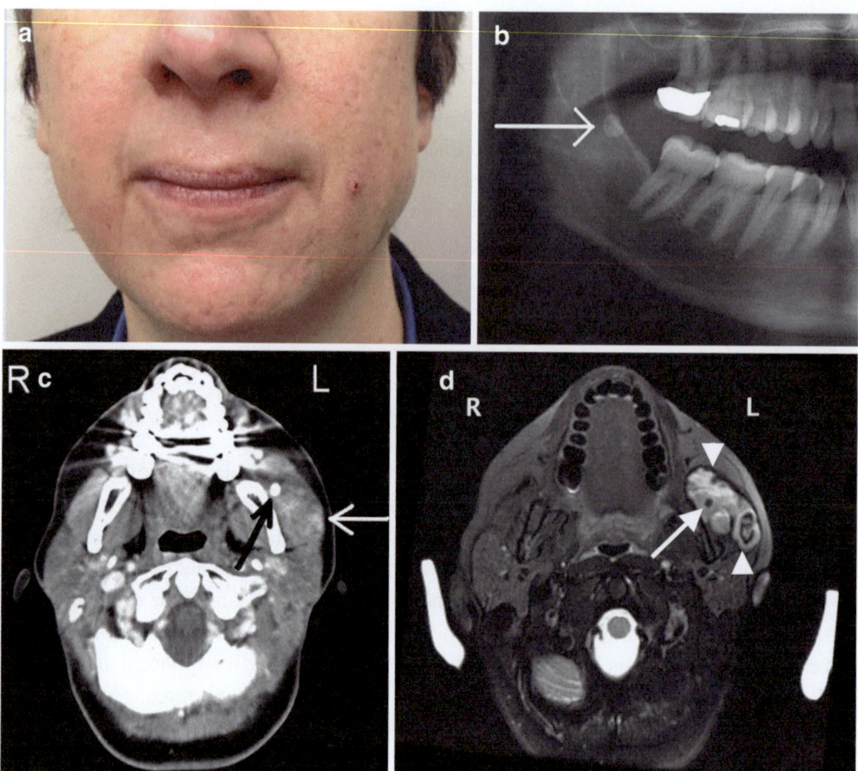

Fig. 19.18 (**a**) Paraglandular. Patient I. Left parotid area swelling from intramasseteric hemangioma (Mandel L, J Oral Maxillofac Surg 2014;72:2192). (**b**) Paraglandular. Patient I. Intramasseteric hemangioma Phlebolith (arrow). (Mandel L, J Oral Maxillofac Surg 2014;72:2192). (**c**) Paraglandular. Patient I. CT scan with contrast. Intramasseteric hemangioma. Vascular component (white arrow) and phlebolith (black arrow) (Mandel L, J Oral Maxillofac Surg 2014;72:2192). (**d**) Paraglandular. Patient I. MRI. Intramasseteric hemangioma. Phlebolith (arrow) and vascular component (arrow heads) (Mandel L, J Oral Maxillofac Surg 2014;72:2192)

The diagnosis of a head and neck IMH can be aided by the presence of the wattle sign [38] which develops because the IMH accumulates blood and gets larger when the head is prone or in a dependent position. A dependent head discourages a venous return from the vascular lesion to the superior vena cava because of gravity. An increased IMH swelling from vascular retention is the end result. Confirmation can be obtained from patients who often note that the swelling is most marked when awakening after sleep. With the patient's return to a vertical position from the horizontal sleeping position, the increased IMH vascular volume gradually dissipates as gravity takes effect and a reversion to the original swelling size occurs.

Differentiating the masseteric IMH from a PG sialadenitis is facilitated by the absence of the signs and symptoms associated with PG inflammation. Imaging (MRI, CT) will also serve to eliminate a diagnosis of PG pathology. The T2-weighted MRI is the imaging procedure of choice for an IMH because it clearly highlights the free water content of vascular lesions (Fig. 19.18d). The CT scan readily identifies calcified phleboliths but has difficulty in identifying vascular pathology (Fig. 19.18c). Standard radiographs are helpful in recognizing the presence of a phlebolith because these calcifications tend to demonstrate a concentric ring pattern upon X-ray examination rather than the even opacity of a sialolith. Furthermore, VM phleboliths differ from sialoliths in that phleboliths are usually multiple and randomly placed and do not follow the parotid duct's pathway [39]. The concentric ring ovality of the phlebolith can serve as a distinguishing mark when compared with the sialolith whose frequent evenly opaque elliptical shape has been contoured by a salivary duct.

Because the IMH has no defined border and surgery can lead to serious intra- and postoperative bleeding, embolization of the feeding vessel has become the treatment of choice. Sclerotherapy and radiation have also been advocated. Patients often choose to avoid treatment and opt for periodic observations because the lesion is essentially asymptomatic and is very slow growing.

Paraglandular Pathology: Submasseteric Abscess

Although the masseter muscle (MM) inserts along a broad expanse of the lateral surface of the mandibular ramus, Bransby-Zachary [40] found a narrow ramus area devoid of MM insertion, the submasseteric space (SMS). The SMS extends from the anterior border of the midpoint of the ramus upward and backward to the condylar neck region. Infection of the SMS can occur and usually originates from the mandibular third molar region. The somewhat unusual backward extension of infection, from the mandibular molar area along the lateral surface of the ramus, can bring about a submasseteric abscess (SMA) in the SMS with signs and symptoms that simulate a chronic parotitis.

The parotid gland (PG) has a close anatomic relationship to the MM with some overlap on the muscle by the PG. When pus accumulates in the SMS to form the SMA, the lateral wall of the space, the MM, is displaced laterally and causes a visibly diffuse facial parotid area swelling (Fig. 19.19a). Furthermore, because the MM serves as the lateral border of the SMS, the muscle itself inevitably becomes secondarily involved in the inflammatory process and a myositis with trismus develops [41] (Fig. 19.19b, c). The inflammatory infiltrate associated with the myositis thickens the MM and further accentuates the facial swelling that is readily confused with a parotitis.

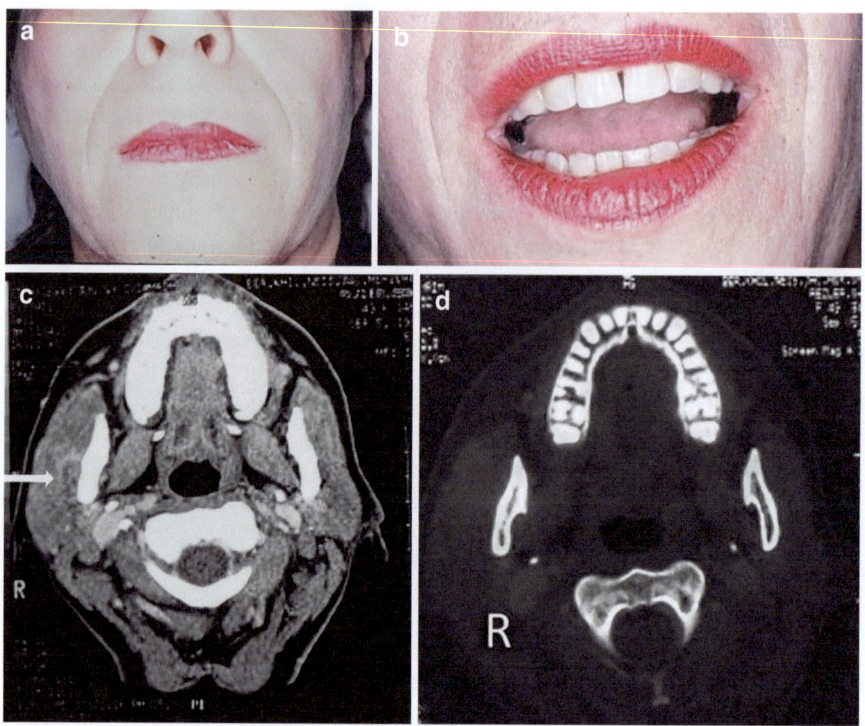

Fig. 19.19 (**a**) Paraglandular. Patient J. Submasseteric abscess. Right parotid area swelling. (**b**) Paraglandular. Patient J. Submasseteric abscess with trismus. (**c**) Paraglandular. Patient J. CT scan. Lucent submasseteric abscess (arrow) and right masseteric myositis. (**d**) Paraglandular. Patient J. CT scan bony window. Submasseteric abscess. Increased bone deposition right ramus

Patients with an SMA have been seen with prolonged recurrent histories of swelling, trismus, and pain. Antibiotic therapy, to combat these symptoms, often is the first line of defense. However, any relief is temporary and recurrences of symptoms are to be expected. The recurrent exacerbations are a result of the limited effect of antibiotic therapy on a closed space infection replete with anaerobic organisms [42].

An initial diagnosis of chronic parotitis because of recurrent parotid area swellings can be avoided with a detailed history and examination. A pre-existing mandibular molar problem (pericoronitis, infected molar or infection following a molar extraction) or even a misdirected mandibular block needle injection [41] all point away from a PG etiology. Extraorally, the bulk of the facial SMS swelling will occupy an area slightly anterior to the PG's pre-auricular position. Palpation of the extraoral swelling causes some discomfort while no pain will be elicited with palpation of the uninvolved PG. Of great significance is the presence of the trismus that is caused by the MM myositis, originating from the muscle's direct contact with the SMA. Trismus is not a significant feature of a parotitis. Although the recurrent SMS swellings can be confused with the presence of a chronic parotitis, the swellings are not associated with meals. Furthermore, saliva exiting from the PG's intraoral duct orifice will be seen to be clear rather than the cloudy saliva caused by contained pus seen in patients with a parotitis.

Imaging (CT, MRI) is most helpful in clinching an SMA diagnosis, because of the ability of the CT scan (Fig. 19.19c, d) and the MRI [43, 44] to define tissue densities. Diagnosis of an inflammatory process is facilitated with these imaging tools. A myositis can be recognized by heightened muscle enhancement and by an increased muscle density and bulk resulting from the infiltration of inflammatory products. The areas of increased density may alternate with zones of decreased density that reflect abscess formation and muscle necrosis (Fig. 19.19c). MRI is the preferred method for evaluating soft tissue lesions, but CT scanning is useful for imaging bone. Because the ramus represents the limiting medial wall of the SMS infection and because the juxtaposed infection has usually been present for a prolonged period, bony changes in the abutting ramus in the form of a hyperostosis responding to a persistent low-grade osteitis can be expected (Fig. 19.19d). Osteomyelitis does not usually develop because the bacterial virulence is not sufficient to overcome host resistance.

Successful treatment of the infectious process is achieved with adequate drainage of pus from the SMS. A surgical incision, intraorally and/or extraorally, into the SMS along the lateral border of the ramus represents the best therapeutic option. The surgical incision and drainage must be supplemented with appropriate antibiotics and supportive care.

Paraglandular Pathology: HIV-Associated Lipodystrophy Syndrome

The HIV/AIDS disease morphed into a chronic manageable condition when highly active antiretroviral therapy (HAART) was introduced for its treatment. This therapeutic regimen usually included two nucleoside reverse transcriptase inhibitors (NRTI) and a protease inhibitor (PI) or a non-NRTI. Consequently, disease progression has been inhibited and the patient's quality of life has improved. Unfortunately, patients have experienced collateral damage from the medications in the form of the lipodystrophy syndrome (LS), whose prevalence in HIV patients who are receiving HAART has been reported to have a 10–80% range [45].

The LS is defined as a significant body fat redistribution that is often accompanied by a hyperlipidemia and insulin resistance. The fat redistribution may manifest itself as lipohypertrophy (LH) (fat accumulation), lipoatrophy (LA) (fat wasting), or a mixture of both LA and LH [46]. The NRTIs, particularly stavudine, as well as the PIs, have been documented as significant factors in the development of LS [46, 47]. The exact mechanisms by which these HAART agents play a role in the development of LS are not fully understood. However, it has been suggested that LA results when the synergistic activity of the HAART medications inhibits proliferation and maturation of the preadipocytes [48]. Besides the use of NRTIs and the PIs, other risk factors for the development of LA include HIV disease activity and host factors such as age [45]. Risk factors for LH development include increasing age, female sex, and elevated triglycerides [45]. Lipoatrophy tends to occur in the buttocks, malar area of the face, and arms and legs. In contrast, LH is usually manifest along the abdominal waist, in the breast, and in the cervicofacial areas [45].

Bilateral parotid gland (PG) swelling is not an unusual finding in HIV patients and is often associated with the diffuse infiltrative CD8 lymphocytosis syndrome (DILS). The swellings mostly reflect the presence of lymphoepithelial cysts whose elimination can be achieved with HAART. Nevertheless, despite the successful PG swelling eradication with HAART, HIV patients who have been on long-term therapy have been seen in the Salivary Gland Center with apparent bilateral PG swellings. Histories indicate that the swellings are persistent, do not fluctuate in size, and are painless. Palpation will reveal that the swellings generally follow the anatomic outline of the PG, have a normal tissue tone, and are painless. Intraorally, normal salivary returns are observed at the orifices of the parotid duct when the PG is extraorally massaged.

If HIV patients are being successfully treated with HAART, why then would some present themselves with supposed PG swellings? Imaging, whether it be a CT scan or MRI, will clearly reveal the source of the parotid area swellings in these HIV patients (Fig. 19.20a, c). Paraparotid accumulations of subcutaneous fat will be distinctly depicted in some HIV patients who are receiving long-term HAART that includes NRTIs and PIs. Simultaneously, these patients may have a thick neck, buffalo hump (Fig. 19.20b), and an increased abdominal girth, all serving as signs of the effects of LH. Malar soft tissue wasting and thinned buttocks and extremities also are present as result of the effect of LA.

Therapeutically, attempts to modify the adipose changes in LS by altering the medication regimen have resulted in only moderate success [49] and should be weighed against the possibility that any new regimen will impact HIV treatment by not adequately controlling HIV replication.

Paraglandular Pathology: Submandibular Space Infection

The suprahyoid segment of the anterior neck triangle can be divided into two triangular subdivisions, the submandibular triangle (SMT), a triangle of major interest, and the submental triangle. Superiorly, the SMT is bordered by the body of the mandible. Anteriorly and posteriorly, the SMT is limited by the anterior and posterior bellies of the digastric muscle, respectively. The chief structures located in this triangle are the large main body of the submandibular salivary gland (SMSG) and the submandibular lymph nodes.

The submandibular fascial space (SMS) is a potential space whose borders correspond to the anatomic outline of the SMT. Because this space contains the SMSG, infection of the space can readily be interpreted as originating from an infected SMSG. However, SMS infection is usually caused by an infected mandibular molar (Fig. 19.21) whose root apex is lingually positioned below the mylohyoid muscle's insertion, as the muscle slants upward toward its posterior attachment to the lingual

Fig. 19.20 (a)
Paraglandular. Patient
K. Lipodystrophy
syndrome. HIV
associated. Bilateral
parotid area swelling.
(b) Paraglandular. Patient
K. Lipodystrophy
syndrome. HIV
associated. Buffalo hump.
(c) Paraglandular. Patient
K. CT scan. Lipodystrophy
syndrome. HIV associated.
Bilateral paraparotid fat
deposition (arrows)

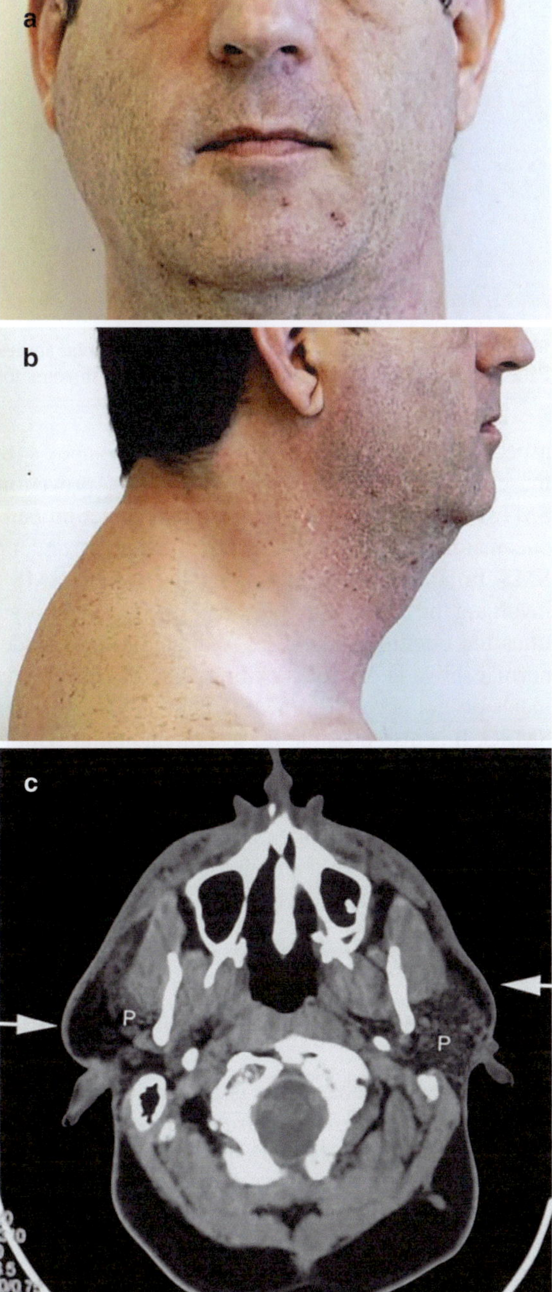

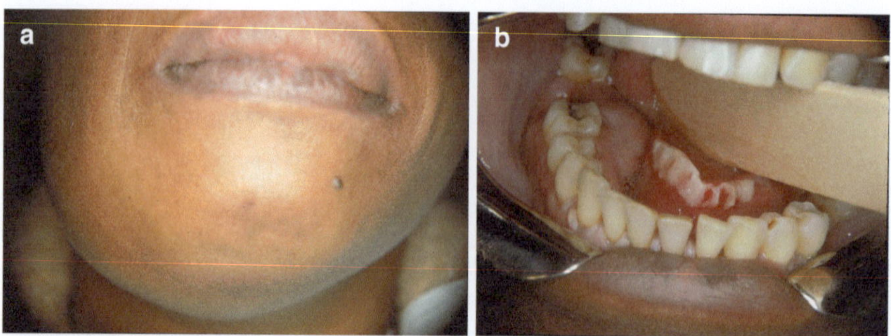

Fig. 19.21 (**a**) Paraglandular. Patient L. Submandibular abscess (dental origin). (**b**) Paraglandular. Patient L. Submandibular abscess originating from infected tooth root #31

aspect of the mandible. Because of the root apex's inferior position, the mylohyoid muscle no longer serves as a barrier preventing infectious spread to the SMT. Alternatively, mandibular molar infection can move buccally inferior to the buccinator muscle's mandibular attachment and enter the inferiorly positioned SMS. In both cases, infection localized in the SMS [50] causes pain and swelling involving the area occupied by the SMSG. A cursory oral examination usually identifies the odontogenic cause. A diagnosis of sialadenitis can be eliminated when normal saliva is observed exiting from the duct orifice of the SMSG. The fact that meals do not accentuate SMSG pain and swelling is further evidence of a normal SMSG. It is also possible for a submandibular lymphadenitis to develop secondary to an oral infection that drains into the lymphatics of the submandibular lymph nodes.

Radiographs (periapical, panoramic), supplemented by a CT scan or MRI when indicated, will disclose the offending tooth. Dental care is required and when necessary, a surgical incision and drainage of the SMS. Antibiotics, analgesics, and supportive care are integral aspects of therapy.

Paraglandular Pathology: Sublingual Space Infection

The sublingual space (SLS) is anatomically located in the mouth floor. The oral surface of the mylohyoid muscle (MyM) serves as the space's inferior limitation, while the oral mucosa beneath the tongue functions as the roof of the SLS. Anteriorly and laterally, the SLS is limited by the lingual aspect of the mandible. Posteriorly, it is bordered by the muscles along the base of the tongue. The genioglossus muscle serves to separate the SLS into two halves. Infections of mandibular teeth usually track buccally to cause a clinical buccal swelling. However, on occasion, the odontogenic infection may move lingually superior to the MyM and locate between the oral mucosa and the oral surface of the MyM [51]. The consequent inflammatory reaction in the SLS inevitably envelops the sublingual salivary gland, a major

Fig. 19.22 Paraglandular. Sublingual space cellulitis

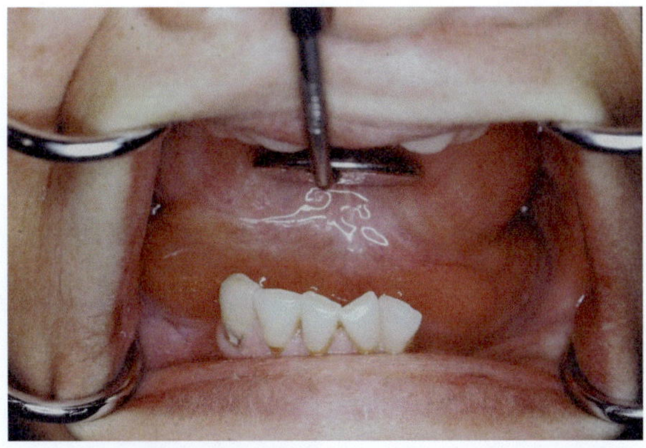

inhabitant of the SLS, and a diffuse mouth floor edematous inflammatory swelling that is painful and erythematous becomes evident (Fig. 19.22).

A superficial examination of the mouth floor in a SLS infection with its extensive edematous inflammation can suggest the presence of the fluid containing ranula. Differentiation rests in the fact that the SLS swelling is inflammatory in origin while ranulas are non-inflammatory painless cyst-like swellings. Ranulas create problems associated with their physical presence, whereas a SLS infection demonstrates classic inflammatory symptomatology and has the potential to spread and cause serious systemic problems.

An intraoral examination can usually pinpoint the offending tooth, with imaging serving as a major diagnostic aid in identifying the infected tooth that is causing the SLS infection. Intraoral periapical films, panoramic radiographs, or CT scanning and MRI, when indicated, are essential aids.

Standard treatment requires dental care for the offending tooth. Surgical incision and drainage of the SLS, to evacuate any accumulated pus, are mandatory. Antibiotics, analgesics, and supportive care must be included in the therapeutic regimen.

Paraglandular Pathology: Lymphatic Malformation

Lymphatic malformations (LMs) are thought to develop embryologically from sequestrations of lymphatic tissue during the fetal development of the lymphaticovenous sacs. If these sacs fail to communicate with the developing lymphatic or venous systems, they will go on to form a LM [52]. The congenital LM manifests itself as a slow growing fluid-filled cyst-like lesion. Growth results from both the accumulation of lymph and the development of endothelial sprouts that infiltrate and migrate through adjacent tissue planes [53].

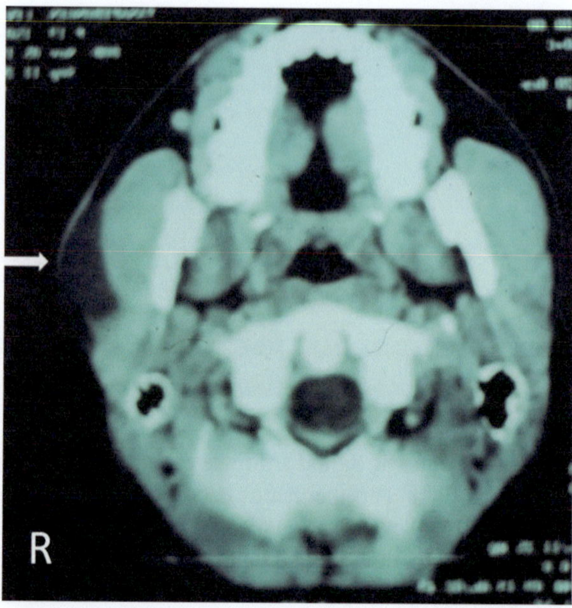

Fig. 19.23 Paraglandular. CT scan. Lucent lymphatic malformation parotid area (arrow)

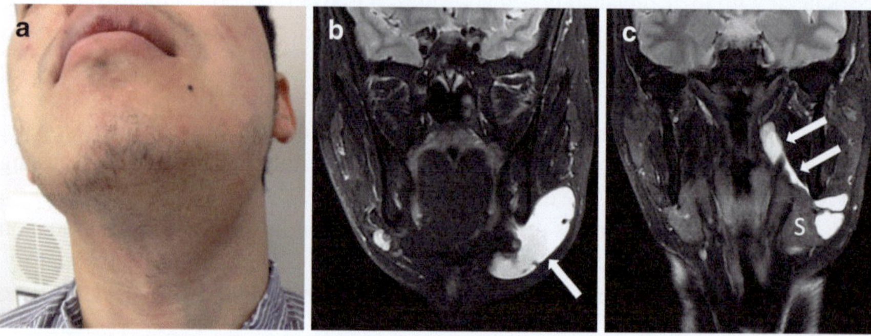

Fig. 19.24 (**a**) Paraglandular. Patient M. Extraoral view. Lymphatic malformation (left submandibular area). (**b**) Paraglandular. Patient M. MRI. Lymphatic malformation. Submandibular area (arrow). (**c**) Paraglandular. Patient M. MRI. Lymphatic malformation extending into tissue planes (arrows). Submandibular salivary gland (S)

Although mostly seen in children, LMs in adults are not an unusual occurrence. Trauma or an upper respiratory infection can cause a LM to arise de novo, or it can activate congenitally dormant abnormal lymphatic tissue to form a clinically visible LM [54]. Most LMs involve the lymphatic rich head and neck region, often the parotid area (Fig. 19.23) [55] and the submandibular triangle (Fig. 19.24) [56]. The growth of an LM is commensurate with the growth of the patient. Clinically, the LM is poorly encapsulated and has the ability to infiltrate adjacent tissue planes (Fig. 19.24c). When palpated, the LM is noted to be painless, soft, and compressible. The LM varies in size from a few millimeters (microcystic) to several centimeters (macrocystic) with a tendency for intermittent exacerbations of pain and swelling incited by infection or a traumatic episode. Clinically, the LM is observed either in a localized cyst-like form or as an extensive infiltrating cervicofacial lesion (Fig. 19.24b, c) [57].

Imaging has become the key method utilized for the diagnosis of an LM. The MRI has proven to be the primary diagnostic imaging modality because it has the superior ability to enhance the LM's fluid content. Consequently, the extent of the LM and its anatomic relation to surrounding structures will be clearly revealed (Fig. 19.24b, c).

Microscopic study of an LM reveals cyst-like spaces that may or may not communicate with each other. The spaces are surrounded by a thin one-layer endothelial cell lining infiltrated by a scattering of lymphocytes and macrophages. The cyst-like spaces contain an eosinophilic protein rich fluid, a critical diagnostic clue obtained when performing a fine-needle aspiration biopsy. The connective tissue intervening between the spaces includes collections of lymphocytes [58].

Because of their frequent proximity to the salivary glands, differential diagnosis of a head and neck LM must incorporate salivary gland pathology. Patients with a LM in the parotid or submandibular salivary gland areas have been referred to the Salivary Gland Center with diagnoses of salivary gland disease (Figs. 19.23 and 19.24). Close scrutiny and investigation indicated that the problem was an extraglandular LM. Differential diagnosis from the relatively common sialadenitis is mandatory. Clinically, the LM differs from a sialadenitis by the absence of the symptomatology associated with the inflammation that occurs in a sialadenitis (pain, episodic swelling, cloudy saliva). Neoplasms can be differentiated from a LM when the aspirate obtained from a fine-needle biopsy reveals characteristic neoplastic cells.

If the LM is localized and does not infiltrate around vital anatomic structures, surgery is the preferred treatment approach. Sclerotherapy has become the most widely used therapeutic procedure for those infiltrating LMs whose surgical removal would be problematic. A variety of sclerotherapeutic agents is available, but doxycycline appears to be the safest and most effective [59]. Recently sirolimus, a medication that inhibits lymphogenesis by reducing lymphatic synthesis, has been utilized with some success [60].

Paraglandular Pathology: Dermoid Cyst

The dermoid cyst (DC) is usually observed in the midline of the mouth floor (Fig. 19.25). It is believed to result from congenitally included ectoderm that has been trapped during the bilateral embryologic fusion of the developing mandibular or hyoid arches, respectively, the first and second branchial arches [61]. A review of 1495 cases of DC indicated that most head and neck dermoids occur in the orbital region because of the complex fusion lines present in the orbital area that are available to trap

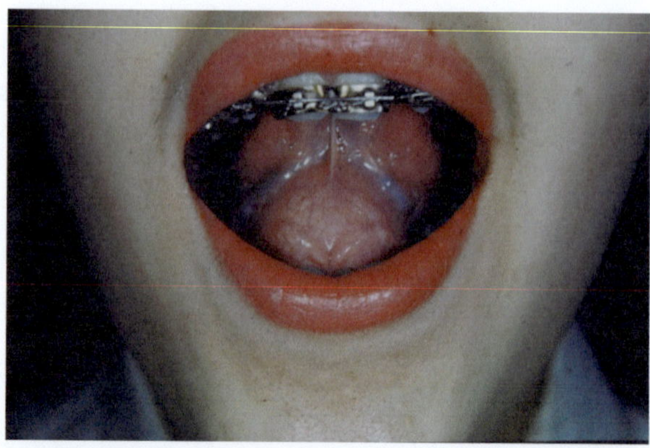

Fig. 19.25 Paraglandular. Dermoid cyst. Intraoral. Midline

ectoderm [62]. The oral region, particularly the midline of the mouth floor, represents the next most frequent location for the head and neck DC. Although most DC occur in the midline of the mouth floor, some are present in the submandibular area (Fig. 19.26). These laterally positioned DCs presumably originate in the midline of the oral cavity above the mylohyoid muscle. Subsequently, the DC probably migrates laterally during its expansion and extends inferiorly into the submandibular triangle either through a dehiscence in the mylohyoid muscle or around the muscle's posterior border. With the DC's lateral-inferior shift and growth, the swelling that develops in the submandibular triangle is frequently misinterpreted as submandibular salivary gland (SMSG) pathology or even a plunging ranula (Fig. 19.26a, b).

The DC may go unnoticed for prolonged periods because it is asymptomatic. With growth, it becomes clinically apparent during the second and third decades of life. The DC grows slowly and is a well-circumscribed unilocular mass. Palpation indicates that the DC is painless and has a doughy consistency because of its contained keratin. The lateral DC, located in the submandibular triangle, tends to be larger than the intraoral variety, possibly because its growth is not impeded by surrounding mandibular bone.

A CT scan will reveal that the migrated DC is unilocular and has a smooth margin and a developed cystic wall (Fig. 19.26b). The contents are homogeneous and low in attenuation [63], reflecting the presence of keratin. Displacement of the neighboring SMSG will also be evident.

Histologically, the wall of the DC consists of stratified squamous epithelium and contains dermal appendages such as hair follicles, sebaceous, and sweat glands (Fig. 19.26c). An epidermoid variety also exists and is devoid of these appendages, but otherwise it is identical to the appendage-containing DC. The delineation of a DC from the epidermoid cyst has no clinical significance and is dependent only on the microscopic findings.

Because the DC has a well-defined cystic wall with a doughy keratin content, it lends itself to a blunt surgical dissection and removal in toto. Recurrence is not a concern.

Fig. 19.26 (**a**) Paraglandular. Dermoid cyst. Patient N. Laterally positioned in submandibular gland area. (**b**) Paraglandular. Dermoid cyst. Patient N. CT scan (coronal view). Cyst extends into submandibular area. (**c**) Paraglandular. Microscopic view of dermoid cyst with hair follicle (arrow A) and sebaceous gland (arrow B)

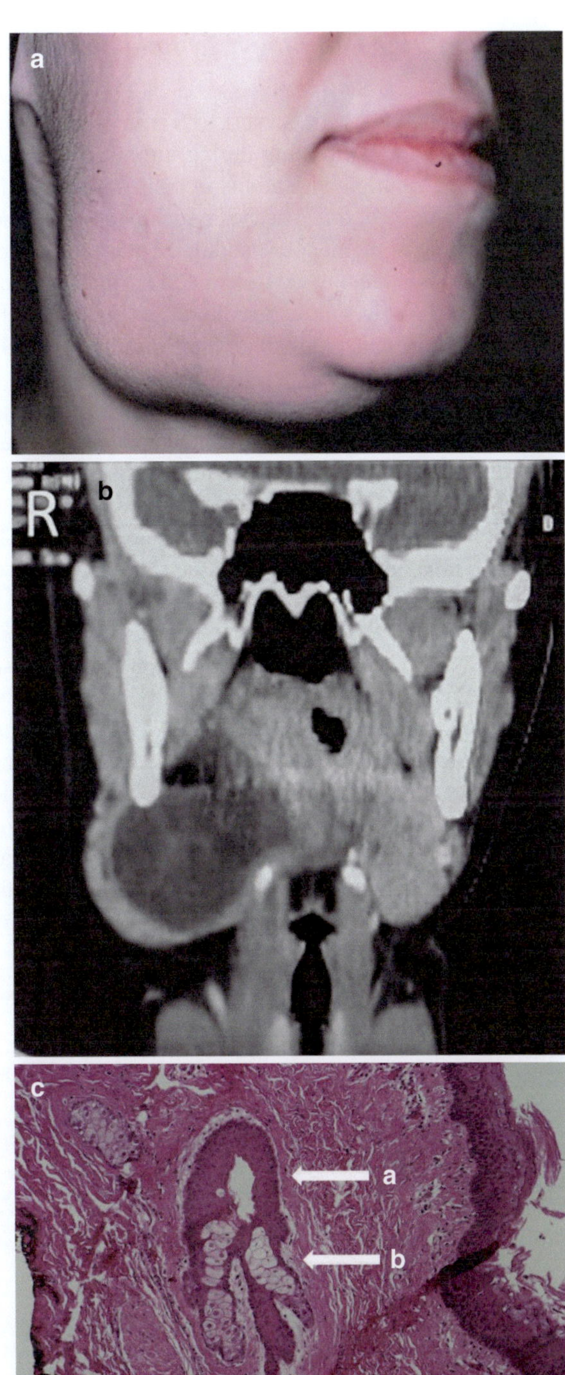

Paraglandular Pathology: Lymphoepithelial Cyst

The oral lymphoepithelial cyst (LEC) is an uncommon lesion that is usually discovered as an incidental finding during a routine dental examination. The LEC has a wide age distribution with adults in their fourth decade of life (mean age 39 years) most often affected [64]. The cyst typically presents itself as a freely movable dome-shaped painless submucosal nodule in the mouth floor or ventral surface of the tongue. It has a smooth non-ulcerated surface, a firm consistency when palpated, and a characteristic yellow discoloration (Fig. 19.27a). Although it can vary in size from a few millimeters to 2.0 cm, it generally is less than 1.0 cm in diameter.

Etiologically, the LEC develops in ectopic tonsillar tissue. Ectopic tonsillar tissue represents tonsillar tissue that occurs outside of the major tonsil groups (palatine, lingual, adenoids, and tubal tonsils). Small nodular aggregates of ectopic lymphoid tissue are scattered throughout the mouth, most frequently in the mouth floor and the undersurface of the tongue. The LEC may have its origin during the embryologic period if epithelium becomes entrapped in the developing oral ectopic lymphoid tissue. Subsequently, trauma or inflammation may act as the stimulus for the embryologically included epithelium to proliferate and form a LEC. Alternatively, the LEC may result from obstruction of an epithelially lined ectopic tonsillar crypt. These crypts are normal anatomic structures associated with groupings of tonsillar tissue. A stimulus such as trauma or inflammation may trigger cryptal epithelial proliferation with LEC formation.

Microscopically, the LEC is usually lined by a parakeratinized stratified squamous epithelium. The cystic cavity mostly contains keratin and desquamated epithelial cells. Lymphoid tissue, often containing follicles, surrounds the cyst and is based on a fibrous connective tissue wall (Fig. 19.27b).

Clinically, a mouth floor LEC has a close resemblance to a submandibular duct sialolith. Its location, color, and configuration create the confusion. Differentiation is facilitated by the absence of the signs and symptoms associated with an

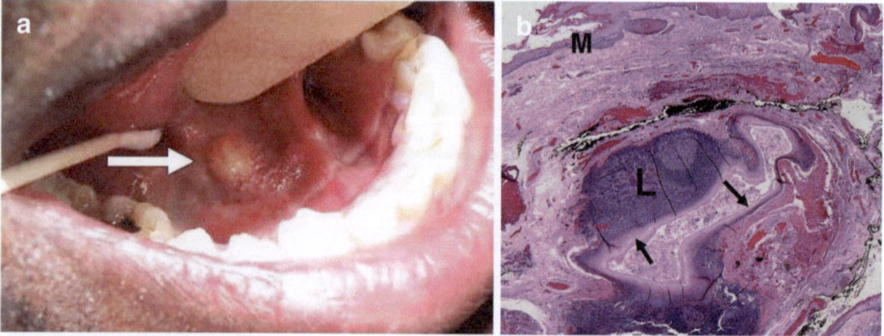

Fig. 19.27 (**a**) Paraglandular. Lymphoepithelial cyst (arrow). Patient O. (**b**) Paraglandular. Lymphoepithelial cyst. Patient O. Cyst lumen lined by stratified squamous epithelium (arrows) with lymphoidal nodules (L) in cyst wall. Oral mucosal epithelium present (M)

obstructive sialadenitis. Furthermore, imaging fails to reveal the calcification associated with a sialolith.

The LEC, because of its size, delineation, and superficial location, lends itself to local surgical excision. Healing is rapid and recurrences have not been reported. Final diagnosis awaits the microscopic examination.

Paraglandular Pathology: Facial Angioedema

Orofacial angioedema (AE) is an adverse reaction that can develop from the use of commonly prescribed antihypertensives such as an angiotensin-converting enzyme (ACE) inhibitor or an angiotensin receptor blocker (ARB). The AE caused by ACE inhibitors or ARBs usually involves the head and neck areas including the location of the parotid gland (PG). Patients have been referred to the Salivary Gland Center because swellings in the parotid/cheek areas defied accurate diagnoses. Tentative diagnoses of a PG problem were made and prompted the referral.

The areas of AE swelling caused by these drugs, in order of frequency, are the oral mucosa, tongue, lips, facial cheek, and neck [65]. The average age of AE onset is 52–62 years with 65% being female [66]. Clinically, the AE is a painless non-inflammatory, non-pitting, non-pruritic asymmetric edema that can involve the skin and subcutaneous tissues overlying the PG. Initially, the edema is mild and resolves rapidly (Fig. 19.28). Regardless, multiple transient recurrences can occur, and there is some tendency for the AE to increase in severity with time. Progression to airway obstruction and a fatal outcome are possible.

The causations of AE from an ACE inhibitor or an ARB are different. The ACE inhibitor, after a series of interactions, prevents the inactivation of bradykinin. Because bradykinin is not inactivated, tissue edema from vasodilation and an increase in capillary permeability are significantly enhanced. The exact role of the ARB in producing AE is not fully understood, but it may be related to its ability to block the vascular angiotensin 1 receptor [66]. The incidence of AE with ACE

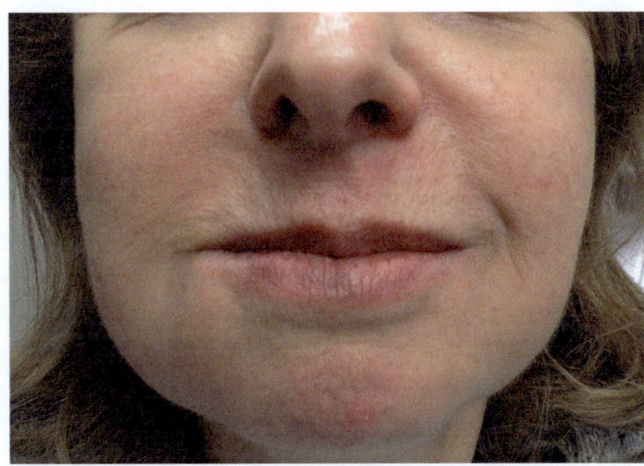

Fig. 19.28 Paraglandular. Right facial angioedema. Swelling peaked 24 h previously. Note absence of right nasolabial fold

inhibitor has been reported to range from 0.1 to 0.7%, while its incidence is somewhat lower with the ARBs [67]. The AE may become manifest within a few hours or weeks following either medication's ingestion, or its appearance may be delayed for many years following prolonged medication use.

The orofacial AE symptomatology associated with an ACE inhibitor or ARB can be mild or severe. Mild transient episodes require reassurance and a referral for medication re-evaluation. The treatment protocol for the more severe cases requires the use of intravenous steroids, diphenhydramine, and epinephrine.

Dental Conditions

Because saliva is recognized as an essential component in the prevention of dental caries, many patients with extensive dental damage have been referred to the Salivary Gland Center (SGC) based on the assumption that some salivary issue has caused their dental problem. Undoubtedly, hyposalivation will lead to extensive caries, but the hyposalivation is only significant enough to cause major dental deterioration in patients who have Sjögren syndrome (SS) and in patients who have received cancericidal doses of radiation in the head and neck area that incorporated the salivary glands and when aplasia affects multiple salivary glands. Although antisialogogic medications (psychotherapeutics, many cardiovascular drugs, antihistamines, etc.) have been implicated as causative agents for increased caries, the SGC has failed to confirm their guilt. It must be remembered that these medications individually can cause a mild salivary diminution when the glands are at rest. However, when stimulated (eating, etc.), the effect of the drug is overcome, a normal salivary return is obtained and apparently is sufficient to protect dental structures. Nevertheless, it is possible that patients receiving multiple antisialogogues may become prone to dental caries from the cumulative hyposalivary effect of the multiple drugs being used.

Rampant caries in patients who do not have SS, histories of radiation, or salivary gland aplasia usually is dietary in origin [68]. The high sucrose intake from soft drinks combined with their acid (phosphoric) levels in the range of pH 2.4 are the usual culprits [69]. Candy bars, fruit juices, sucking on hard candies, and the continuous use of sugar-containing chewing gum are also prime offenders that promote caries (Fig. 19.29). Methamphetamine abusers also develop rampant caries resulting from a decreased salivation, sugar craving, and poor oral hygiene (Fig. 19.30).

The loss of surface tooth substance by a chemical process (acidity) that does not involve bacteria has been referred to as dental erosion [70]. Because it is a chemical, not a physical, process, a more accurate term is corrosion. Loss of dental structure, particularly the enamel at pH 5.5 from acidic salivary contact, has been observed many times in patients referred to the SGC. Regurgitation of gastric acids (pH 1.5–2.0) from the multiple episodes associated with gastroesophageal reflux or from bulimic emesis also can cause significant loss of enamel structure. Similar dental destruction is seen in wine (pH 2.5) sippers and professional wine tasters [71] because the wine is

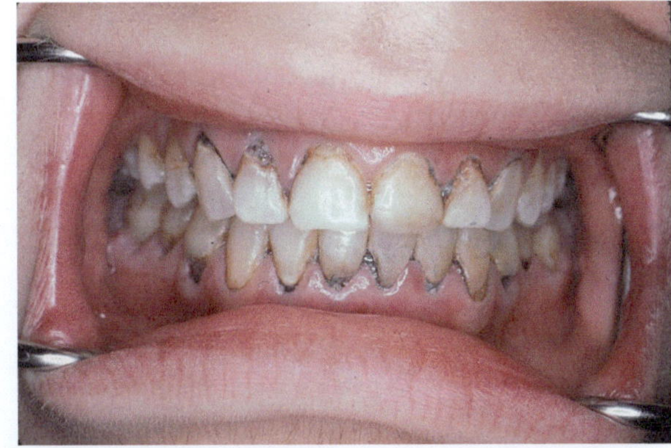

Fig. 19.29 Dental conditions. Extensive cervical caries from excessive sucking on mint candies

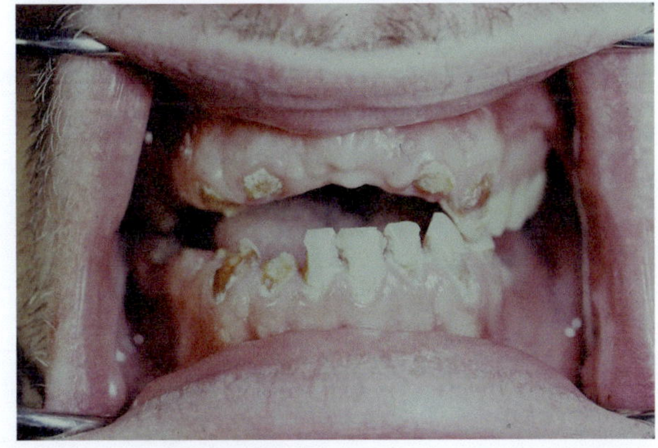

Fig. 19.30 Dental conditions. Dental destruction. Methamphetamine abuser ("meth mouth")

orally maintained, rather than swallowed, for prolonged periods and allowed to have its deleterious acidic effect on dental surfaces (Fig. 19.31). Overuse of acidic foods (citrus fruits and juices) will produce a similar dental reaction.

Dental attrition (Fig. 19.4), another cause of dental damage, is characterized by excessive physical wear on enamel and/or dentin. It is observed in awake bruxers/clenchers where the parafunctional activity is thought to be initiated by anxiety and/or stress [72]. Bruxism also occurs during sleep, and a relationship with obstructive sleep apnea (OSA) has been noted with 33–50% of OSA patients also suffering from sleep bruxism [73].

In contrast, abrasion is the physical wearing away of tooth structure by an extraoral foreign object such as a toothbrush (Fig. 19.32) or by an abrasive dentifrice. Patients have been referred to the SGC because their observed dental attrition/abrasion was believed to have a salivary origin. Such flawed diagnoses can be avoided only with a complete history and a thorough visual oral examination of the pattern of dental structure loss.

Therapy for reflux disease has been reviewed in Chap. 2. Therapy for bruxism has been reviewed in this chapter under the section "Masseteric Hypertrophy." Dietary adjustments are advised when indicated, while toothbrush instruction should solve the problem related to dental abrasion.

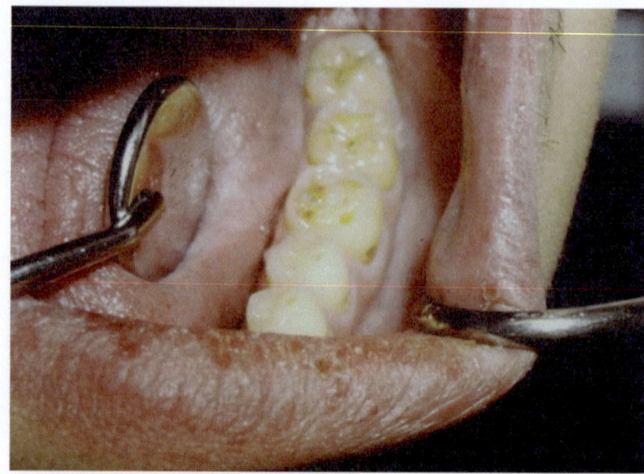

Fig. 19.31 Dental conditions. Wine sipper. Loss of occlusal enamel with dentin exposure and presence of white enamel rim

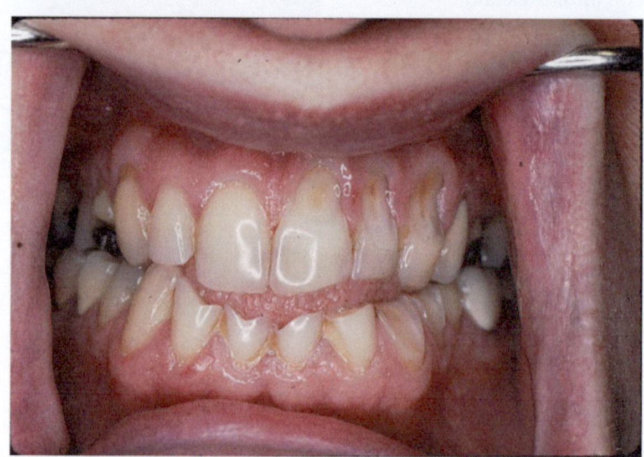

Fig. 19.32 Dental conditions. Toothbrush trauma

Drooling

Hypersalivation is defined as an excessive production of saliva that can lead to salivary accumulations in the mouth floor. If an increased salivary flow or normal accumulations of saliva are not functionally managed by swallowing, drooling of saliva will occur. Drooling leads to problems associated with perioral macerations, bad hygiene, and the social stigmata associated with an individual's appearance and the soiling of the person's clothing.

Swallowing begins when masticated food reaches the posterior oral cavity. It is an involuntary complex reflex that involves both the pharynx and larynx. A wide variety of disorders can cause a swallowing dysfunction that results in a failure of the clearance of oral saliva. Drooling develops and has proven to be a common problem present in the neurologically and motor impaired patient. Dysphagia with salivary collection and drooling are often observed in patients with Parkinson's disease (PD) (Fig. 2.4), Alzheimer's disease (Fig. 2.3), cerebral palsy, and amyotrophic lateral sclerosis (ALS) [74]. In these patients, saliva will pool in the anterior mouth floor because it cannot be effectively transported backward in the oral cavity and swallowed due to the patient's impaired neuromuscular function. Although the salivary accumulation and drooling are mainly caused by failure of posterior movement and by dysphagia, the drooling is further amplified by the fact that the head, in patients with PD and ALS, is usually in a forward leaning position. In addition, many of these patients demonstrate a facial hypokinesia with a failure to close the mouth and seal the lips [75, 76]. They also may have a sensory dysfunction which impedes the recognition of the presence of pooling and/or drooling [77].

Other causes of dysphagia-instigated drooling have been reported to occur in muscular dystrophies, poliomyelitis, and in patients who have received cancericidal doses of cervical irradiation that may have damaged the swallowing musculature [78, 79]. Drooling is also an issue that is frequently seen in the intellectually disabled. Regardless of the cause, it is essential to recognize the fact that these drooling patients are not producing excessive saliva, their drooling problem represents a management quandary.

Patients with drooling complaints have been referred to the Columbia University Salivary Gland Center because their drooling was misinterpreted as a manifestation of hypersalivation. Treatment for these patients must be focused first on recognizing the underlying medical condition and then alleviating the symptom (drooling) of the systemic condition. Therapeutically, antisialogogic agents can be prescribed to reduce the normal but unmanageable salivary volume. Scopolamine, glycopyrrolate, and atropine have been utilized with some success. Botulinum toxin A injections into multiple salivary glands are successful but must be repeated after several months [80]. Conservative therapy that involves biofeedback and observation is always an acceptable approach. The key to successful therapy is a team approach whose membership includes the family, the physician, the dentist, speech therapist, occupational therapist, and neurologist.

A further review of drooling can be found in Chap. 2.

References

1. Simon GE, VonKorff M, Piccinelli M, Fullerton C, Ormel J. An international study of the relation between somatic symptoms and depression. N Engl J Med. 1999;341(18):1329–35. https://doi.org/10.1056/NEJM199910283411801.
2. Preboth M. Clinical review of recent findings on the awareness, diagnosis and treatment of depression. Am Fam Physician. 2000;61(10):3158–68.
3. Cui Y, Zhang H, Wang S, et al. Stimulated parotid saliva is a better method for depression prediction. Biomedicines. 2022;10(9):2220. Published 2022 Sep 7. https://doi.org/10.3390/biomedicines10092220.
4. Votta TJ, Mandel L. Somatoform salivary complaints. Case reports. N Y State Dent J. 2002;68(1):22–6.
5. Christmas WA. La maladie du petit papier. J Am Coll Health. 1999;47(6):289–91. https://doi.org/10.1080/07448489909595661.
6. Legg J. Enlargement of the temporal and masseter muscles on both sides. Trans Pathol Soc Lond. 1880;31:361–6.

7. Kuhn M, Türp JC. Risk factors for bruxism. Swiss Dent J. 2018;128(2):118–24.

8. Ahlgren J, Omnell KA, Sonesson B, Toremalm NG. Bruxism and hypertrophy of the masseter muscle. A clinical, morphological and functional investigation. Pract Otorhinolaryngol (Basel). 1969;31(1):22–9. https://doi.org/10.1159/000274876.

9. Pary A, Pary K. Masseteric hypertrophy: considerations regarding treatment planning decisions and introduction of a novel surgical technique. J Oral Maxillofac Surg. 2011;69(3):944–9. https://doi.org/10.1016/j.joms.2010.06.205.

10. Balaji SM, Balaji P. Square face correction by gonial angle and masseter reduction. Ann Maxillofac Surg. 2020;10(1):66–72. https://doi.org/10.4103/ams.ams_22_20.

11. Choe SW, Cho WI, Lee CK, Seo SJ. Effects of botulinum toxin type A on contouring of the lower face. Dermatol Surg. 2005;31(5):502–8. https://doi.org/10.1111/j.1524-4725.2005.31151.

12. Bayer S, Helfgen EH, Bös C, Kraus D, Enkling N, Mues S. Prevalence of findings compatible with carotid artery calcifications on dental panoramic radiographs. Clin Oral Investig. 2011;15(4):563–9. https://doi.org/10.1007/s00784-010-0418-6.

13. Jain K, Arun Prasad B, Sreedharan SE, Kannath S, Varma RP, Sylaja PN. Studying plaque characteristics in extracranial carotid artery disease using CT angiography—risk predictors beyond luminal stenosis. Clin Neurol Neurosurg. 2022;222:107420. https://doi.org/10.1016/j.clineuro.2022.107420.

14. Maia PRL, Tomaz AFG, Maia EFT, Lima KC, Oliveira PT. Prevalence of soft tissue calcifications in panoramic radiographs of the maxillofacial region of older adults. Gerodontology. 2022;39(3):266–72. https://doi.org/10.1111/ger.12578.

15. Friedlander AH, Gratt BM. Panoramic dental radiography as an aid in detecting patients at risk for stroke. J Oral Maxillofac Surg. 1994;52(12):1257–62. https://doi.org/10.1016/0278-2391(94)90047-7.

16. Friedlander AH, Baker JD. Panoramic radiography: an aid in detecting patients at risk of cerebrovascular accident. J Am Dent Assoc. 1994;125(12):1598–603. https://doi.org/10.14219/jada.archive.1994.0237.

17. Friedlander AH, Friedlander IK. Identification of stroke prone patients by panoramic radiography. Aust Dent J. 1998;43(1):51–4. https://doi.org/10.1111/j.1834-7819.1998.tb00153.x.

18. Takahashi A, Sugawara C, Kudoh T, et al. Prevalence and imaging characteristics of palatine tonsilloliths detected by CT in 2,873 consecutive patients. ScientificWorldJournal. 2014;2014:940960. https://doi.org/10.1155/2014/940960.

19. Kim MJ, Kim JE, Huh KH, et al. Multidetector computed tomography imaging characteristics of asymptomatic palatine tonsilloliths: a retrospective study on 3886 examinations. Oral Surg Oral Med Oral Pathol Oral Radiol. 2018;125(6):693–8. https://doi.org/10.1016/j.oooo.2018.01.014.

20. Aspestrand F, Kolbenstvedt A. Calcifications of the palatine tonsillary region: CT demonstration. Radiology. 1987;165(2):479–80. https://doi.org/10.1148/radiology.165.2.3659369.

21. Lee KC, Mandel L. Lingual (not palatine) tonsillolith: case report. J Oral Maxillofac Surg. 2019;77(8):1650–4. https://doi.org/10.1016/j.joms.2019.03.006.

22. Sano K, Ogawa A, Inokuchi T, Takahashi H, Hisatsune K. Buccal hemangioma with phleboliths. Report of two cases. Oral Surg Oral Med Oral Pathol. 1988;65(2):151–6. https://doi.org/10.1016/0030-4220(88)90156-9.

23. Gooi Z, Mydlarz WK, Tunkel DE, Eisele DW. Submandibular venous malformation phleboliths mimicking sialolithiasis in children. Laryngoscope. 2014;124(12):2826–8. https://doi.org/10.1002/lary.24758.

24. Sato S, Takahashi M, Takahashi T. A case of multiple phleboliths on the medial side of the right mandible. Case Rep Dent. 2020;2020:6694402. Published 2020 Dec 27. https://doi.org/10.1155/2020/6694402.

25. Kato H, Ota Y, Sasaki M, Arai T, Sekido Y, Tsukinoki K. A phlebolith in the anterior portion of the masseter muscle. Tokai J Exp Clin Med. 2012;37(1):25–9. Published 2012 Apr 20.

26. Eisenkraft BL, Som PM. The spectrum of benign and malignant etiologies of cervical node calcification. AJR Am J Roentgenol. 1999;172(5):1433–7. https://doi.org/10.2214/ajr.172.5.10227533.

27. Marchiori E, Hochhegger B, Zanetti G. Lymph node calcifications. J Bras Pneumol. 2018;44(2):83. https://doi.org/10.1590/s1806-37562018000000003.
28. Lindeboom JA, Smets AM, Kuijper EJ, van Rijn RR, Prins JM. The sonographic characteristics of nontuberculous mycobacterial cervicofacial lymphadenitis in children. Pediatr Radiol. 2006;36(10):1063–7. https://doi.org/10.1007/s00247-006-0271-6.
29. Mandel L, Surattanont F, Miremadi R. Cat-scratch disease: considerations for dentistry. J Am Dent Assoc. 2001;132(7):911–4. https://doi.org/10.14219/jada.archive.2001.0303. PMID: 11480644.
30. Fletcher RH, Malamud SC, Slap GB, Tsevat J, et al. When you find lymphadenopathy. Patient Care. 1992;26:83–103.
31. Lee IK, Liu JW. Tuberculous parotitis: case report and literature review. Ann Otol Rhinol Laryngol. 2005;114(7):547–51. https://doi.org/10.1177/000348940511400710. PMID: 16134352.
32. Chen HC, Kang BH, Lai CT, Lin YS. Sarcoidal granuloma in cervical lymph nodes. J Chin Med Assoc. 2005;68(7):339–42. https://doi.org/10.1016/S1726-4901(09)70172-8. PMID: 16038376.
33. Petrovic I, Ahmed ZU, Hay A, et al. Sarcomas of the mandible. J Surg Oncol. 2019;120(2):109–16. https://doi.org/10.1002/jso.25477.
34. Tseng CH, Wang WC, Chen CY, Hsu HJ, Chen YK. Retrospective analysis of primary intraosseous malignancies in mandible and maxilla in a population of Taiwanese patients. J Formos Med Assoc. 2022;121(4):787–95. https://doi.org/10.1016/j.jfma.2021.08.024.
35. Magat G, Sener SO, Cetmili H. Metastatic breast cancer to bilateral mandibular ramus regions. J Cancer Res Ther. 2019;15(5):1177–80. https://doi.org/10.4103/jcrt.JCRT_447_17.
36. Zengin AZ, Celenk P, Sumer AP. Intramuscular hemangioma presenting with multiple phleboliths: a case report. Oral Surg Oral Med Oral Pathol Oral Radiol. 2013;115(1):e32–6. https://doi.org/10.1016/j.oooo.2012.02.032.
37. Mulliken JB, Glowacki J. Hemangiomas and vascular malformations in infants and children: a classification based on endothelial characteristics. Plast Reconstr Surg. 1982;69(3):412–22. https://doi.org/10.1097/00006534-198203000-00002.
38. Mandel L, Surattanont F. Clinical and imaging diagnoses of intramuscular hemangiomas: the wattle sign and case reports. J Oral Maxillofac Surg. 2004;62(6):754–8. https://doi.org/10.1016/j.joms.2003.05.022.
39. Gordon JS, Mandel L. Masseteric intramuscular hemangioma: case report. J Oral Maxillofac Surg. 2014;72(11):2192–6. https://doi.org/10.1016/j.joms.2014.06.001.
40. Bransby-Zachary GM. The sub-masseteric space. Br Dent J. 1948;84(1):10–7.
41. Mandel L. Diagnosing protracted submasseteric abscess: the role of computed tomography. J Am Dent Assoc. 1996;127(11):1646–50. https://doi.org/10.14219/jada.archive.1996.0101.
42. Rai A, Rajput R, Khatua RK, Singh M. Submasseteric abscess: a rare head and neck abscess. Indian J Dent Res. 2011;22(1):166–8. https://doi.org/10.4103/0970-9290.79990.
43. Balatsouras DG, Kloutsos GM, Protopapas D, Korres S, Economou C. Submasseteric abscess. J Laryngol Otol. 2001;115(1):68–70. https://doi.org/10.1258/0022215011906867.
44. Jones KC, Silver J, Millar WS, Mandel L. Chronic submasseteric abscess: anatomic, radiologic, and pathologic features. AJNR Am J Neuroradiol. 2003;24(6):1159–63.
45. Guzman N, Vijayan V. HIV-associated lipodystrophy. In: StatPearls. Treasure Island: StatPearls Publishing; 2021.
46. Njelekela M, Mpembeni R, Muhihi A, Ulenga N, Aris E, Kakoko D. Lipodystrophy among HIV-infected patients attending care and treatment clinics in Dar es Salaam. AIDS Res Treat. 2017;2017:3896539. https://doi.org/10.1155/2017/3896539.
47. Alikhani A, Morin H, Matte S, Alikhani P, Tremblay C, Durand M. Association between lipodystrophy and length of exposure to ARTs in adult HIV-1 infected patients in Montreal. BMC Infect Dis. 2019;19(1):820. Published 2019 Sep 18. https://doi.org/10.1186/s12879-019-4446-9.

48. Kobayashi N, Nakahara M, Oka M, Saeki K. Additional attention to combination antiretroviral therapy-related lipodystrophy. World J Virol. 2017;6(3):49–52. https://doi.org/10.5501/wjv.v6.i3.49.

49. Martin A, Smith DE, Carr A, et al. Reversibility of lipoatrophy in HIV-infected patients 2 years after switching from a thymidine analogue to abacavir: the MITOX extension study. AIDS. 2004;18(7):1029–36. https://doi.org/10.1097/00002030-200404300-00011.

50. Ariji Y, Gotoh M, Kimura Y, Naitoh M, Kurita K, Natsume N, Ariji E. Odontogenic infection pathway to the submandibular space: imaging assessment. Int J Oral Maxillofac Surg. 2002;31(2):165–9. https://doi.org/10.1054/ijom.2001.0190. PMID: 12102414.

51. Gupta M, Singh V. A retrospective study of 256 patients with space infection. J Maxillofac Oral Surg. 2010;9(1):35–7. https://doi.org/10.1007/s12663-010-0011-1.

52. Colbert SD, Seager L, Haider F, Evans BT, Anand R, Brennan PA. Lymphatic malformations of the head and neck-current concepts in management. Br J Oral Maxillofac Surg. 2013;51(2):98–102. https://doi.org/10.1016/j.bjoms.2011.12.016. Epub 2012 Feb 22. PMID: 22360972.

53. Adams MT, Saltzman B, Perkins JA. Head and neck lymphatic malformation treatment: a systematic review. Otolaryngol Head Neck Surg. 2012;147(4):627–39. https://doi.org/10.1177/0194599812453552. Epub 2012 Jul 11. PMID: 22785242.

54. Biasotto M, Clozza E, Tirelli G. Facial cystic lymphangioma in adults. J Craniofac Surg. 2012;23(4):e331–4. https://doi.org/10.1097/SCS.0b013e31825435bd. PMID: 22801170.

55. Lerat J, Mounayer C, Scomparin A, Orsel S, Bessede JP, Aubry K. Head and neck lymphatic malformation and treatment: clinical study of 23 cases. Eur Ann Otorhinolaryngol Head Neck Dis. 2016;133(6):393–6. https://doi.org/10.1016/j.anorl.2016.07.004. Epub 2016 Aug 3. PMID: 27497629.

56. Curran AJ, Malik N, McShane D, Timon CV. Surgical management of lymphangiomas in adults. J Laryngol Otol. 1996;110(6):586–9. https://doi.org/10.1017/s0022215100134334. PMID: 8763385.

57. Wiegand S, Zimmermann AP, Eivazi B, Sesterhenn AM, Werner JA. Lymphatic malformations involving the parotid gland. Eur J Pediatr Surg. 2011;21(4):242–5. https://doi.org/10.1055/s-0031-1271810.

58. Elluru RG, Balakrishnan K, Padua HM. Lymphatic malformations: diagnosis and management. Semin Pediatr Surg. 2014;23(4):178–85. https://doi.org/10.1053/j.sempedsurg.2014.07.002. Epub 2014 Jul 15. PMID: 25241095.

59. Jamal N, Ahmed S, Miller T, Bent J, Brook A, Parikh S, Ankola A. Doxycycline sclerotherapy for pediatric head and neck macrocystic lymphatic malformations: a case series and review of the literature. Int J Pediatr Otorhinolaryngol. 2012;76(8):1127–31. https://doi.org/10.1016/j.ijporl.2012.04.015. Epub 2012 May 7. PMID: 22572407.

60. Gallant SC, Chewning RH, Orbach DB, Trenor CC 3rd, Cunningham MJ. Contemporary management of vascular anomalies of the head and neck—part 1: vascular malformations: a review. JAMA Otolaryngol Head Neck Surg. 2021;147(2):197–206. https://doi.org/10.1001/jamaoto.2020.4353. PMID: 33237296.

61. Leveque H, Saraceno CA, Tang CK, Blanchard CL. Dermoid cysts of the floor of the mouth and lateral neck. Laryngoscope. 1979;89(2 Pt 1):296–305. https://doi.org/10.1288/00005537-197902000-00012.

62. New GB, Erich JB. Dermoid cyst of the head and neck. Surg Gynecol Obstet. 1937;65:48–56.

63. Kurabayashi T, Ida M, Sasaki T. Differential diagnosis of submandibular cystic lesions by computed tomography. Dentomaxillofac Radiol. 1991;20(1):30–4. https://doi.org/10.1259/dmfr.20.1.1884850.

64. Khelemsky R, Mandel L. Lymphoepithelial cyst of mouth floor. J Oral Maxillofac Surg. 2010;68(12):3055–7. https://doi.org/10.1016/j.joms.2010.07.048.

65. Tisch M, Lampl L, Groh A, Maier H. Angioneurotic edemas of the upper aerodigestive tract after ACE-inhibitor treatment. Eur Arch Otorrinolaringol. 2002;259(8):419–21. https://doi.org/10.1007/s00405-002-0481-y.

66. Grant NN, Deeb ZE, Chia SH. Clinical experience with angiotensin-converting enzyme inhibitor-induced angioedema. Otolaryngol Head Neck Surg. 2007;137(6):931–5. https://doi.org/10.1016/j.otohns.2007.08.012.
67. Irons BK, Kumar A. Valsartan-induced angioedema. Ann Pharmacother. 2003;37(7–8):1024–7. https://doi.org/10.1345/aph.1C520.
68. Burt BA, Pai S. Sugar consumption and caries risk: a systematic review. J Dent Educ. 2001;65(10):1017–23. PMID: 11699972.
69. Reddy A, Norris DF, Momeni SS, Waldo B, Ruby JD. The pH of beverages in the United States. J Am Dent Assoc. 2016;147(4):255–63. https://doi.org/10.1016/j.adaj.2015.10.019. Epub 2015 Dec 2. PMID: 26653863; PMCID: PMC4808596.
70. Schroeder PL, Filler SJ, Ramirez B, Lazarchik DA, Vaezi MF, Richter JE. Dental erosion and acid reflux disease. Ann Intern Med. 1995;122(11):809–15. https://doi.org/10.7326/0003-4819-122-11-199506010-00001. PMID: 7741364.
71. Mandel L. Dental erosion due to wine consumption. J Am Dent Assoc. 2005;136(1):71–5. https://doi.org/10.14219/jada.archive.2005.0029. PMID: 15693499.
72. Lavigne GJ, Khoury S, Abe S, Yamaguchi T, Raphael K. Bruxism physiology and pathology: an overview for clinicians. J Oral Rehabil. 2008;35(7):476–94. https://doi.org/10.1111/j.1365-2842.2008.01881.x.
73. Wieczorek T, Michałek-Zrąbkowska M, Więckiewicz M, et al. Sleep bruxism contributes to motor activity increase during sleep in apneic and nonapneic patients—a polysomnographic study. Biomedicines. 2022;10(10):2666. Published 2022 Oct 21. https://doi.org/10.3390/biomedicines10102666.
74. Hockstein NG, Samadi DS, Gendron K, Handler SD. Sialorrhea: a management challenge. Am Fam Physician. 2004;69(11):2628–34. PMID: 15202698.
75. Abdo WF, van de Warrenburg BP, Burn DJ, Quinn NP, Bloem BR. The clinical approach to movement disorders. Nat Rev Neurol. 2010;6(1):29–37. https://doi.org/10.1038/nrneurol.2009.196.
76. Kalf JG, Munneke M, van den Engel-Hoek L, et al. Pathophysiology of diurnal drooling in Parkinson's disease. Mov Disord. 2011;26(9):1670–6. https://doi.org/10.1002/mds.23720.
77. Dray TG, Hillel AD, Miller RM. Dysphagia caused by neurologic deficits. Otolaryngol Clin North Am. 1998;31(3):507–24. https://doi.org/10.1016/s0030-6665(05)70067-0. PMID: 9628947.
78. Stathopoulos P, Dalakas MC. Autoimmune neurogenic dysphagia. Dysphagia. 2022;37(3):473–87. https://doi.org/10.1007/s00455-021-10338-9. Epub ahead of print. PMID: 34226958; PMCID: PMC8257036.
79. Logemann JA, Bytell DE. Swallowing disorders in three types of head and neck surgical patients. Cancer. 1979;44(3):1095–105. https://doi.org/10.1002/1097-0142(197909)44:3<1095::aid-cncr2820440344>3.0.co;2-c. PMID: 476587.
80. Lagalla G, Millevolte M, Capecci M, Provinciali L, Ceravolo MG. Botulinum toxin type A for drooling in Parkinson's disease: a double-blind, randomized, placebo-controlled study. Mov Disord. 2006;21(5):704–7. https://doi.org/10.1002/mds.20793. PMID: 16440332.

Chapter 20
Benign Salivary Gland Neoplasms

Kevin C. Lee

Abstract Benign salivary gland neoplasms are uncommon; however, providers treating conditions of the head, neck, and oral cavity are almost guaranteed to encounter these lesions in clinical practice. Benign salivary tumors all harbor a similar prototypical appearance depending on their location. Given their rarity and nondescript presentation, the difficulty with salivary tumors lies in the diagnosis which often requires a healthy level of clinical suspicion. The purpose of this chapter is to provide an overview of the epidemiology, diagnosis, and management of benign salivary tumors.

Introduction

Benign salivary neoplasms comprise a heterogenous group of lesions that may arise within various subsites of the mouth, face, and neck. Because these lesions are uncommon in the general population, the proper diagnosis of salivary gland tumors requires the clinician to have a high level of suspicion. There are certain clinical findings that may hint to the presence of a salivary tumor; however, identifying salivary gland pathology remains challenging even for the experienced provider because it often mimics other more common processes. The purpose of this chapter on benign salivary neoplasms is to provide a foundational understanding of the clinical symptomatology as it relates to pathology and to illustrate the spectrum of clinico-radiologic presentations. Seeing a range of manifestations will assist the reader in recognizing these lesions in their practice.

© The Author(s), under exclusive license to Springer Nature Switzerland AG 2024

L. Mandel, *Clinical Management of Salivary Gland Disorders*, https://doi.org/10.1007/978-3-031-50012-1_20

Etiology and Epidemiology

Salivary gland tumors comprise approximately 5% of all head and neck tumors [1]. The estimated global incidence is fewer than 15 per 100,000 people [1]. Fortunately, over 70% of these tumors are benign [1]. The World Health Organization (WHO) has recognized more than ten histological subtypes of benign epithelial salivary tumors, and a female predilection has been observed for most of these entities [2]. The intention of this chapter is to focus on the clinical aspects of the most commonly encountered neoplasms.

The etiology of most salivary tumors is unknown, and nearly all lesions occur sporadically. As a result, most tend to be diagnosed in the fifth decade of life. There is some thought that prior radiation effect on a salivary gland may subsequently induce the development of a pleomorphic adenoma, which is a benign mixed tumor composed of epithelial and myoepithelial elements [3]. Radiation and smoking increase the risk of developing a Warthin's tumor. However, with the exception of Warthin's tumor, which is a characteristically cystic tumor with lymphatic deposits, there do not appear to be any universally accepted environmental or genetic risk factors for benign salivary tumors [4].

Salivary tissue is distributed throughout the aerodigestive tract, and the bulk of salivary mass is found within the major salivary glands. The parotid is the largest salivary gland by volume, and the "Rule of 80's" is often quoted when discussing parotid tumors. This rule states that 80% of salivary neoplasms arise in the parotid, of which 80% are histologically benign, of which 80% are ultimately diagnosed as pleomorphic adenomas [5]. Another axiom states that as the size of the involved gland decreases, the incidence of neoplasm likewise decreases, while the risk of malignancy increases. The proportion of neoplasms that are benign in the parotid, submandibular, and sublingual glands is approximately 80%, 50%, and 20%, respectively [6]. Although these rules almost certainly represent an oversimplification, and should not be used in isolation, it is hard to calculate more precise estimates for salivary neoplasms given their uncommon incidence.

Minor salivary glands exist throughout the submucosa of the head and neck region. They are present in the paranasal sinuses, nasopharynx, oral cavity, oropharynx, and even larynx. Tumors of the minor salivary glands comprise only 10–20% of all salivary tumors, with the majority arising in the hard or soft palate [6]. The labial glands are the second most common site for minor salivary tumors, and the upper lip is more often involved than the lower lip. Minor salivary tumors are typically malignant, and this is concordant with the aforementioned relationship between gland size and histologic behavior. The exception to this generalization is the labial salivary glands, where tumors of the upper lip are usually benign [7]. As in major salivary neoplasms, middle-aged females tend to be more often affected for unclear reasons.

Pleomorphic adenomas are by far the most common benign tumor regardless of subsite. In terms of common tumor locations, Warthin's tumors occur almost exclusively in the parotid glands. Canalicular adenomas have a predilection for the minor labial salivary glands of the upper lip, but they are still infrequently seen there given their rarity [8]. Other tumors may occur at various sites, but location alone is not enough to clinch a diagnosis.

History

A careful and accurate history of present illness, with a pertinent review of symptoms, provides the foundation for differentiating a benign from a malignant mass. Any prior treatment for salivary neoplasms should be ascertained. Local recurrence may be due to inadequate surgery or tumor spillage during prior attempts at removal. For the pleomorphic adenoma, intraoperative capsule rupture is thought to occur in up to 5% of cases, and it can take as long as 15 years for tumor recurrence [9]. In general, neoplasms occur unilaterally with the exception of oncocytomas and Warthin's tumor (Fig. 20.1). Warthin's tumor can uniquely present with metachronous lesions that present in a multifocal and/or bilateral distribution. As such, it may be difficult to distinguish a recurrent primary from a second primary lesion. As discussed, salivary tissue is present throughout the oral, head, and neck region. When a patient presents with a facial or oral mass, it is important to obtain the duration of the lesion and any associated size changes over time. Rapid growth is indicative of a more aggressive biology. Typically, a benign neoplasm will be completely asymptomatic, slow growing, and only discovered when it reaches a visible or bothersome size. Salivary tumors do not fluctuate in size. Episodic swelling argues against a neoplastic process and should prompt additional infectious and inflammatory studies.

The symptoms of benign salivary tumors largely stem from mass effect on the neighboring structures. For gradually enlarging benign parotid lesions, facial nerve compression can occasionally result in a unilateral palsy. A history of chronic, long-standing symptoms that have been present for years to decades is highly suggestive of a benign process. Spontaneous pain is only reported with 2–5% of benign neoplasms and is much more commonly observed in the setting of malignancy [10]. It is important to realize that the presence of pain is not diagnostic and therefore cannot be used to rule out a benign process. Other symptoms that may be elicited through careful questioning include dysphagia and trismus. These are generally present with large deep lobe parotid tumors.

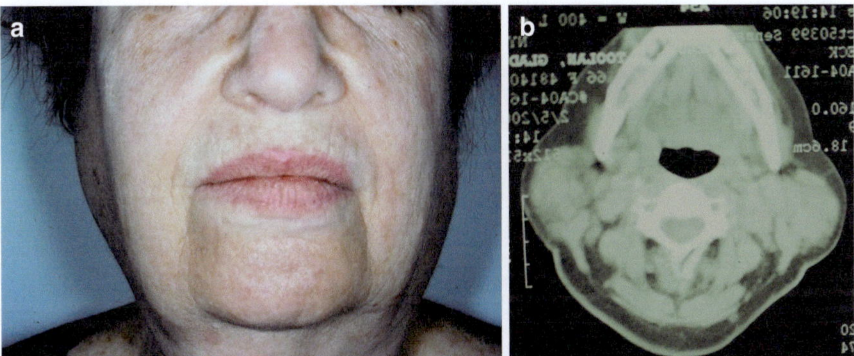

Fig. 20.1 Oncocytomas of the bilateral parotid glands. (**a**) Bilateral preauricular facial swelling. (**b**) CT face axial view demonstrating symmetric enlargement of the parotid glands

Physical Examination

The physical examination for suspected salivary tumors incorporates many of the tenants of the basic head and neck examination. Careful attention should be paid to the location of the swelling. The parotid gland sits below and anterior to the tragal pointer and posterior to the mandibular angle. It wraps medially around the mandibular ramus anterior to the mastoid tip and adjacent to the styloid process. Parotid body tumors present as preauricular masses, whereas parotid tail tumors occur below the lobule of the ear (Fig. 20.2). The facial nerve divides the substance of the parotid gland into both superficial and deep lobes. The deep lobe is situated in the parapharyngeal space which abuts the oropharynx and nasopharynx more medially. A facial process of the parotid duct exists in some individuals. This anterior extension is directly attached to the parotid body and follows the course of the Stenson's duct. In up to 50% of the population, when the anterior extension is detached, it is considered accessory parotid tissue [11]. Tumors of the facial process of the parotid or the accessory parotid tissue can present as mid-cheek swellings that may mimic cutaneous pathology [12] (Fig. 20.3). The submandibular glands sit beneath the mandibular angle over top of the digastric tendon. The mylohyoid muscle divides the submandibular gland into a superficial and a deep lobe, and the bulk of tissue exists in the superficial lobe. Like with the parotid gland, this designation is entirely nominal since the gland does not have a natural cleavage plane separating the two lobes. The Wharton duct travels intimately with the lingual nerve into the floor of mouth where it crosses medial and superior to the lingual nerve at the level of the first and second mandibular molar. The sublingual glands are paired structures that reside in the floor of mouth lateral to the Wharton duct and the lingual nerve. Unlike the other major glands, the sublingual glands are drained by multiple ducts of Rivinus. The Bartholin duct, not always present, is the most dominant of these many sublingual ducts, and it unites with the distal portion of the Wharton duct to drain saliva out of the sublingual caruncle.

Size, measured in the largest diameter, should be documented in addition to any changes to the overlying skin or mucosa. The mass in question should be evaluated for pain, mobility, and fixation to the surrounding tissues. A lesion that glides easily between the fingertips is more likely to be well-encapsulated and benign. A movable

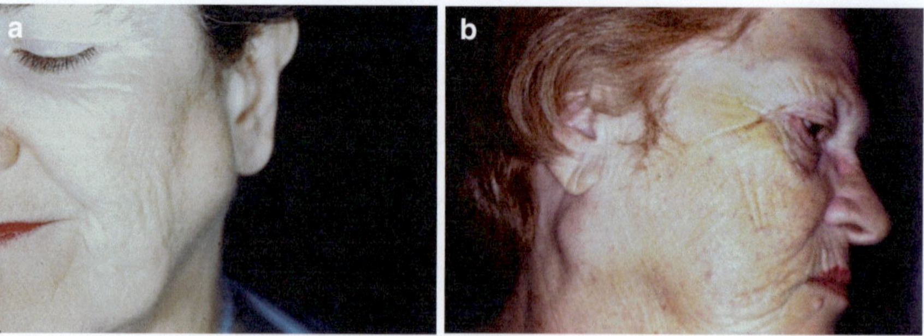

Fig. 20.2 The superficial lobe of the parotid is divided into two regions. (**a**) Parotid body tumors are located in the preauricular space which is immediately anterior to the tragus. (**b**) Parotid tail tumors are located at the inferior portion of the parotid gland overlying the mandibular angle

Fig. 20.3 (**a**) Swellings of the mid-cheek may represent tumors of a facial extension of the parotid or accessory parotid tissue. (**b**) Axial T2-weighted magnetic resonance image showing a well-defined nodular mass (arrow). (**c**) Final histopathology confirmed pleomorphic adenoma of accessory parotid tissue (hematoxylin and eosin, 100 magnification)

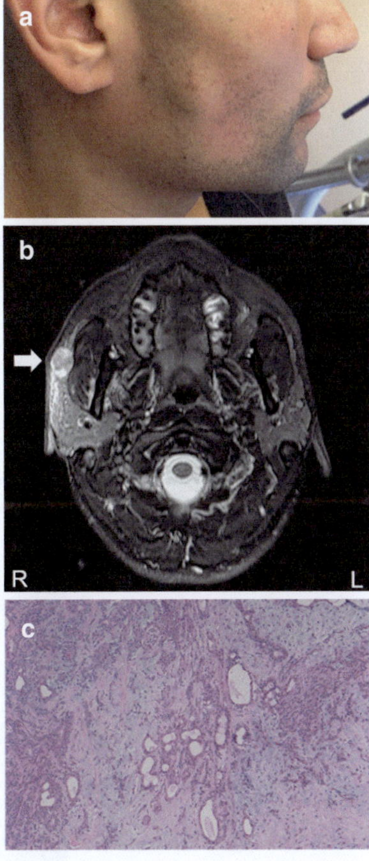

mass with a lobulated surface architecture is often suggestive of a pleomorphic adenoma (Fig. 20.4). When examining parotid masses, facial nerve function must be evaluated and compared for symmetry. Any focal weakness should be localized to one of the five branches to determine which trunk or branch is involved. Although perineural invasion does not occur, benign masses can still cause a compression neuropraxia. In such cases, patients should be counseled that facial nerve weakness may not improve even with tumor extirpation. Submandibular gland masses may visually present with many of the same characteristics of submandibular space infections (Fig. 20.5). However, on physical exam, benign submandibular tumors do not demonstrate the hallmarks of inflammation. That is to say, they are nontender and do not have erythematous skin changes. Like with that of the parotid, benign submandibular tumors are circumscribed and moveable. The submandibular sialolith, or salivary stone, may also mimic a neoplastic growth given that it is firm to palpation and enlarges gradually through calculus deposition.

The oral cavity should still be inspected for patients with external facial swellings. Flow from the Stensen and Wharton ducts should be visualized bilaterally with gentle massage of the respective glands. Inability to express saliva suggests an obstructive process which can be secondary to compression. Compression can also

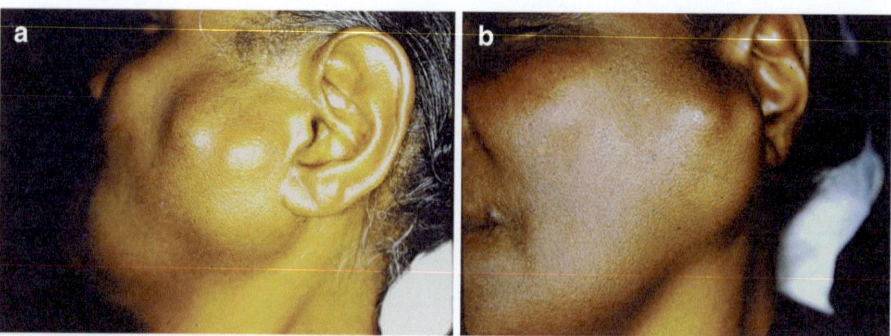

Fig. 20.4 Pleomorphic adenoma of the left parotid body. Lobulated surface architecture appreciated on (**a**) lateral and (**b**) frontal views

Fig. 20.5 Left submandibular gland tumor presenting as a (**a**) swelling beneath the mandibular body and anterior to the mandibular angle. (**b**) Sialogram demonstrating mass effect of the tumor and inferior displacement of the submandibular duct

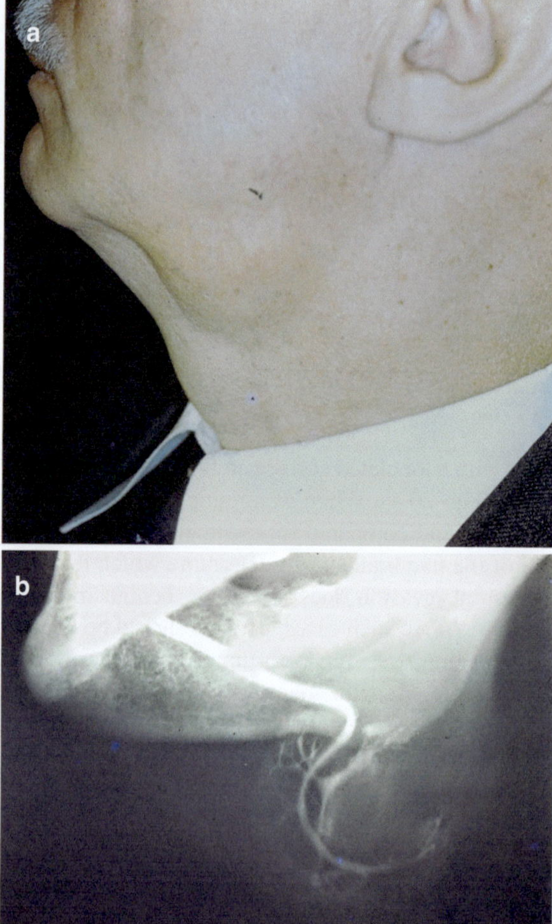

occur more distally from sublingual pathology as the sublingual gland sits immediately lateral to the course of the Wharton duct and the lingual nerve. The pharyngeal tissues should be inspected for symmetry and midline deviation. Deep lobe parotid tumors can push centrally along the tonsillar pillars and cause a shift in the soft palate. This should be distinguished from primary masses of the soft palate which do not involve expansion of the tonsillar pillars. Palatal tumors of the minor salivary glands often appear along the posterolateral surface and can mimic the appearance of an odontogenic abscess (Fig. 20.6). Fluctuance and tenderness of the mass in

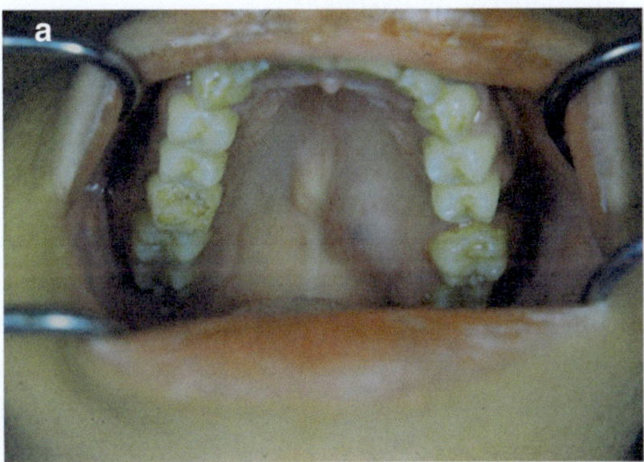

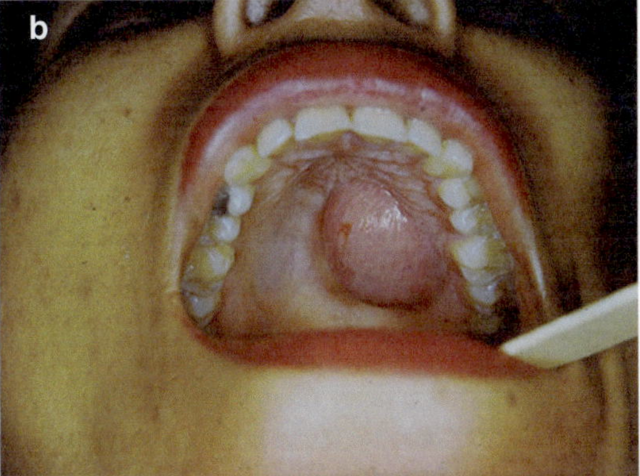

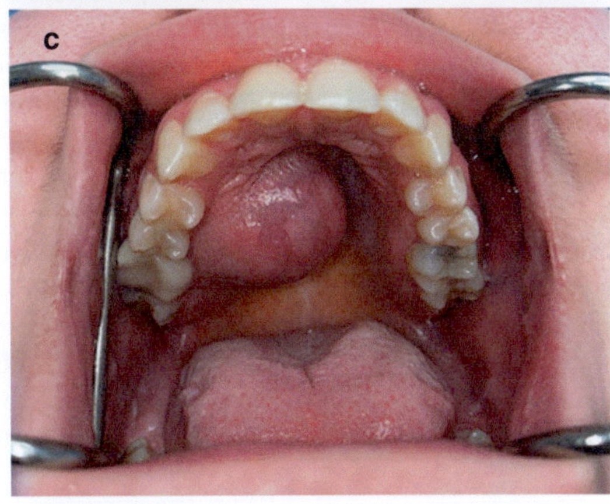

Fig. 20.6 Minor salivary gland tumors of hard palate tend to occur along the posterolateral palate adjacent to the alveolus. (**a**) Concomitant midline torus with a lateral palatal pleomorphic adenoma. (**b**) Lateral palatal pleomorphic adenoma with more superficial location and well-defined clinical boundaries. (**c**) Lateral palatal pleomorphic adenoma with a more vascular and slightly lobulated appearance

question as well as dental mobility and vitality should be assessed to identify possible dental disease.

Cervical lymph nodes should be checked for regional metastases even when malignancy is unlikely. Parotid lymphatics drain into the nodal basins along the anterior border of the sternocleidomastoid muscle. Lymphatic drainage from intraoral, submandibular, and sublingual tissues first passes just beneath the mandibular angle, before reaching the cervical lymphatics. Again, palpation of lymph nodes should proceed bilaterally and any discernable asymmetries or masses should be inspected for alarming features such as skin changes, pain, and fixation to the underlying tissues.

Imaging and Diagnostic Tests

There are a variety of imaging modalities to characterize the location and features of suspected salivary tumors. Prior to the advent of cross-sectional imaging, radiographic sialograms were used by some to evaluate the salivary ducts and parenchyma. For space-occupying lesions within or adjacent to salivary glands, such as salivary tumors, a "ball-in-hand" pattern can be appreciated (Fig. 20.7). In this manner, the duct system is displaced but remains intact, and there is no extravasation of the contrast. The sialographic criteria for malignancy are controversial and are often of minimal assistance when trying to determine the behavior of a tumor [13]. Ultrasound (US) can be used to visualize superficial structures such as the parotid, submandibular, and sublingual glands. It can also be used to image the cervical lymph nodes. On US, cystic structures appear hypoechoic whereas solid structures appear hyperechoic. Tissues that are well-defined and homogenous are more likely to be benign, although dystrophic calcifications and hemorrhage, which occur in long-standing lesions, may muddy the picture. Doppler signals can be superimposed to evaluate vascular patterns. Benign tumors generally demonstrate lower grades of vascularity given their indolent growth. The interpretation of these dynamic doppler images requires specialized training and is not routinely obtained. Furthermore, real-time ultrasound imaging is a helpful adjunct for guiding fine needle aspiration cytology (FNAC) of deep lobe and parapharyngeal lesions.

Presently, computed tomography (CT) and/or magnetic resonance imaging (MRI) scans are the standard first-line choices for imaging salivary tumors. Both modalities will give insight into the tumor location, presence of extraglandular extension, whether the edges are well-defined, internal lesion homo/heterogeneity, and nodal enlargement [14]. CT scans are superior for detecting bony changes and therefore should be considered in all minor salivary gland tumors of the palate. They can also readily identify salivary calculi of the submandibular gland which can be mistaken for neoplasms on physical exam. MRIs are the initial investigation of choice because they offer better visualization of the soft tissue planes and assessment of the perineural environment (Fig. 20.8). Like CT, MRI cannot be relied on to make a final diagnosis as there is considerable overlap in features among lesions [15]. The drawbacks of MRI are the greater cost and time for data acquisition.

Fig. 20.7 "Ball-in-hand" appearance of benign salivary tumor. The ball represents the tumor (red circle) and the hand represents the ductal system visualized using radiopaque contrast. Sialogram of parotid tumor as demonstrated on (**a**) frontal and (**b**) oblique views

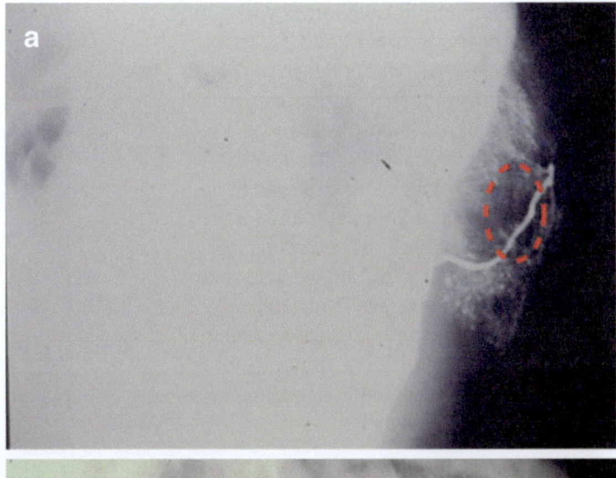

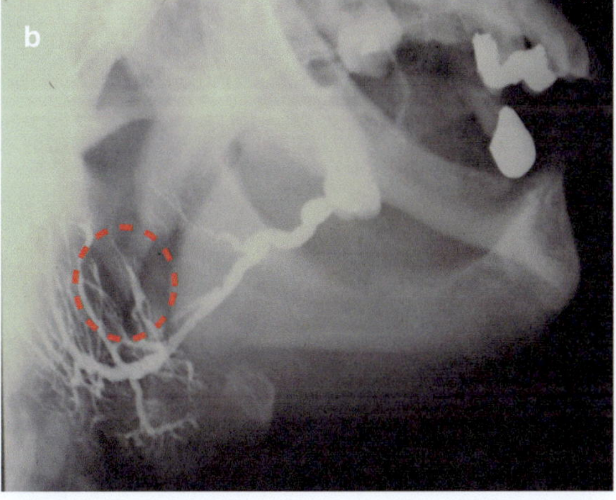

FNAC is a minimally invasive, cost-effective procedure for sampling cells that theoretically avoids seeding tumor into the overlying skin. It is recommended that every patient presenting with a suspected salivary neoplasm be investigated with an FNAC as it gives the greatest diagnostic yield [16]. Cellular characteristics are able to predict the risk of malignancy with excellent (over 80%) sensitivity and specificity [16, 17]. The main pitfall to FNAC, which is common to any biopsy technique, is sampling error. However, this is more common in the setting of low-grade malignancy or in the case of malignant transformation of a benign tumor. Both the American Society of Cytopathology and the International Academy of Cytology endorse the Milan System for Reporting Salivary Gland Cytopathology. The Milan System stratifies FNAC samples by the risk of malignancy and gives recommendations for clinical management. Open transcutaneous incisional biopsy should never be performed for suspected salivary neoplasm because of the aforementioned risk of tumor seeding and spillage [18]. If a tissue specimen is desired prior to proceeding to the operating room, a percutaneous core needle biopsy can be performed. This has the advantages of an FNAC as well as the benefits and accuracy of a tissue diagnosis [19]. For oral lesions, transmucosal incisional biopsies are routinely

Fig. 20.8 Pleomorphic adenomas will enhance on post-contrast T1 and T2 series, whereas simple cysts will enhance on T2 but not post-contrast T1. Benign tumors generally have high T2 signal intensity, whereas malignant tumors generally have low-to-intermediate T2 signal. This is a case of an MRI face with and without contrast for an accessory lobe pleomorphic adenoma. (**a**) Non-contrast T1-weighted image with tumor appearing hypointense. (**b**) Post-contrast T1-weighted image with fat suppression showing enhancement of the tumor. (**c**) Non-contrast T2-weighted image showing enhancement of the image

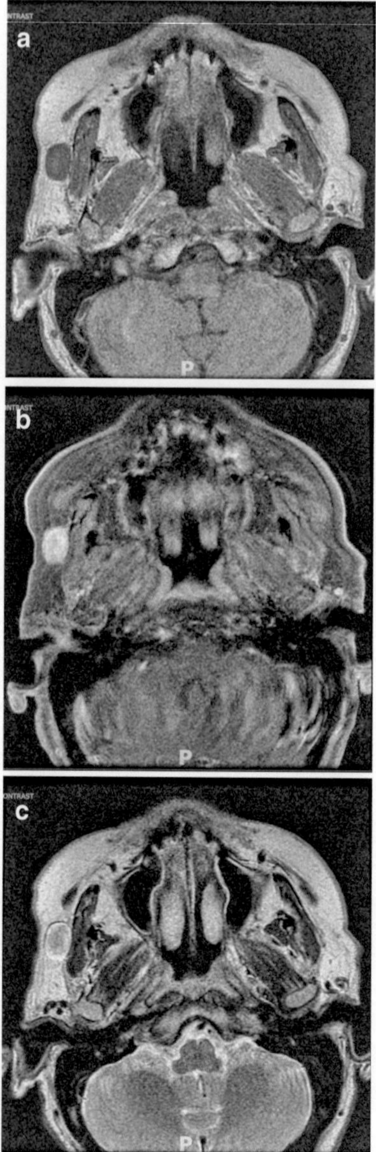

performed with the understanding that the overlying mucosa will generally be taken en bloc with the tumor to reduce the probability of recurrence.

The primary goal of preoperative tumor sampling is to differentiate benign from malignant entities. Unfortunately, cytology is not always reliable. Despite this understanding, patients are often taken to the operating room based on the FNAC report especially for parotid lesions where transcutaneous sampling is not advised.

If the exam and imaging show suspicion for a cancerous process but the FNAC argues against malignancy, intraoperative frozen biopsies may be taken off the explanted specimen to assist with the diagnosis and surgical decision making. Based on the frozen section analysis, the surgeon can proceed with either risk-stratified care or stage the oncologic surgery for when the patient is amenable and the final pathology is released. For lesions that are known to be benign, it is not necessary to obtain intraoperative frozen sections as knowledge of the exact histopathology will not alter the final management.

Treatment

Benign salivary tumors are managed surgically, but because most are slow-growing, urgency is not required. Nevertheless, deferring treatment is associated with further enlargement and possible malignant transformation. The extent of resection depends on the regional anatomy as well as the surgical philosophy. For benign salivary neoplasms, it is not necessary to remove a margin of uninvolved tissue; however, the planned resection almost always extends beyond the tumor boundary to avoid an incomplete removal since subclinical excrescences may be present. When the tumor impinges upon extraglandular tissues, it is recommended to remove one uninvolved anatomic boundary with the specimen. For example, in the case of a palatal tumor of the minor salivary glands that does not erode into the bone, one should resect the periosteum with the tumor as a composite specimen. Warthin's tumors are the exception and may be managed expectantly given the extreme rarity of malignant transformation and difficulty to achieve complete surgical cure.

Laterally located parotid tumors are treated with either a superficial lobe parotidectomy or extracapsular dissection. Extracapsular dissection is a form of partial parotidectomy whereby the tumor is separated and removed from the gland using a dissection plane immediately superficial to the tumor capsule. As previously discussed, the facial nerve serves as a potential plane that separates the superficial lobe from the deep lobe. A superficial lobe parotidectomy is the standard approach for removing such tumors. The main drawback to this technique is the risk of postoperative facial weakness because the facial nerve needs to be identified and exposed along its entire length. Extracapsular dissection of the parotid does not necessitate identification of the facial nerve and is appropriate for most benign tumors that are distinct and well-encapsulated. This technique involves tumor enucleation with a variable cuff of healthy uninvolved parotid tissue. The concern with a less radical surgery is that low-grade malignancies may be misdiagnosed as benign tumors on FNAC and be indistinguishable from benign tumors on preoperative workup. Therefore, most would agree that a superficial lobe parotidectomy is the standard approach; however, when there is a confident diagnosis of a benign laterally located parotid tumor, the preference for superficial lobe parotidectomy versus extracapsular dissection remains surgeon-dependent [20]. Recent meta-analyses have shown similar rates of disease control with both; however, surgeon experience likely plays an influential role in quality of outcome [21]. It should be noted that the role of extracapsular dissection for pleomorphic adenomas is hotly debated. This is because inadvertent violation of the capsule from a close dissection produces spillage and field tumorization. There may also be incomplete removal of microscopic outgrowths or excrescences. For tumors of the deep lobe, the choice of surgery is less equivocal. Most surgeons advocate for a total parotidectomy. This is because access to the deep lobe is provided through an antecedent superficial lobectomy. It is difficult, if not impossible, to remove the deep lobe in isolation without disturbing the overlying superficial glandular tissue. Removing larger volumes of glandular tissues increases the risks of facial palsy, Frey's syndrome, and facial contour deformity. In the case of deep lobe extirpation, there is also a risk of first bite syndrome [22].

Unlike those of the parotid, tumors of the other major salivary glands generally necessitate removal of the entire gland. The greatest risks of submandibular gland excision include injury to the marginal mandibular branch of the facial nerve as it dips below the mandible, the hypoglossal nerve, and the lingual nerve. The lingual nerve runs intimately with the submandibular duct, and intraoperatively the two structures often appear similar in caliber and texture. There have been instances where a partial sialoadenectomy has been performed for submandibular tumors [23]. The submandibular glands produce the majority of resting salivary flow, and preservation surgery is thought to conserve basal salivary production. This technique is only possible with benign disease that is located peripherally and away from the Wharton duct. The sublingual gland is likewise associated with the lingual nerve and Wharton's duct, both of which run medial to the gland.

Adjuvant treatment is not necessary for benign disease. Some have proposed adjuvant radiotherapy for recurrent pleomorphic adenomas given their propensity for further recurrence [24]. The available evidence supports lower recurrence rates in these cases with upfront surgery and subsequent radiation [25]. Prospective data is pending, and this practice has not been routinely adopted across centers.

Prognosis

Patients should be reassured that the prognosis of benign salivary tumors is excellent. The recurrence rate is low for benign salivary neoplasms following adequate surgery. An estimated 5% risk of recurrence is often quoted for newly diagnosed and treated pleomorphic adenomas [26]. The roughly 5% recurrence rate is also quoted for other salivary neoplasms such as surgically treated canalicular adenomas [27]. The risk of reappearance increases dramatically with subsequent attempts at removal as prior recurrence is a predictor of future recurrence. Recurrent pleomorphic adenomas have an estimated 40% risk of reoccurrence at 5 years after reoperation [28]. Among the subset of pleomorphic adenomas that do recur, only 5% will become malignant [26, 29]. The risk is directly proportional to the duration of the lesion. Approximately 10% of pleomorphic adenomas will show cancerous changes after 15 years of nontreatment [30]. With Warthin's tumor there is a 3% risk of recurrence following adequate surgery, and most alleged recurrences likely represent second metachronous lesions arising out of the prior resection bed [31]. Recently, there has been a push to treat Warthin's tumors with active surveillance if the location and size are not clinically problematic since malignant transformation is exceedingly rare [31].

Conclusion

In conclusion, benign salivary gland tumors are uncommon lesions that may masquerade as other more frequently encountered head and neck pathologies. Many neoplastic entities may sporadically arise from the salivary gland tissue; however, nearly all benign tumors share a commonality in presentation and clinical course that is a function of location and duration. The diagnostician's primary task is to ensure that the tumor is benign because malignant tumors, while less prevalent, carry a more complicated treatment paradigm.

References

1. Seethala RR. Salivary gland tumors: current concepts and controversies. Surg Pathol Clin. 2017;10(1):155–76.
2. El-Naggar AK, Chan JK, Grandis JR, Takata T, Slootweg PJ. World Health Organization classification of head and neck tumours. Lyon: IARC; 2017.
3. Rice DH, Batsakis JG, McClatchey KD. Postirradiation malignant salivary gland tumor. Arch Otolaryngol. 1976;102(11):699–701.
4. Guzzo M, Locati LD, Prott FJ, Gatta G, McGurk M, Licitra L. Major and minor salivary gland tumors. Crit Rev Oncol Hematol. 2010;74(2):134–48.
5. Pinkston JA, Cole P. Incidence rates of salivary gland tumors: results from a population-based study. Otolaryngol Head Neck Surg. 1999;120(6):834–40.
6. Liao WC, Chih-Chao C, Ma H, Hsu CY. Salivary gland tumors: a clinicopathologic analysis from Taipei Veterans General Hospital. Ann Plast Surg. 2020;84(1S Suppl 1):S26–33.
7. Neville BW, Damm DD, Weir JC, Fantasia JE. Labial salivary gland tumors. Cancer. 1988;61(10):2113–6.
8. Daley TD. The canalicular adenoma: considerations on differential diagnosis and treatment. J Oral Maxillofac Surg. 1984;42(11):728–30.
9. Mantsopoulos K, Iro H. Tumour spillage of the pleomorphic adenoma of the parotid gland: a proposal for intraoperative measures. Oral Oncol. 2021;112:104986.
10. Venkatesh S, Srinivas T, Hariprasad S. Parotid gland tumors: 2-year prospective clinicopathological study. Ann Maxillofac Surg. 2019;9(1):103–9.
11. Ahn D, Yeo CK, Han SY, Kim JK. The accessory parotid gland and facial process of the parotid gland on computed tomography. PLoS One. 2017;12(9):e0184633.
12. Lee KC, Mandel L. Persistent midcheek nodule. J Am Dent Assoc. 2018;149(11):990–4.
13. Kushner DC, Weber AL. Sialography of salivary gland tumors with fluoroscopy and tomography. AJR Am J Roentgenol. 1978;130(5):941–4.
14. Lee YY, Wong KT, King AD, Ahuja AT. Imaging of salivary gland tumours. Eur J Radiol. 2008;66(3):419–36.

15. Zaghi S, Hendizadeh L, Hung T, Farahvar S, Abemayor E, Sepahdari AR. MRI criteria for the diagnosis of pleomorphic adenoma: a validation study. Am J Otolaryngol. 2014;35(6):713–8.
16. Salgarelli AC, Capparè P, Bellini P, Collini M. Usefulness of fine-needle aspiration in parotid diagnostics. Oral Maxillofac Surg. 2009;13(4):185–90.
17. Liu CC, Jethwa AR, Khariwala SS, Johnson J, Shin JJ. Sensitivity, specificity, and post-test probability of parotid fine-needle aspiration: a systematic review and meta-analysis. Otolaryngol Head Neck Surg. 2016;154(1):9–23.
18. Zbären P, Triantafyllou A, Devaney KO, Poorten VV, Hellquist H, Rinaldo A, et al. Preoperative diagnostic of parotid gland neoplasms: fine-needle aspiration cytology or core needle biopsy? Eur Arch Otorrinolaringol. 2018;275(11):2609–13.
19. Heidari F, Heidari F, Rahmaty B, Jafari N, Aghazadeh K, Sohrabpour S, et al. The role of core needle biopsy in parotid glands lesions with inconclusive fine needle aspiration. Am J Otolaryngol. 2020;41(6):102718.
20. Martin H, Jayasinghe J, Lowe T. Superficial parotidectomy versus extracapsular dissection: literature review and search for a gold standard technique. Int J Oral Maxillofac Surg. 2020;49(2):192–9.
21. Albergotti WG, Nguyen SA, Zenk J, Gillespie MB. Extracapsular dissection for benign parotid tumors: a meta-analysis. Laryngoscope. 2012;122(9):1954–60.
22. Houle A, Mandel L. First bite syndrome after deep lobe parotidectomy: case report. J Oral Maxillofac Surg. 2014;72(8):1475–9.
23. Ge N, Peng X, Zhang L, Cai ZG, Guo CB, Yu GY. Partial sialoadenectomy for the treatment of benign tumours in the submandibular gland. Int J Oral Maxillofac Surg. 2016;45(6):750–5.
24. Nicholas SE, Fu W, Liang AL, DeLuna R, Vujaskovic L, Bishop J, et al. Radiation therapy after surgical resection improves outcomes for patients with recurrent pleomorphic adenoma. Adv Radiat Oncol. 2021;6(3):100674.
25. Mc Loughlin L, Gillanders SL, Smith S, Young O. The role of adjuvant radiotherapy in management of recurrent pleomorphic adenoma of the parotid gland: a systematic review. Eur Arch Otorrinolaringol. 2019;276(2):283–95.
26. Valstar MH, de Ridder M, van den Broek EC, Stuiver MM, van Dijk BAC, van Velthuysen MLF, et al. Salivary gland pleomorphic adenoma in the Netherlands: a nationwide observational study of primary tumor incidence, malignant transformation, recurrence, and risk factors for recurrence. Oral Oncol. 2017;66:93–9.
27. Peraza AJ, Wright J, Gómez R. Canalicular adenoma: a systematic review. J Craniomaxillofac Surg. 2017;45(10):1754–8.
28. Wittekindt C, Streubel K, Arnold G, Stennert E, Guntinas-Lichius O. Recurrent pleomorphic adenoma of the parotid gland: analysis of 108 consecutive patients. Head Neck. 2007;29(9):822–8.
29. Maxwell EL, Hall FT, Freeman JL. Recurrent pleomorphic adenoma of the parotid gland. J Otolaryngol. 2004;33(3):181–4.
30. Kligerman MP, Jin M, Ayoub N, Megwalu UC. Comparison of parotidectomy with observation for treatment of pleomorphic adenoma in adults. JAMA Otolaryngol Head Neck Surg. 2020;146(11):1027–34.
31. Quer M, Hernandez-Prera JC, Silver CE, Casasayas M, Simo R, Vander Poorten V, et al. Current trends and controversies in the management of warthin tumor of the parotid gland. Diagnostics. 2021;11(8):1467.

Chapter 21
Malignant Salivary Gland Neoplasms

Kevin C. Lee

Abstract Neoplasms of the salivary gland are rare, and fortunately the overwhelming majority are benign. Salivary gland malignancies are extremely uncommon and only comprise a small portion of all salivary neoplasms. While clinicians of the head, neck, and oral cavity may diagnose a handful of salivary tumors in their career, many will never encounter a salivary gland cancer. As such, an even higher index of suspicion is required to recognize the presence of a salivary carcinoma. The purpose of this chapter is to provide an overview of the epidemiology, diagnosis, and management of malignant salivary tumors.

Introduction

Similar to their benign counterparts, malignant salivary gland neoplasms comprise a heterogenous group of lesions that can present throughout the aerodigestive tract. There are at least 20 distinct histologic subtypes of salivary cancer recognized by the 2017 World Health Organization (WHO) classification [1]. A tissue diagnosis is always required to confirm the pathology; however, there are certain antecedent clinical clues that may alert the provider to the presence of a malignant process. A healthy suspicion for cancer will inform the necessary diagnostic work-up and ensure that such a diagnosis is not overlooked. Unlike benign tumors, the prognosis and natural course of salivary malignancies vary considerably with the histological subtype and the tumor stage. The purpose of this chapter is to highlight the diagnostic and therapeutic differences that clinicians must appreciate when confronted with a malignant salivary tumor.

© The Author(s), under exclusive license to Springer Nature
Switzerland AG 2024

L. Mandel, *Clinical Management of Salivary Gland Disorders*,
https://doi.org/10.1007/978-3-031-50012-1_21

Etiology and Epidemiology

Approximately, 20% of all salivary tumors are malignant [2]. Although the malignancy risk is greater with masses of the submandibular and sublingual glands, the majority of malignant salivary tumors are located in the parotid. This is because the number of parotid tumors far outweighs that of other subsites despite the understanding that only 15–30% of parotid tumors are ultimately malignant [2, 3]. Sublingual gland tumors are uncommon but nearly all are malignant and therefore should be assumed to be cancer until proven otherwise. As with benign tumors, there is also a slight female predilection seen with most salivary malignancies. The exception is with submandibular malignancies which have a slight male predilection for unclear reasons. The typical age of diagnosis is in the fifth or sixth decade of life. Salivary neoplasms are uncommon in children; however, there is some data to suggest that the probability of malignancy is greater when they arise in pediatric populations [3]. As is typical of most pediatric solid cancers, pediatric salivary cancers generally present with a higher grade and a more aggressive behavior.

The most common salivary cancer is the mucoepidermoid carcinoma (MEC). The MEC is the most frequently encountered salivary cancer across all subsites with the exception of the submandibular gland and the minor salivary glands of the sinonasal passages where the adenoid cystic carcinoma (AdCC) predominates. There is a potential association of MEC formation with ionizing radiation exposure [4]. Although its occurrence is sporadic, a unique chromosomal translocation has been found to be present in over half of MEC lesions [5]. A description of the specific pathologic features is outside of the scope of this chapter; however, it is important to distinguish between low-grade and high-grade MEC variants. The low-grade MEC can mimic the features and behavior of a pleomorphic adenoma, whereas the high-grade MEC is more aggressive and akin to a conventional cancer.

Other salivary parenchymal cancers are less commonly encountered. At the parotid and the sublingual glands, the AdCC is the second most common salivary malignancy. The AdCC is neurotropic and has a tendency for early perineural invasion; however, it does not typically enter the regional lymphatics until the later stages despite being a carcinoma. As such, it is described as being both indolent and relentless. The AdCC should not be confused with the acinic cell carcinoma (ACC) which arises almost exclusively within the parotid gland in up to 90% of cases. The ACC can present bilaterally, which is a unique feature that is very uncharacteristic of neoplasms in general. In contrast, the polymorphous low-grade adenoma (PLGA) rarely involves the parotid gland and occurs almost exclusively in the minor salivary glands of the palate. It is the second most common intraoral minor salivary gland cancer following the MEC. The carcinoma ex-pleomorphic adenoma (CExPA) can occur at any subsite and is the malignant counterpart to the pleomorphic adenoma. As previously discussed in the context of benign neoplasms, the risk of malignant transformation increases with lesion duration and recurrence.

Finally, there are cancers that are located within the glandular tissues but that do not originate from parenchyma. In addition to the secretory and ductal elements, salivary glands harbor immunologic components that can evolve into non-Hodgkin lymphomas. Patients with Sjogren's syndrome can classically develop extranodal mucosa-associated lymphoid tissue (MALT) lymphomas from chronic immune stimulation. Mirroring the pattern of Sjogren's syndrome, these MALT lymphomas usually involve the parotid followed by the submandibular glands and can arise bilaterally [6]. MALT lymphomas are indolent and generally accompanied by excellent rates of survival, but when left untreated they can progress to become diffuse large B-cell lymphomas (DLBCLs) which carry a more guarded prognosis. Squamous cell carcinoma (SCC) is the most common form of head and neck cancer. Primary salivary SCC is extremely rare and often a misdiagnosis because salivary SCC nearly always represents direct extension or a metastatic deposit of a mucosal or cutaneous primary [7]. Similarly, salivary melanomas are never primary in origin. The presence of SCC or melanoma in the salivary gland should prompt an investigation for an unknown primary.

History

The intake history for any head and neck mass should include the aforementioned elements that have been outlined for benign lesions (duration, size, associated symptoms). Because malignancies do not respect the anatomic boundaries and will infiltrate the surrounding structures, early neuropathies and pain can be seen even with small volume disease. This is in contrast to benign tumors where nerve deficits occur secondary to mass effect and tumor compression. When malignancy is suspected, it is prudent to further inquire about systemic symptoms related to recent weight loss or fatigue as well as any other constitutional symptoms such as fevers and night sweats. Involuntary weight loss is a nonspecific finding that can result from the increased metabolic demands of the body and/or tumor microenvironment. In the setting of carcinomatosis or even localized cancer, prolonged inflammatory cytokine production can precipitate cachexia and malaise. Just as with other head and neck cancers, the lungs are typically the first echelon of distant metastatic deposits outside of the cervical lymphatics. Therefore, new onset cough, dyspnea, and hemoptysis should be worked-up with appropriate imaging.

The presence of an autoimmune exocrinopathy or a history of other head and neck tumors should be documented. Unexplained fevers may be a part of the cancer metabolic syndrome, but intense fevers and night sweats may signal the presence of B-symptoms which are the constitutional symptoms associated with disseminated lymphoma. Because the major salivary glands harbor intraglandular lymphatics, both parotid and submandibular swellings may represent in-transit metastases from a regional skin or oral cancer. It is therefore important to inquire about prior skin cancers on the scalp or face as well as any history of oral cancers. Familial and social history should be obtained as part of the standard work-up; however, there are no strong links between salivary cancer and hereditary or environmental exposures as salivary gland malignancies occur sporadically.

Physical Exam

The physical exam to investigate any salivary tumors should proceed in an identical fashion regardless of potential malignancy status. However, there are certain clinical findings that will increase the pretest probability of a salivary malignancy. The location and size (largest linear diameter) are vital for the purposes of cancer staging. The location will guide the exam of the lymphatic drainage patterns which is important for salivary carcinomas. The superficial lobe of the parotid contains the majority of the intraparotid lymph nodes, and palpable nodules around a dominant parotid mass may represent intraglandular nodal spread. This is important because cancers with proven lymphovascular invasion have substantially increased risk of clinical or occult cervical nodal disease. Immobility and fixation, pain and/or bleeding on palpation, and ulceration are all concerning for malignancy. Cancer arises from rapid and unregulated cell division. As a result, friable capillary networks form through neovascularization to match the metabolic demand of the tumor environment. When the malignant cells outgrow their blood supply, necrosis and ulceration occur. Cancer cells can erode through the skin or mucosa when the growth pattern is exophytic. With sublingual gland and floor of mouth malignancies, sometimes the surface changes may underestimate the true tumor burden if the growth pattern is endophytic. Minor salivary gland cancers of the oral cavity can erode the palatal bone causing an oronasal communication or burrow into the alveolus and mimic signs of periodontitis. As previously mentioned, spontaneous or evoked pain arises from perineural invasion of the tumor. Similarly, facial nerve involvement should be carefully assessed with all parotid tumors. Any deficits in the setting of malignancy are likely secondary to tumor invasion rather than compression neuropraxia. The parapharyngeal space contains the cranial nerves 9, 10, 11, and 12. Deep lobe parotid malignancies that extend posteriorly into the post-styloid compartment can present with odynophagia from glossopharyngeal nerve (cranial nerve 9) invasion.

Imaging and Diagnostic Tests

As with benign tumors, transcutaneous biopsies are generally avoided when planning for the preservation of the overlying skin. Parotid and submandibular gland tumors are therefore investigated preoperatively with fine needle aspiration cytology (FNAC). Intraorally, any suspicious lesions can be directly sampled with an incisional biopsy. Seeding through a transmucosal biopsy is less of a concern because a composite mucosal resection is the standard treatment for minor and sublingual salivary cancers. For sinonasal tumors, a Caldwell Luc approach, or an intraoral antrostomy, is ill-advised when cancer is suspected because doing so may theoretically seed tumor through the antrostomy into the overlying buccal tissues.

Most centers with endoscopic capability will elect to biopsy sinonasal lesions transnasally through a medial maxillectomy approach.

The preferred initial choice of imaging for suspected salivary gland malignancy is a magnetic resonance imaging (MRI) scan. Compared to a computed tomography (CT) study, a contrast-enhanced MRI of the primary tumor provides superior soft tissue anatomic detail and permits the evaluation of extraglandular extension and perineural invasion. CT scans are additionally obtained to delineate the resection boundaries if there is extensive bony destruction in case of sinonasal and palatal disease. CT scans of the neck and chest are also the preferred imaging modality for completing the staging work-up and evaluating regional lymphadenopathy. When there is locally or regionally advanced disease and further concern for disseminated metastases, many centers will obtain a full body positron emission tomography (PET) scan. This study evaluates hypermetabolic activity using a positron-emitting glucose analog (fluorine-18-2-fluoro-2-deoxy-D-glucose; FDG) that localizes areas of rapid cell division. Unlike conventional head and neck squamous cell carcinoma, low-grade and slow growing salivary cancers, such as the low-grade MEC and the AdCC, may lack FDG avidity. In these instances, when a low-grade salivary malignancy is present, a PET scan may produce a false negative result. Furthermore, PET scans cannot be relied on to discriminate between benign and malignant salivary tumors. Certain benign lesions, such as Warthin's tumor, have increased glucose metabolism and will generate false positive PET results. Therefore, a histopathologic evaluation remains the gold standard for diagnosis.

Treatment

Although there may be slight practice variations at different institutions, the guidelines for head and neck cancer treatment are largely based upon the parameters outlined by the National Comprehensive Cancer Network (NCCN) [8]. Nearly all of the NCCN management recommendations for salivary cancers are derived from data pertaining to parotid cancers. As such, the management of other subsites (submandibular, sublingual, minor salivary) is largely extrapolated from that of parotid cancer. The histologic subtypes of salivary cancer are classified as either low-grade or high-grade depending on the growth rate and metastatic potential. The tumor grade and the propensity for spread will dictate the choice of the treatment algorithm. Low-grade tumors include ACC, oncocytic carcinoma, and myoepithelial carcinoma. High-grade tumors include salivary duct carcinoma, primary squamous cell carcinoma, and CExPA. As previously discussed, MEC has both low-grade and high-grade varieties.

As with oral squamous cell carcinoma, the mainstay of salivary cancer treatment is surgery. Carcinoma surgery generally entails (1) local treatment of the tumor with an en-bloc resection that includes a cuff of normal tissue and (2) regional lymphadenectomy on an as needed basis. Ideally, the removal of a carcinoma should be accompanied by a 1 cm visual clinical margin and a 5 mm microscopic margin of uninvolved tissue. Given the dense network of structures in the head and neck region, these surgical margins are usually unattainable without excessive morbidity. All resectable primary salivary cancers must be treated with complete excision of the involved gland. The exception lies with parotid cancers, where there is consideration for preserving the deep lobe when the malignancy is laterally located and isolated to the superficial lobe. Furthermore, the recommended practice is to preserve a functional facial nerve at all costs even if the tumor abuts the nerve and the final pathology will reveal a close or positive margin. Facial nerve preservation is supported by the existing evidence which shows equivalent local control rates with a less radical surgery [9]. If the overlying skin is adherent to the parotid or submandibular tumor, it must be included in the composite resection. For cancers of the submandibular and sublingual glands, if there is no gross tumor spread into the adjacent lingual or hypoglossal nerves, most surgeons will elect to exclude the nerve from the tumor specimen even if they are contained within the imaginary 1 cm margin. Similarly, for minor salivary gland malignancies, the deep margin of the resection can stop after removal of the next uninvolved anatomic boundary. These exceptions allow surgeons to reduce the defect size in oncologic surgery.

The surgical management of the regional lymph nodes can be addressed either at the time of tumor extirpation or in a staged fashion if the preoperative pathology is equivocal. Due to FNAC sampling error and the preference against transcutaneous open biopsy, it is not uncommon to take a patient to the operating room with the presumption of benign disease only to have the final pathology significant for a low-grade malignancy. When there is clinical evidence of lymphadenopathy in the setting of a cancer diagnosis, a neck dissection is always indicated to clear the disease. For early stage (T1 or T2) cancers that have both a low-grade histology and no clinical evidence of nodal spread, a surgical lymphadenectomy can be deferred for observation. When the cancer pathology is high-grade or when the tumor is locally advanced (greater than 4 cm in diameter or invades tissues outside of the salivary gland), the NCCN recommends a prophylactic (or elective) neck dissection of the at-risk lymphatic drainage basins because of the higher likelihood of occult nodal disease. For parotid cancers, an elective neck dissection entails removal of the upper and middle deep cervical lymph nodes (levels 2 and 3). For submandibular, sublingual, and intraoral minor salivary glands, an elective neck dissection entails removal of the submental and submandibular lymph nodes (level 1) in addition to the upper and middle deep cervical nodes (levels 2 and 3). Some providers recommend routinely offering an elective neck dissection to all patients with sublingual, submandibular, or minor salivary gland cancers regardless of tumor grade given the anatomic proximity of these glands to the cervical nodes [3].

Based on the final pathology report, a multidisciplinary discussion will determine the need for risk-stratified adjuvant therapy. Postoperative radiation therapy to the tumor bed and/or at-risk cervical nodal levels is recommended when there is microscopic evidence of perineural invasion, lymphovascular invasion, high-grade histology, or locally advanced disease. The addition of concurrent chemotherapy to radiation is indicated in the presence of unresectable positive margins and metastatic disease extending beyond the lymph node capsule. With recurrent disease, the choice of salvage therapy varies considerably across different institutions.

Prognosis

The overall prognosis of major salivary cancers is better than that of minor salivary cancers [10]. Among major salivary cancers, those involving the parotid have the best prognosis. The favorable survival with parotid cancers is a direct function of their earlier detection. Common to all cancers, the extent of disease is the strongest predictor of survival. Cancer is considered incurable once there is evidence of distant metastatic deposits beyond the regional lymphatics.

Since salivary cancers are heterogenous, it is also important to consider the biology of the tumor when counseling patients. Certain low-grade histologic subtypes will tend to remain localized and behave similarly to benign pathology. Low-grade MEC, PLGA, and ACC all have roughly 90% 5-year survival rates with adequate surgical treatment [11–13]. On the other hand, the group of high-grade tumors have less than a 50% 5-year survival due to early and aggressive spread [14]. AdCC is unique in that patients universally experience distant recurrence from migration along the perineural lymphatics; however, failures will typically occur late, up to 10–20 years after treatment [15]. Therefore, these patients will have good intermediate 5-year survival but require long-term follow-up beyond the standard 5- to 10-year window of most cancer patients [15].

Conclusion

Salivary gland cancers comprise a small minority of all oral, head, and neck cancers. Because of their uncommon incidence, salivary malignancies may be overlooked for other more likely processes. As with all cancers, early detection provides the best opportunity to improve survival. Salivary cancers are heterogenous, and the tumor grade is an important determinant of treatment response. With the exception of parotid cancers, most of the management guidelines for salivary cancers are borrowed from the experiences at the other head and neck anatomic subsites. Future collaborative efforts are needed to enhance the quality of evidence for this rare disease (Figs. 21.1, 21.2, 21.3, 21.4, 21.5, and 21.6).

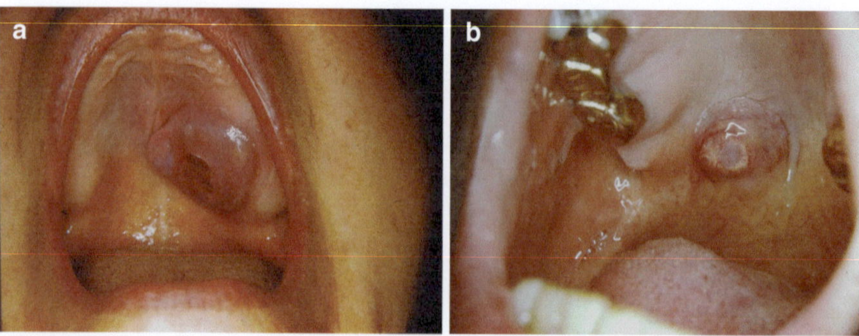

Fig. 21.1 Malignant salivary gland tumors of the palate. (**a**) Similar to that of benign disease, there is a tendency for salivary malignancies to occupy a posterolateral location along the hard palate. The central ulceration raises the clinical concern for a cancer diagnosis. (**b**) Minor salivary malignancy with central ulceration occupying the junction of the hard and soft palate. It is important to recognize that salivary tissue is not limited to the hard palate and is present in the submucosa of the soft palate as well

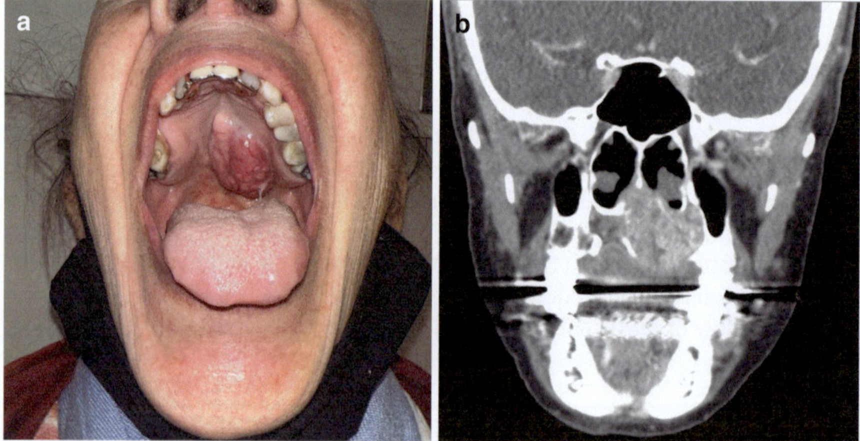

Fig. 21.2 Polymorphous low-grade adenoma of the hard palate. (**a**) Clinical appearance demonstrating a lobulated appearance with nonspecific surface vascular changes and a lack of frank ulceration. (**b**) CT maxillofacial demonstrating bony destruction and invasion into the nasal cavity. Despite the smooth lobulated appearance on physical examination, the aggressive behavior on imaging raises the suspicion for malignancy

Fig. 21.3 Adenoid cystic carcinoma of the deep lobe of the parotid. (**a**) Flaccid paralysis indicating invasion of the right facial nerve. (**b**) MRI T2-weighted coronal view showing an enhancement of the entire right parotid gland with abnormal architecture of the deep lobe situated medial to the mandibular ramus. (**c**) High-power microscopic view of excised specimen. Cellular infiltrate (A) surrounding nerve fiber (N) (hematoxylin and eosin, ×400 magnification)

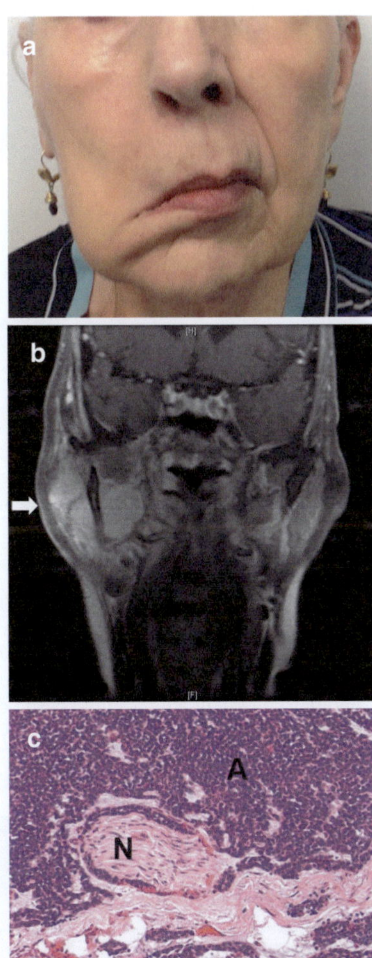

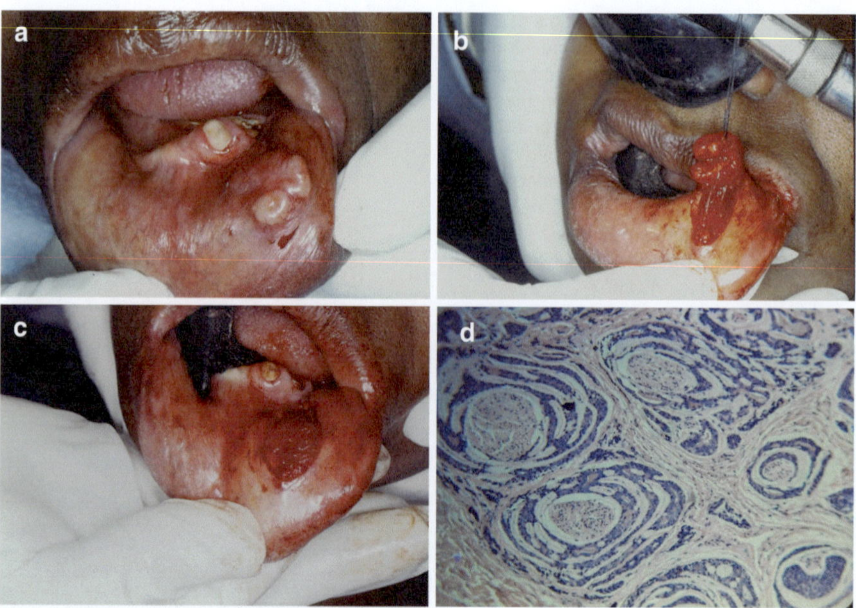

Fig. 21.4 (**a**) Clinical appearance of lesion suspicious for salivary neoplasms. (**b**) Excisional biopsy performed due to size. (**c**) Excision taken to the depth of the orbicularis oris. (**d**) Final pathology consistent with adenoid cystic carcinoma. Despite a nodular, well-demarcated appearance, as with other subsites, minor salivary tumors of the lower lip are typically malignant

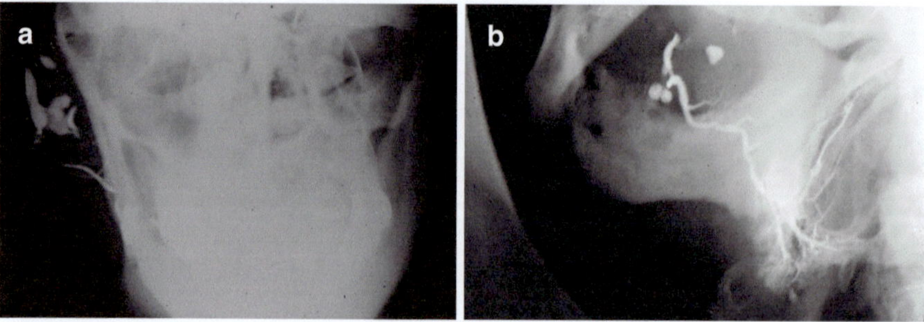

Fig. 21.5 Sialogram of parotid malignancy showing "puddling" or intraparenchymal spillage of contrast. (**a**) Frontal and (**b**) oblique views

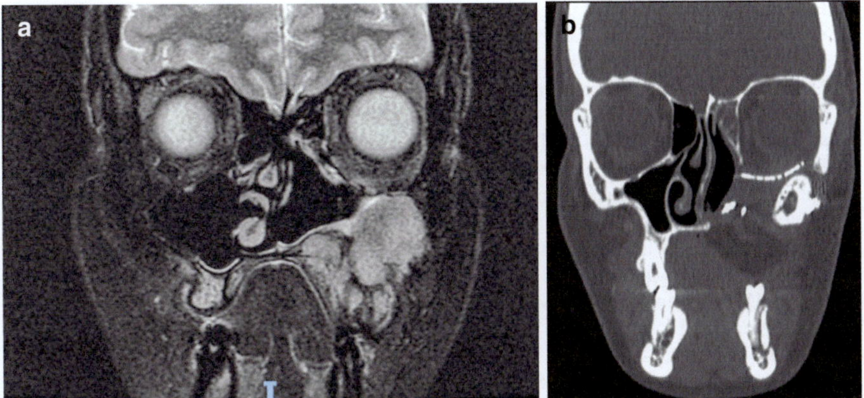

Fig. 21.6 Adenoid cystic carcinoma of left maxilla. (**a**) MRI T2-weighted coronal view demonstrating tumor extension superiorly toward the orbit. (**b**) Postoperative CT scan showing hemimaxillectomy defect following reconstruction with preservation of the left orbital contents. The intact periorbita serves as an anatomic boundary that allows the surgeon to reduce the reliance on 1 cm deep surgical margins

References

1. El-Naggar AK, Chan JK, Grandis JR, Takata T, Slootweg PJ. World Health Organization classification of head and neck tumours. Lyon: IARC; 2017.
2. Seethala RR. Salivary gland tumors: current concepts and controversies. Surg Pathol Clin. 2017;10(1):155–76.
3. Carlson ER, Schlieve T. Salivary gland malignancies. Oral Maxillofac Surg Clin North Am. 2019;31(1):125–44.
4. Dzul S, Jaenisch H, Nagle C, Joiner M, Miller S. Radiation induced mucoepidermoid carcinoma of the parotid gland following post-operative radiotherapy to the earlobe for keloid prophylaxis. Ear Nose Throat J. 2022:1455613221099998.
5. O'Neill ID. t(11;19) translocation and CRTC1-MAML2 fusion oncogene in mucoepidermoid carcinoma. Oral Oncol. 2009;45(1):2–9.
6. Mandel L, Surattanont F. Bilateral parotid swelling: a review. Oral Surg Oral Med Oral Pathol Oral Radiol Endod. 2002;93(3):221–37.
7. Edafe O, Hughes B, Tsirevelou P, Goswamy J, Kumar R. Understanding primary parotid squamous cell carcinoma—a systematic review. Surgeon. 2020;18(1):44–8.
8. Caudell JJ, Gillison ML, Maghami E, Spencer S, Pfister DG, Adkins D, et al. NCCN guidelines® insights: head and neck cancers, version 1.2022: featured updates to the NCCN guidelines. J Natl Compr Cancer Netw. 2022;20(3):224–34.

9. Guntinas-Lichius O, Silver CE, Thielker J, Bernal-Sprekelsen M, Bradford CR, De Bree R, et al. Management of the facial nerve in parotid cancer: preservation or resection and reconstruction. Eur Arch Otorrinolaringol. 2018;275(11):2615–26.
10. Dos Santos ES, Rodrigues-Fernandes CI, Speight PM, Khurram SA, Alsanie I, Costa Normando AG, et al. Impact of tumor site on the prognosis of salivary gland neoplasms: a systematic review and meta-analysis. Crit Rev Oncol Hematol. 2021;162:103352.
11. Biron VL, Lentsch EJ, Gerry DR, Bewley AF. Factors influencing survival in acinic cell carcinoma: a retrospective survival analysis of 2061 patients. Head Neck. 2015;37(6):870–7.
12. Patel TD, Vazquez A, Marchiano E, Park RC, Baredes S, Eloy JA. Polymorphous low-grade adenocarcinoma of the head and neck: a population-based study of 460 cases. Laryngoscope. 2015;125(7):1644–9.
13. Chen MM, Roman SA, Sosa JA, Judson BL. Histologic grade as prognostic indicator for mucoepidermoid carcinoma: a population-level analysis of 2400 patients. Head Neck. 2014;36(2):158–63.
14. Haderlein M, Scherl C, Semrau S, Lettmaier S, Uter W, Neukam FW, et al. High-grade histology as predictor of early distant metastases and decreased disease-free survival in salivary gland cancer irrespective of tumor subtype. Head Neck. 2016;38(Suppl 1):E2041–8.
15. Ellington CL, Goodman M, Kono SA, Grist W, Wadsworth T, Chen AY, et al. Adenoid cystic carcinoma of the head and neck: incidence and survival trends based on 1973-2007 surveillance, epidemiology, and end results data. Cancer. 2012;118(18):4444–51.

Index